WHO CAN USE THIS BOOK?

1.   Anyone interested in osteopathic (manual) medicine

Practicing clinicians (M.D. or D.O.), occupational or physical therapists can utilize the information and techniques in this book to further their knowledge in osteopathic medicine.

2.   1ST and 2ND year medical students

OMT Review is an excellent quick reference for medical students during the first two years of medical school. Many students find the high yield facts helpful when studing for their OMT exams. The outline format is easier than sifting through pages of text, making studying more efficient.

3.   Medical students studying for COMLEX Steps 1, 2 and 3

This book is designed to eliminate the need of sifting through old OMT notes when studying for the COMLEX boards. For those students comfortable with their knowledge of OMT, it may prove beneficial to start with the COMLEX examinations. Hone in on weak areas, then study those chapters in the book. Also, focus on the autonomic reflexes in chapter 10, "Facilitation". Many board questions will stem from this area.

4.   Last minute cramming

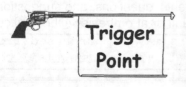

Trigger Point

The information contained in the gray shaded box following this symbol is important. Trigger Points are main concepts. For those individuals cramming for exams, Trigger Points help the reader to pull out key information quickly.

NOTE: The information contained in the gray shaded box following this symbol does not have any relation to Travell's triggerpoint (see chapter 11). The Trigger Point symbol in this text is a method of highlighting important information.

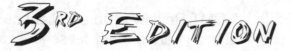

OMT REVIEW

3RD EDITION

Copyright © 1998, 1999, 2003, 2009 by Robert G. Savarese, D.O.
Chapter 13 "Lymphatics" Copyright © by John D. Capobianco, D.O. F.A.A.O. printed with permission.

For any comments, questions, and suggestions,
please send e-mail to the author at omtreview@hotmail.com

Reprints of chapters may be purchased from
Robert Savarese at omtreview@hotmail.com

ISBN: 0-9670090-0-6
Printed in the United States of America

Notice: The authors of this volume have taken care to make certain that the information contained herein is correct and compatible with the standards generally accepted at the time of the publication. As new information becomes available, changes in treatment modalities invariably follow; therefore when choosing a particular treatment, the reader should consider not only the information provided in this manual but also any recently published medical literature on the subject. The nature of this text is to be a comprehensive review, but due to the extraordinary amount of material it is beyond the scope of this text to include all aspects of osteopathic medicine. It is advised that the reader familiarizes himself with the information contained in one of the excellent osteopathic texts that form the cornerstone of osteopathic medical education. Lastly, the authors and distributors disclaim any liability, loss, injury, or damage incurred as a consequence, directly or indirectly, of the use and application from any of the contents of this volume.

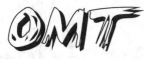
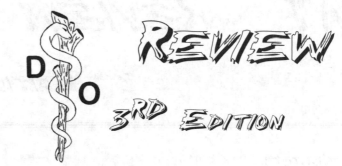

OMT REVIEW
3RD EDITION

Editor-in-chief

Robert G. Savarese D.O.
Jacksonville Orthopaedic Institute
Jacksonville, Florida

Former Chief Resident
Kessler Institute for Rehabilitation, Newark, NJ

Interventional Spine/Pain Management Fellowshlp
Florida Spine Institute, Clearwater, Fl

Chapter Editor	*COMLEX Question Editor*

John D. Capobianco, D.O., F.A.A.O.
Clinical Associate Professor
Department of Osteopathic Medicine
New York College of Osteopathic
   Medicine
Old Westbury, NY

General Practice of Osteopathy
Sea Cliff, NY

James J.Cox, Jr., D.O.
Contributing Editor/Author COMLEX
Basic Sciences
Kaplan Medical, COMLEX Division
New York, NY

Professor
Department of Osteopathic Medicine
LECOM College of Osteopathic
Medicine
Bradenton, FL

Medical Illustration by
Robert Savarese,D.O.

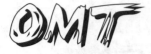 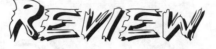 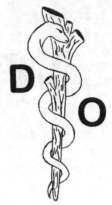

3RD EDITION

Contributors

Arjang Abassi, D.O.
Private Practive Interventional Physiatry/Pain Management
Long Island Spine Specialists
Commack, New York

Daniel Berson, D.O.
Private Practice Anesthesiology
Cardiovascular & Anesthesiology Associates
Austin, Texas

John D. Capobianco, D.O., F.A.A.O.
Clinical Associate Professor
Department of Osteopathic Medicine
New York College of Osteopathic Medicine
Old Westbury, NY
General Practice of Osteopathy
Glen Cove, New York

James J. Cox, Jr., D.O.
Director of Osteopathic Medicine
Contributing Editor/Author COMLEX Basic
Sciences
Kaplan Medical, COMLEX Division
New York, NY
Professor
Department of Osteopathic Medicine
LECOM
College of Osteopathic Medicine
Bradenton, FL

Glenn S. Fuoco, D.O.
Private Practice Interventional Physiatry/Pain Management
Tampa Bay Orthopedics
St. Petersburg, Florida

Marc Kaprow, D.O.
Clinical Assistant Professor
Internal Medicine
Nova Southeastern University
Ft. Lauderdale, Florida
General Practice Internal Medicine
Hollywood, Florida

Robert G. Savarese D.O.
Private Practice Interventional Physiatry/Pain Management
Jacksonville Orthopaedic Institute
Jacksonville, Florida

Osteopathic Fellow Editors

Lisa Preston (NYCOM)
Amy Schram (NYCOM)
Jonas Sokolof (NYCOM)
David Wang (WVCOM)

Peer Reviewers

Todd Berry, B.S. (WVSOM)
Shirley Chen B.S (NSUCOM)
David Choi (NYCOM)
Jim Cox D.O. (NSUCOM)
Bradley Marcus, D.O. (NSUCOM)
Matt Stine (TUCOM)
Jenica Rose (TUCOM)

DEDICATION

===================

To Haylie and Brielle
- for filling life with laughter and smiles

Acknowledgments

The third edition of OMT Review is a compilation of the knowledge and ideas from colleagues, experts, and friends. I wish to extend special thanks to the following people:

The editors, John Capobianco, D.O.,F.A.A.O. and Jim Cox, D.O. John's extensive knowledge in osteopathic medicine ensured the future readers of this book correct information in a concise format. Jim's extraordinary knowledge regarding COMLEX format and frequently tested COMLEX material will undoubtedly help many osteopathic medical students studying for the boards.

All the contributors, who demonstrated enthusiasm and determination toward their contribution to this book. Thank you very much for the long hours spent putting together your chapters.

Melissa Savarese, O.T.R., for the many hours spent revising the final manuscripts.

Scott Nadler, D.O. and Gerard Malanga, M.D. who have both played an integral role in my development as a resident.

The Department of Physical Medicine and Rehabilitation at UMDNJ/Kessler. The comprehensive didactics, coupled with excellent faculty and their willingness to teach, established a foundation upon which all residents can build a healthy and rewarding career in physiatry. I would like to personally thank the faculty and residents who have imparted their knowledge upon myself and others, in order to improve health care and further medical education.

The entire OMM faculty at Nova Southeastern University, whose wisdom, insight and guidance sparked my interest in osteopathic medicine.

Robert G. Savarese, D.O.

During the first two years of my medical training, the need for a comprehensive OMT review book became increasingly apparent. Every year, thousands of osteopathic medical students are left sifting through two years of OMT notes, or reading various texts, in order to study for the OMT section of the boards.

This book was written to reflect the current understanding and knowledge of osteopathic medicine as written in the Foundations for Osteopathic Medicine and the many other texts which form the cornerstone of osteopathic medical education. This book reflects some of the changes made to the recently published second edition of the Foundations for Osteopathic Medicine as well.

OMT Review is in not intended to substitute for any of the excellent osteopathic reference texts. It is intended to be used as quick reference as well as a board review. A combination of basic osteopathic principles along with important clinical points makes this book useful for osteopathic medical students as well as anyone interested in osteopathic medicine. It is hoped that the concise style, tables, and illustrations help summarize and enhance the readers' recollection of principle points. The comprehensive examination at the end of the book will help students gauge their progress, and focus their efforts with maximum efficiency.

It is my sincere wish that this book will serve as a source through which its readers can rapidly grasp the fundamental principles of osteopathic medicine.

Robert G. Savarese D.O.

COMMITTMENT TO OUR READERS

If any reader of OMT Review needs clarification on a topic in the book, I would like to extend an invitation for you to e-mail the author at **omtreview@hotmail.com**. I would be glad to answer any of your questions.

Robert G. Savarese, D.O.

TABLE OF CONTENTS

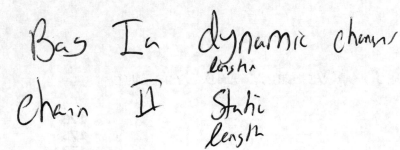

Bas In dynamic chains onulospral

Chain II Static   length

Ymate Abd for spndla

CHAPTER 1

THE BASICS

I. Somatic dysfunction

A. Definition - *"Somatic dysfunction is an impairment or altered function of related components of the somatic (body framework) system: skeletal, arthroidial, and myofascial structures and related vascular, lymphatic and neural elements."*[1 p.1138]

<u>In simpler terms</u>: Somatic dysfunction is a restriction that can occur in bones joints, muscle, and fascia. Blood supply, lymph flow and nervous function may be altered in somatic dysfunction.

B. Diagnostic criteria

A somatic dysfunction can present as:

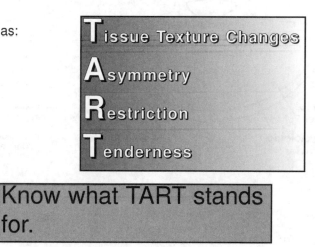

Tissue Texture Changes
Asymmetry
Restriction
Tenderness

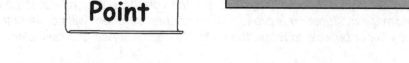

Trigger Point

Know what TART stands for.

1. <u>Tissue texture changes</u> - may present in many ways. The surrounding tissue may be edematous, tender, fibrosed, atrophied, rigid, or hypertonic.

2. <u>Asymmetry</u> - bones, muscles, or joints may feel asymmetric to the corresponding structures.

3. <u>Restriction</u> (see fig 1.1a and 1.1b) - a joint with a somatic dysfunction will have restricted motion. Under normal physiologic conditions a joint has two barriers:
   a. **Physiologic barrier** - a point at which a patient can actively move any given joint. For example, a person may actively rotate his head 80° to either side.
   b. **Anatomic barrier** - a point at which a physician can passively move any given joint. For example, a physician may passively rotate the same patient's head 90° to either side. <u>NOTE</u>: any movement beyond the anatomical barrier will cause ligament, tendon, or skeletal injury.

1

c. In somatic dysfunction, a joint will have a **restrictive (or pathologic) barrier** (see fig 1.1b). A restrictive barrier lies before the physiologic barrier, and prevents full range of motion of that joint. For example, a patient may have a full range of motion for rotation of the neck to the right. However, the patient may only be able to turn his head to the left approximately 70°. Therefore, a restrictive barrier is met when turning the head to the left.

Trigger Point

Know the difference between physiologic, anatomic and restrictive barriers.

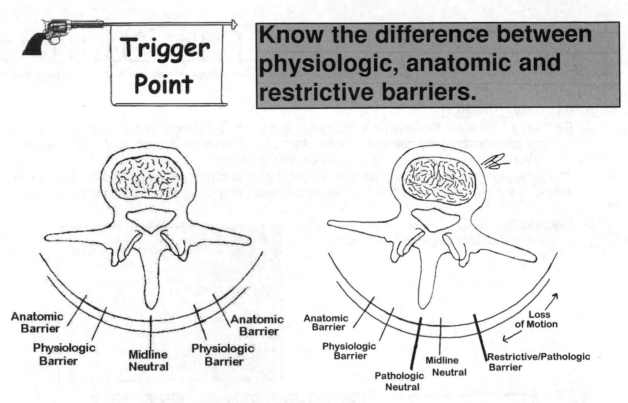

Fig 1.1a (left): In a vertebral segment without somatic dysfunction, the vertebrae may rotate equally to either side. Fig 1.1b (right): If somatic dysfunction is present, the vertebral segment will not lie in the midline position, and the patient will not be able to rotate the vertebral segment past the restrictive (or pathologic) barrier.

4. <u>Tenderness</u> - A painful sensation may be produced during palpation of tissues where it should not occur if there was no somatic dysfunction. This is the only subjective component of TART.

C. **Differences between acute and chronic somatic dysfunction**
TART findings will be altered as an injury changes from acute to chronic. Table 1.1 describes findings in acute vs. chronic somatic dysfunction. [1 p.476, 2 p.9]

Table 1.1

Acute Inflammation (handwritten)

Findings	Acute	Chronic
Tissue texture changes	Edematous, erythematous, boggy with increased moisture. Muscles hypertonic.	Decreased or no edema, no erythema, cool dry skin, with slight tension. Decreased muscle tone, flaccid, ropy, fibrotic.
Asymmetry	Present	Present with compensation in other areas of the body.
Restriction	Present, painful with movement	Present, decreased or no pain.
Tenderness	Severe, sharp	Dull, achy, burning

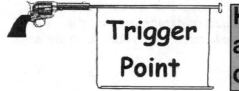

Trigger Point

Know the findings regarding acute vs. chronic somatic dysfunction.

II. Fryette's Laws

A. Law I

In 1918 Harrison Fryette noted, with the use of the Halladay spine, that there were certain rules to spinal motion in the thoracic and lumbar regions. Fryette combined the principles of somatic dysfunction and these rules to establish what are now regarded as Fryette's laws. Fryette's laws act as guidelines for physicians to discriminate different types of dysfunctions, and to determine diagnoses.

Fryette noticed that *if the spine is in the neutral position (no flexion or extension), and if sidebending is introduced, rotation would then occur to the opposite side (fig 1.2)*. This typically applies to more than two vertebral segments (i.e. a group of vertebrae). For example, if a person were to sidebend at T6 - L2, the bodies of the vertebrae would rotate in the opposite direction. He noticed that if a group of vertebrae is in the neutral position and was restricted in left rotation, then the group of vertebrae is rotated right and sidebent left. Although Fryettes Law I typically applies to a group of vertebral segments, some authors believe that sidebending and rotation *may* occur to opposite sides in single vertebral dysfunctions. [1 p.514] However, for the purposes of the board exams, Fryette's law I will apply to a group of vertebrae.

Summary of Law I (fig 1.2)
  In the neutral position:
  sidebending precedes rotation,
  sidebending and rotation occur to opposite sides.

Fryette used this principle for nomenclature of somatic dysfunction:

  e.g.: NS_LR_R = neutral, sidebent left, rotated right.

Memory Tool:
"N", the arrows point in the opposite directions, therefore sidebending and rotation are in opposite directions.

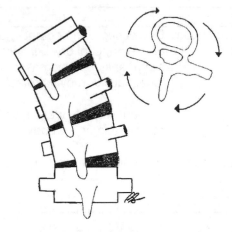

Fig 1.2: Fryette's Law I: Left sidebending without flexion or extension will cause right rotation of all vertebrae.

Fig 1.3: Fryette's Law II: Left sidebending **with flexion or extension** will cause one vertebrae to rotate and sidebend to the same side.

B. Law II

Fryette noticed that if the *spine is in the non-neutral position (either flexed or extended), and rotation is introduced, sidebending would then occur to the same side (fig 1.3)*. This typically applies to a single vertebral segment, however some authors believe it *may* include up to two vertebrae. [1 p.514] For the purposes of the board exams, Fryette's law II will apply to a single vertebral segments. For example, if a person were to rotate to the left in the flexed or extended position at the lumbar spine, one vertebral segment would rotate and sidebend in the same direction. He applied this rule to somatic dysfunction, and noticed if L2 is either flexed or extended and restricted in left rotation, then L2 is rotated right and sidebent right. This became Fryette's second law of spinal motion.

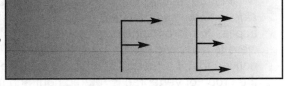

Memory Tool:

In "F"lexed or "E"xtended lesions, the arrows point in the same direction therefore rotation and sidebending are in the same direction.

Summary of Law II (fig 1.3)
    In a non-neutral (flexed or extended) position:
    rotation precedes sidebending, sidebending and rotation occur to the same side.

    Fryette used this principle for nomenclature of somatic dysfunction:
        <u>e.g.</u>: FR_RS_R or FRS_R = flexed, rotated and sidebent right.

Law I is typical of group dysfunctions.
    <u>For example</u>: L2-L5 NS_RR_L or NSR_L.
Law II is typical of a single vertebral dysfunction.
    <u>For example</u>: T5 FR_RS_R or FRS_R.

> # NOTE:
> Fryette's laws I and II only apply to the thoracic and lumbar vertebrae!!
> Not the cervical vertebrae!!

C. Law III:
    This was proposed by C.R. Nelson in 1948. He stated that initiating motion at any vertebral segment in any one plane of motion will modify the mobility of that segment in the other two planes of motion. [1 p.1138] For example, forward bending will decrease the ability to sidebend and rotate.

III. Naming and evaluating somatic dysfunction
A. Naming somatic dysfunctions
    As mentioned above, somatic dysfunction is diagnosed by **TART** (tenderness, asymmetry, restriction, and tissue texture changes). When evaluating somatic dysfunction the physician will examine all of these components, especially restriction. Evaluation of restriction will allow the physician to diagnose and name the somatic dysfunction.

    In the case of vertebral segments, motion will occur in flexion/extension, rotation and sidebending to either side. Therefore, restriction can occur in any of these three planes. When referring to segmental motion, or restriction, *it is traditional to refer to excessive motion (or restriction) of the vertebra **above** in a functional vertebral unit (two vertebrae).* For example, when describing the excessive motion (or restriction) of L2, it is this motion (or restriction) of L2 on L3.

Somatic dysfunctions of the spine are always named for their freedom of motion.

Three examples of nomenclature:

1. If L2 is restricted in the motions of flexion, sidebending to the right and rotation to the right, then L2 is said to be extended, rotated and sidebent to the left on L3. This is denoted as L2 ER_LS_L or ERS_L.
2. If T5 is restricted in the motions of extension, sidebending to the left and rotating to the left then, T5 is said to be flexed, rotated and sidebent to the right on T6. This is denoted as T5 FR_RS_R or FRS_R.
3. If T5 - T10 is not restricted in flexion or extension, but is restricted in sidebending to the left and rotating to the right, then T5 is said to be neutral, sidebent right and rotated left. The nomenclature is denoted as T5 - T10 NS_RR_L.

B. Evaluating somatic dysfunctions

<u>Cervical spine</u>
See chapter 2 Cervical Spine section II D "Motion testing".

<u>Thoracic and lumbar spine</u>
1. **Assess rotation by placing the thumbs over the transverse processes of each segment.**
    If the right thumb is more posterior than the left, then the segment is rotated right.
2. **Check the rotation of the segment in flexion.**
    If the rotation gets better (i.e. the right thumb is no longer posterior), this suggests that the segment is flexed, sidebent and rotated right FR_RS_R.
3. **Check the segment in extension.**
    If the rotation gets better in extension, this suggests that the segment is extended, sidebent and rotated right ER_RS_R.

    If the rotation remains the same in flexion and extension, then the segments are neutral sidebent left and rotated right NS_LR_R.

Algorithm for evaluating somatic dysfunction

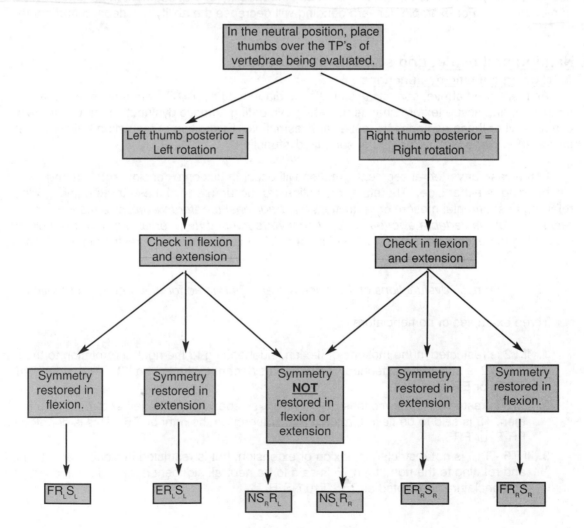

IV. Facet orientation and spinal motion

A. Orientation of SUPERIOR facets

Facet orientation will determine the motion of the vertebral segments. For example, if a pair of facets were to face backward and medial, then sagittal plane motion would be favored (flexion and extension). An easy mnemonic to remember the orientation of superior facets in the axial skeleton is shown in table 1.2.

Table 1.2 [1 p.564]

Region	Facet Orientation	Mnemonic
Cervical	Backward, upward, medial	**BUM**
Thoracic	Backward, upward, lateral	**BUL**
Lumbar	Backward, medial	**BM**

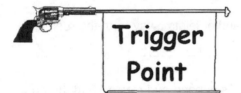

Trigger Point

Know the superior facets orientation.

B. Physiologic motion of the spine

The human spine can move in three planes or any combination thereof. Each plane corresponds with a particular axis and motion as shown in table 1.3.

Table 1.3

Motion	Axis	Plane
Flx'n/ext'n	Transverse	Sagittal
Rotation	Vertical	Transverse
Sidebending	Anterior - posterior	Coronal

V. Muscle contraction

A. **Isotonic contraction** - Muscle contraction that results in the approximation of the muscle's origin and insertion without a change in its tension. In such a case the operator's force is less than the patient's force. [1 p.693, p.1129]

B. **Isometric contraction** - Muscle contraction that results in the increase in tension without an approximation of origin and insertion. In such a case the operator's force and the patient's force are equal. [1 p.693 p.1129]

C. **Isolytic contraction** - Muscle contraction against resistance while forcing the muscle to lengthen. In such a case the operator's force is more than the patient's force. [1 p.693 p.1129]

D. **Concentric contraction** - Muscle contraction that results in the approximation of the muscle's origin and insertion. [1 p.693 p.1129]

E. **Eccentric contraction** - Lengthening of muscle during contraction due to an external force. [1 p.693 p.1129]

VI. Osteopathic Treatment

A. Direct vs. Indirect treatment

As mentioned earlier, all somatic dysfunctions will have a restrictive (pathologic) barrier. This restrictive barrier will inhibit movement in one direction thus causing asymmetry within the joint or tissue. The goal of osteopathic treatment is to eliminate this restrictive barrier, thus restoring symmetry.

Osteopathic practitioners use a variety of treatments to achieve this goal. All of these treatments fall into two categories, **direct treatment** and **indirect treatment**.

In a <u>direct treatment</u>, the practitioner "engages" the restrictive barrier. This means that the body tissues and/or joints are eventually moved through the restrictive barrier. This can be done by direct palpation of the dysfunctional tissues or using a body part as a lever.

For example:
1. If T3 was FR_RS_R, the practitioner would extend, rotate and sidebend T3 to the left.
2. If the abdominal fascia moved more freely cephalad than caudad, the practitioner would hold the tissue caudad (toward the barrier) allowing the tissues to stretch.

In an <u>indirect treatment</u> the practitioner moves tissues and/or joints away from the restrictive barrier into the direction of freedom.

For example:
1. If T3 was FR_RS_R, the practitioner would flex, sidebend and rotate T3 to the right.
2. If the abdominal fascia moved more freely cephalad than caudad, the practitioner would hold the tissue cephalad (away from the barrier) allowing the tissues to relax.

B. Passive vs. Active Treatment

In an active treatment, the patient will assist in the treatment, usually in the form of isometric or isotonic contraction.

In a passive treatment, the patient will relax and allow the practitioner to move the body tissues.

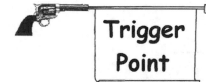

Trigger Point

Direct Treatment: ⟶ Towards the barrier.
Indirect Treatment: ⟶ Away from the barrier
Active Treatment: ⟶ Patient assists during treatment.
Passive Treatment: ⟶ Patient relaxes during treatment.

Table 1.4

Treatment Type	Direct or Indirect	Active or Passive
Myofascial Release	Both	Both
Counterstrain	Indirect	Passive
Facilitated Positional Release	Indirect	Passive
Muscle Energy	Direct (rarely indirect)	Active
High Velocity Low Amplitude	Direct	Passive
Osteopathy in the Cranial Field	Both	Passive
Lymphatic treatment	Direct	Passive
Chapman's reflexes	Direct	Passive

(handwritten under table: BLT   Indirect   Passive)

VII. Treatment Plan

A. Choice of Treatment
Precise answers to choice of technique do not exist; there are only general guidelines. [56 p.576-7]
1. Elderly patients and hospitalized patients typically respond better to indirect techniques or gentle direct techniques such as articulatory techniques.
2. The use of HVLA in a patient with advanced osteoporosis or metastatic cancer may lead to a pathologic fracture. [56 p.576-7] → *RA*
3. Acute neck strain/sprains are often better treated with indirect techniques to prevent further strain.

B. Dose and Frequency
Absolute rules for dose and frequency do not exist. Typical guidelines are as follows: [56 p.576-7]
1. For sicker patients, limit the OMT to a few key areas. → *Less time, more frequency*
2. Allow time for the patient's body to respond to the treatment that was given.
3. Pediatric patients can be treated more frequently; whereas geriatric patients may need a longer time to respond to the treatment.
4. Acute cases should have a shorter interval between treatments; as they respond to the treatment, the interval can be increased.

C. Sequencing of Treatment → *Center out, Anterior → Posterior*
There are different opinions regarding what should be treated first. Guidelines on sequencing are not absolute. Each physician after gaining experience develops his or her own approach. The following is a sample sequence: [56 p.576-7]
1. For psoas syndrome, treat the lumbar spine [56 p.577] or thoraco-lumbar spine[58] first.
2. Treat the ribs and upper thoracic spine before treating the cervical spine.
3. Treat the thoracic spine before treating rib dysfunctions.
4. For acute somatic dysfunctions, treating peripheral areas will allow access to the acute area.
5. Cranial treatment can make the patient relax, this will allow OMT to work in other areas.
6. For extremity problems, treat the spine, sacrum and ribs first(axial skeleton).

CHAPTER 1 REVIEW QUESTIONS

1. Which of the following is not an example of a somatic dysfunction?
    A. Acute cholecystitis secondary to gallstones.
    B. Rotator cuff tear secondary to repetitive trauma.
    C. Lumbar strain/sprain.
    D. Osteoarthritis resulting in a decreased range of motion and end range pain.
    E. Adhesive capsulitis.

2. Which one of the following is not a diagnostic characteristic of somatic dysfunction?
    A. Edema.
    B. Temperature change.
    C. Tenderness.
    D. Full range of motion in a joint.
    E. Asymmetry.

3. All of the following are examples of a chronic somatic dysfunction of the right shoulder EXCEPT?
    A. A slight or no increase in temperature of the musculature surrounding the right shoulder.
    B. Asymmetry with noticeable compensation in other areas of the body.
    C. Moist, edematous, erythematous and boggy tissue around the right shoulder.
    D. Restriction with very little or no pain with movement of the right shoulder.

4. In evaluation of a patient with mid-thoracic pain you find that T6 is $ER_L S_L$ (ERS_L). This means that T6 is restricted in?
    A. Flexion, rotation and sidebending to the left in relation to T7.
    B. Flexion, rotation and sidebending to the right in relation to T7.
    C. Flexion, rotation and sidebending to the right in relation to T5.
    D. Extension, rotation and sidebending to the left in relation to T5.
    E. Extension, rotation and sidebending to the right in relation to T5.

5. A point at which a patient can actively move any given joint is defined as?
    A. A physiologic barrier.
    B. A anatomic barrier.
    C. A pathologic/restrictive barrier.
    D. A rotational barrier.
    E. A dysfunctional barrier.

6. While evaluating a patient's upper back pain, you notice that T2 appears to be rotated right. Flexing the patient's head down to T2, causes T2 to further rotate to the right. Extending the patient's head causes T2 to return to the neutral position. Which of the following best describes the somatic dysfunction of T2?
    A. $ER_R S_R$
    B. $FR_R S_R$
    C. $ER_R S_L$
    D. $FR_R S_L$

7. Which of the following statements concerning Fryette's law I is true?
    A. Rotation and sidebending occur to same side when the spine is in the extended position
    B. Sidebending and rotation occur to opposite sides when the spine is in the flexed position.
    C. Rotation and sidebending occur to opposite sides.
    D. Sidebending and rotation occur to the same side when the spine is in the neutral position

8. The orientation of the superior facets of the cervical spine is?
    A. Backward and medial.
    B. Backward, upward and lateral.
    C. Backward, upward and medial.
    D. Forward, upward and lateral.
    E. Forward and medial.

9. Motion of vertebral segments along the sagittal plane can best be described as?
    A. Rotation.
    B. Sidebending.
    C. Rotation and sidebending.
    D. Flexion and extension.

10. Motion of vertebral segments around a vertical axis can best be described as?
    A. Rotation.
    B. Sidebending.
    C. Rotation and sidebending.
    D. Flexion and extension

11. Which of the following treatments is correctly matched?
    A. Myofascial release => Direct technique with passive forces only
    B. Counterstrain => Indirect technique with passive forces only
    C. Muscle Energy => Indirect technique with passive forces only
    D. Facilitated Positional Release => Indirect technique with active forces only
    E. HVLA => Indirect Technique with passive forces only

12. Which of the following statements concerning muscle contraction is correct?
    A. Isotonic contraction results in the approximation of the muscle's origin and insertion with an increase in tension.
    B. Isometric contraction results in the approximation of the muscle's origin and insertion with an increase in tension.
    C. Isotonic contraction results in an increase in muscle tension without an approximation of origin and insertion.
    D. Isometric contraction results in an increase in muscle tension without an approximation of origin and insertion.
    E. Isotonic contraction results in the approximation of the muscle's origin and insertion with a decrease in tension.

ANSWERS

1. A	8. C
2. D	9. D
3. C	10. A
4. B	11. B
5. A	12. D
6. A	
7. C	

CHAPTER 2

CERVICAL SPINE

I. Anatomy

A. Bones

The cervical spine consists of seven vertebral segments (see fig 2.1). C1 and C2 are considered atypical. C1 has no spinous process or vertebral body. C2 has a dens that projects superiorly from its body and articulates with C1. C2 - C6 generally have bifid spinous processes. The articular pillars (or lateral masses) are the portion of bone of the cervical vertebral segments that lie between the superior and inferior facets. The articular pillars are located posterior to the cervical transverse processes, and are used by osteopathic physicians to evaluate cervical vertebral motion. Foramen transversarium are foramina in the transverse process of C1-C6 that allow for the passage of the vertebral artery.

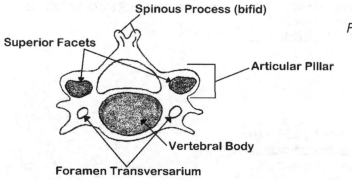

Spinous Process (bifid)

Superior Facets

Articular Pillar

Fig 2.1: A typical cervical vertebrae

Vertebral Body

Foramen Transversarium

B. Muscles

Scalenes (anterior, middle, posterior) - Originates from the posterior tubercle of the transverse processes of the cervical vertebrae and insert onto the rib 1 (anterior and middle) and rib 2 (posterior). [3 p.783] They sidebend the neck to the same side with unilateral contraction, and flex the neck with bilateral contraction. The scalenes also aid in respiration. *The anterior and middle scalene will help elevate the first rib during forced inhalation. The posterior scalene will help elevate the second rib during forced inhalation.* [3 p.793] It is common to have a tender point in one of the scalenes (posterior to the clavicle at the base of the neck) with a first or second inhalation rib dysfunction.

Sternocleidomastoid (SCM) - Originates from the mastoid process and the lateral half of the superior nuchal line. Inserts onto the medial 1/3 of the clavicle and sternum. With unilateral contraction, the SCM will sidebend ipsilaterally and rotate contralaterally (sidebend towards and rotates away). Bilateral contraction will flex the neck. *The SCM divides the neck into anterior and posterior triangles.* [3 p.786] *Shortening or restrictions within the SCM often results in torticollis.*

DART

C. Ligaments

The *alar* ligament extends from the sides of the dens to the lateral margins of the foramen magnum. The *transverse ligament* of the atlas attaches to the lateral masses of C1 to hold the dens in place. Rheumatoid arthritis and Down's syndrome can weaken these ligaments leading to atlanto-axial subluxation. Rupture of this ligament (which may occur with rheumatoid arthritis and Downs syndrome) will result in catastrophic neurological damage. [1 p.541]

D. Joints -

Joints of Luschka - The uncinate processes are superior lateral projections originating from the posterior lateral rim of the vertebral bodies of C3 - C7. [29 p.79] They help support the lateral side of the cervical discs and protect cervical nerve roots from disc herniation. [28 p.210, 29 p.79] *The articulation of the superior uncinate process and the superadjacent vertebrae is known as the Joint of Luschka.* [29 p.373] These joints have also been called uncovertebral joints. [29 p.5] They may or may not be considered true synovial joints, but play an important role in cervical motion, especially sidebending. [28 p.210] *Since the Joints of Luschka are in close proximity to the intervertebral foramina, degenerative changes and hypertrophy can lead to foraminal stenosis and nerve root compression.* [28 p.212] The most common cause of cervical nerve root pressure is degeneration of the Joints of Luschka plus hypertrophic arthritis of the intervertebral synovial (facet) joints. [28 p.214]

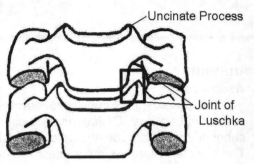

Fig 2.2: Joints of Luschka (a.k.a. uncovertebral joints). Formed by the articulation of the uncinate process and the superadjacent vertebrae.

E. Nerves

There are 8 cervical nerve roots (see fig 2.3). *The upper seven exit above their corresponding vertebrae.* For example, the C7 nerve root will exit between C6 and C7. The last cervical nerve root (C8) will exit between C7 and T1. The brachial plexus is made up of nerve roots from C5 - T1, therefore damage to the lower cervical cord will cause neurological symptoms in the upper extremity.

Fig 2.3: Nerve roots in the cervical region will exit above the corresponding vertebrae.

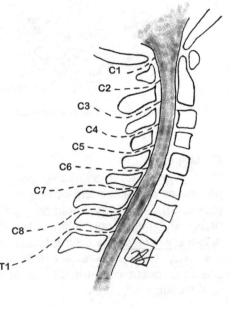

NOTE:
Fryette's laws I and II only apply to the thoracic and lumbar vertebrae!!
Not the cervical vertebrae!!

14

II. Motion and mechanics

A. OA - The OA is considered to be the motion of the occipital condyles on the atlas (C1). *Its primary motion is flexion and extension.* Approximately 50% of the flexion and extension of the cervical spine stems from the OA joint. [28. 188] *Sidebending and rotation occur to opposite sides with either flexion or extension.* Therefore, if the OA is flexed, sidebent left and rotated right, then it means that the occiput on the atlas is flexed, sidebent left and rotated right (FR_RS_L).

B. AA- The AA is considered to be C1 motion on C2. *Its primary motion is rotation (50% of the rotation of the cervical spine occurs here [28.189]). Clinically only rotation occurs at this joint.* [28 p.208] Therefore, if the AA is rotated right it means that the atlas (C1) is rotated right on the axis (C2).

C. Inferior division (C2-C7)- It is generally accepted that *sidebending and rotation occur to the same side. However, recent research by Capobianco et. al.[55] has demonstrated that sidebending and rotation do not always occur to the same side. This research actually demonstrated a higher incidence of sidebending and rotation toward the opposite side thus disproving the common notion that sidebending and rotation occur to the same side. However, for the board exams, C2 - C7 will sidebend and rotate toward the same side.* The inferior division accounts for 50% of the flexion/extension and 50% of the rotation of the entire cervical spine. [28 p.189]

Trigger Point

Segment	Main Motion	Sidebending and rot'n
OA	Flexion and Ext'n	Opposite Sides
AA	Rotation	Opposite Sides
C2-C4	Rotation	Same Sides
C5-C7	Sidebending	Same Sides

D. Motion testing

1. Occipital-atlantal (OA) motion testing -[1 p.544, 28 p.579 - 581]

Translation - Cup the occiput with both hands, with the finger tips and middle finger over the occipito-atlantal articulation. Move the occiput on the atlas by translating to the left then the right. Lateral translation of the occiput to the right (right translation) will produce left sidebending. Therefore, if the OA is restricted in right translation in the flexed position, it suggests an occiput that is extended, rotated left and sidebent right (i.e., restriction of flexion, rotating right and sidebending left).

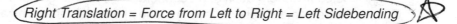

Right Translation = Force from Left to Right = Left Sidebending

Rotation - To detect occipital rotation, stabilize the arch of the atlas with the thumb and index finger. The other hand is placed on top of the skull and rotate to the right and left evaluating freedom and resistance. [28 p.580]

Sidebending - Place finger pads in the occipital sulci and determine the depth of each sulci, left occipital sidebending will seperate the right occipital condyle and atlas, as a result the right sulcus will feel deep. Since sidebending and rotation are toward opposite sides, a right deep sulcus indicates left sidebending, which indicates right rotation.

2. Atlantal-axial (AA) motion testing - [1 p.544-5, 28 p.582-3, 2. 109]

Rotation- Grasp the head with the finger tips contacting the lateral mass of the atlas. Flex the neck to 45° and rotate the head to the right and left. Flexing the cervical spine to 45° will lock out rotation of the typical cervical vertebrae (C2 - C7). A right rotated atlas exhibits restriction in left rotation, and vice versa.

3. C2-C7 motion testing- [1 p.545]

Translation - The translation test is similar to the occiput translation test, except that the physician's finger tips placed over the lateral border of the articular pillars. Lateral translation of the cervical spine to the right (right translation) will produce left sidebending. Therefore, if C3 is restricted in right translation in the flexed position, it suggests that C3 is extended, rotated right and sidebent right.

Rotation - *Method # 1*: With the patient's head supported, place the finger tips of the index finger on the posterior surface of the articular pillars. Rotate to the right and left evaluating freedom or resistance.

Method # 2 [28 p.582]: With the patient's head supported, contact the posterior aspect of the lateral mass with the index finger tips. Push directly anterior with the right finger to induce left rotation, then do the same with the left finger to induce right rotation.

III. Important considerations about the cervical spine

Suboccipital or paravertebral muscle spasms are usually associated with upper thoracic or rib problems on the same side. Therefore, treat these areas first, then treat the cervical spine. [1 p.545]

An acute injury to the cervical spine is best treated with indirect fascial techniques or counterstrain first. [1 p.545]

Cervical foraminal stenosis [28 p.212, 219-20]

Definition - Degenerative changes within the joints of Luschka, hypertrophic changes of the intervertebral (facet) joints, and osteophyte formation associated with arthritis, may result in intervertebral foraminal narrowing. *Degenerative changes within the joints of Luschka and hypertrophy of the intervertebral (facet) joints is the most common cause of cervical nerve root pressure symptoms.* [28 p.211]

Location of pain - Neck pain radiating into the upper extremity.

Quality of pain - Dull ache, shooting pain or paresthesias.

Signs and Symptoms - Increased pain with neck extension, positive Spurling's test (see Chapter 18 - Special tests), paraspinal muscle spasm, posterior and anterior cervical tenderpoints.

Radiology - Osteophyte formation and degenerative joint changes on AP and lateral views. Oblique views demonstrate narrowing of the intervertebral foramina.

Treatment - OMT should be directed at maintaining optimal range of motion of the cervical spine. Articulatory techniques as well as muscle energy can improve segmental range of motion. Myofacial release, counterstrain, and facilitated positional release can improve myofacial restrictions.

CHAPTER 2 REVIEW QUESTIONS

1. Which of the following muscles help elevate the second rib with forced inhalation?
    A. Anterior scalene.
    B. Middle scalene.
    C. Posterior scalene.
    D. Sternocleidomastoid.
    E. Pectoralis minor.

2. Stenosis of the intervertebral foramen between C3 and C4 may effect which nerve root?
    A. C2 nerve root.
    B. C3 nerve root.
    C. C4 nerve root.
    D. C5 nerve root.

3. The primary motion of the occiput on the atlas is?
    A. Flexion/extension.
    B. Sidebending.
    C. Rotation.
    D. Sidebending and rotation.

4. In evaluation of a patient with suboccipital pain you find that his atlanto-axial joint is restricted in right rotation. Which of the following statements is true concerning this somatic dysfunction?
    A. The atlanto-axial joint will be restricted in left sidebending.
    B. C1 on C2 will be restricted in right sidebending.
    C. The occiput on C1 will be restricted in right sidebending.
    D. C2 on C3 will be restricted in right sidebending.
    E. The occiput on C1 will be restricted in flexion.

5. Which one of the following statements concerning the cervical spine is true?
    A. The uncinate process of the cervical spine is located on the spinous process.
    B. The primary motion of the lower cervical spine is rotation
    C. The primary motion of the lower cervical spine is flexion/extension.
    D. Decreased translation to the right at C4 suggests that C4 is restricted in left sidebending.
    E. The C2/C3 vertebral unit is responsible for more than 50% of the overall rotation of the cervical spine.

6. All of the following statements concerning the articular pillars are true EXCEPT:
    A. They are used by the osteopathic physician to evaluate cervical motion.
    B. It is the portion of bone located between the superior and inferior facets.
    C. They are located anterior to the cervical transverse processes.
    D. They are also referred to as the lateral masses.

7. Which cervical segment is best evaluated by flexing the neck to 45° and rotating the head?
    A. OA.
    B. C1.
    C. C2.
    D. C3.
    E. C4.

ANSWERS

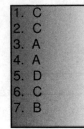

1. C
2. C
3. A
4. A
5. D
6. C
7. B

CHAPTER 3

THORAX AND RIBCAGE

Thorax

I. Anatomy
A. Rule of three's
Spinous processes are large and point increasingly downward from T1-T9, then back to almost an anterior-posterior orientation from T10-T12. [1 p.563]   A useful way to identify the thoracic transverse processes from the location of the corresponding spinous process involves the "**rule of three's**":
1. T1-T3 - the spinous process is *located at the level of the corresponding transverse process.*
2. T4-T6 - the spinous process is *located one-half a segment below the corresponding transverse process.* For example, the spinous process of T5 is located halfway between the tranverse processes of T5 and T6.
3. T7-T9 - the spinous process is *located at the level of the transverse process of the vertebrae below.* For example, the spinous process of T8 is at the level of T9's transverse process.
4. T10-T12 is as follows: [1 p.575]
   T10 follows the same rules as T7-T9.
   T11 follows the same rules as T4-T6.
   T12 follows the same rules as T1-T3.

B. Other anatomical landmarks

The spine of the scapula corresponds with T3.
The inferior angle of the scapula corresponds with the spinous process of T7.
The sternal notch is level with T2.
The sternal angle (angle of Louis) attaches to the 2nd rib and level with T4.
The nipple is at the T4 dermatome.
The umbilicus is at the T10 dermatome.

II. Thoracic motion
A. The motions of the thoracic spine are rotation, sidebending, flexion and extension. Motion is limited by the ribcage. *The main motion of the thorax is rotation.* However, some authors suggest that lower segment (T11 and T12) motion is similar to that of the lumbar region.
These authors report the following: [1 p.572]
Upper and middle thoracic: Rotation > flexion/extension> sidebending.
Lower thoracic: Flexion/extension > sidebending > rotation.

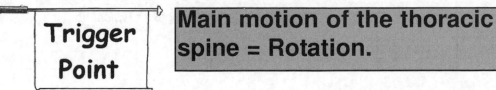

Trigger Point

Main motion of the thoracic spine = Rotation.

B. The thoracic spine follows Fryette's Laws (see chapter 1 for details):
If the spine is in the neutral position (no flexion or extension), and if sidebending is introduced, rotation would then occur to the opposite side.
For example:
T5 - T10 Neutral rotated right and sidebent left = T5 - T10 NR_RS_L

If the spine is in the non-neutral position (either flexed or extended), and rotation is introduced, sidebending would then occur to the same side.
For example:
T5 Flexed rotated right and sidebent right = T5 FR_RS_R

III. Muscles of Respiration

    A. <u>Primary muscles</u>
        1. Diaphragm
          <u>Action</u>:
            a. contracts with inspiration.
            b. causes pressure gradients to help return lymph and venous blood back to the thorax.
          <u>Attachments</u>: xyphoid process, ribs 6-12 on either side, and bodies and intervertebral discs of L1-L3.
          <u>Innervation</u>: Phrenic nerve (C3-C5).

        2. Intercostals (external, internal, innermost, and subcostal)
          <u>Action</u>:
            a. elevate ribs during inspiration
            b. prevent retractions during inspiration

    B. <u>Secondary muscles</u>
        scalenes
        pectoralis minor
        serratus anterior and posterior
        quadratus lumborum
        latissimus dorsi

Ribcage
I. Anatomy

    A. Typical vs. Atypical ribs
      What makes a typical rib typical?
      A typical rib will have all of the following anatomical landmarks:
      1. <u>Tubercle</u>- *articulates with the corresponding transverse process.*
      2. <u>Head</u>- *articulates with the vertebra above and corresponding vertebra.*
      3. <u>Neck</u>
      4. <u>Angle</u>
      5. <u>Shaft</u>

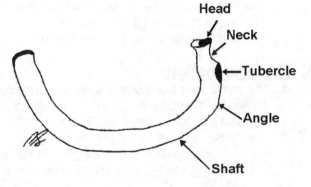

Fig 3.1: Typical rib

A. Typical vs. Atypical ribs (con't)

    Typical ribs: 3-10

    Atypical ribs: 1,2,11and 12

        NOTE: Sometimes rib 10 is considered atypical. [3 p.37]

            Rib 1 - atypical because it articulates only with T1 and has no angle.

            Rib 2 - atypical because it has a large tuberosity on the shaft for the serratus anterior.

            Rib 11 and 12 - atypical because they articulate only with the corresponding vertebrae and lack tubercles.

            Rib 10 - sometimes considered atypical because it articulates only with T10.

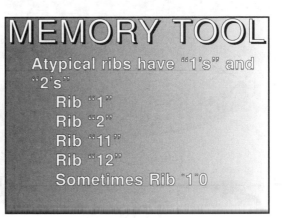

MEMORY TOOL

Atypical ribs have "1's" and "2's"

    Rib "1"

    Rib "2"

    Rib "11"

    Rib "12"

    Sometimes Rib "10"

B. True, False and Floating ribs

    1. Ribs 1-7 attach to the sternum through costal cartilages, therefore they are called **TRUE ribs**.

    2. Ribs 8-12 - do not attach directly to the sternum, therefore they are called **FALSE ribs**. Each of the 8th to 10th ribs is connected by its costal cartilage to the cartilage of the rib superior. For example, the costal cartilage of rib 9 attaches to the costal cartilage of rib 8. Ribs 11-12 remain unattached anteriorly and often further classified as **FLOATING ribs**.

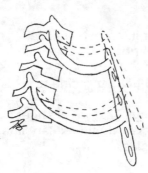

Trigger Point

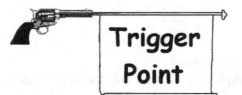

Know the difference between true, floating and false ribs.

II. Rib motion

    There are three classifications of rib movement:

        1. Pump-handle motion

        2. Bucket-handle motion

        3. Caliper motion

    NOTE: All ribs have a varying proportion of these motions depending on their location within the ribcage.

        *The upper ribs (ribs 1-5) move **primarily** in a pump-handle motion.*

        *The middle ribs (ribs 6-10) move **primarily** in a bucket-handle motion.*

        *The lower ribs (ribs 11 and 12) move **primarily** in a caliper motion.*

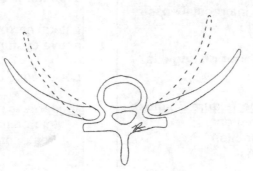

Fig 3.2a: (left) Pump-handle movement of ribs 1-5. The dotted lines show rib position in inhalation.

Fig 3.2b: (right) Caliper motion of floating ribs. The dotted lines represent rib position in exhalation.

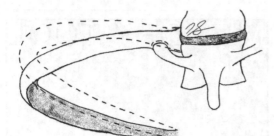

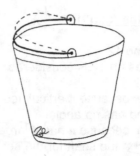

Fig 3.2c: Bucket-handle movement. A posterior-anterior view of a mid-thoracic rib. Note, that with inspiration, the rib moves up, similar to a bucket-handle

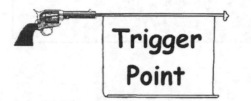

Trigger Point

Know the three different classifications of rib movement

III. Rib dysfunctions:

Definition - A somatic dysfunction in which movement or the position of one rib is altered or disrupted. [1 p.1136]

The most common types of rib dysfunction are:
> **Inhalation Dysfunctions**
> **Exhalation Dysfunctions**

A. Inhalation dysfunction (older terminology: exhalation restriction)
> The dysfunctional rib will move cephalad during inhalation, however the dysfunctional rib will not move caudad during exhalation.
> The rib will therefore appear to be "held up".

Diagnostic Findings Inhalation Dysfunction: [33 p.123, 129]

Pump-Handle Ribs	Bucket-Handle Ribs

Rib elevated: Anteriorly
 	
Anterior part of rib moves cephalad on inspiration and restricted on expiration.
 	
Anterior narrowing of intercostal space above dysfunctional rib.
 	
Superior edge of posterior rib angle is prominent.
 	
Tenderness and Tissue Texture Changes
   Costochondral junction
   Chondrosternal junction
   Posterior rib angles
	Rib elevated: Laterally
	
	Lateral part (shaft) of rib moves slightly upward on inspiration and restricted on expiration.
	
	Lateral narrowing of intercostal space above dysfunctional rib.
	
	Lower edge of rib shaft is prominent.
	
	Tenderness and Tissue Texture changes:
	   Intercostal muscles at mid-axillary line
	   Posterior rib angles

B. <u>Exhalation dysfunction</u> (older terminology: inhalation restriction)

> The dysfunctional rib will move caudad during exhalation, however the dysfunctional rib will not move cephalad during inhalation.
> The rib will therefore appear to be "held down".

BITE

<u>Diagnostic Findings:</u> Exhalation Dysfunction: [33 p.126, 131]

Pump-Handle Ribs

<u>Rib depressed:</u> Anteriorly

Anterior part of rib moves caudad on expiration and restricted on inspiration.

Anterior narrowing of intercostal space below dysfunctional rib.

Inferior edge of posterior rib angle is prominent.

<u>Tenderness and Tissue Texture Changes:</u>
    Costochondral junction
    Chondrosternal junction
    Posterior rib angles

Bucket-Handle Ribs

<u>Rib depressed:</u> Laterally

Lateral part (shaft) of rib moves slightly downward on expiration and restricted on inspiration.

Lateral narrowing of intercostal space below dysfunctional rib.

<u>Tenderness and Tissue Texture Changes:</u>
    Intercostal muscles at mid-axillary line
    Posterior rib angles

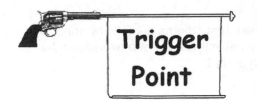

Trigger Point

Know the difference between inhalation and exhalation rib dysfunctions.

C. <u>Group dysfunctions</u>

<u>Definition</u> - An inhalation or exhalation rib dysfunction in which the movement or the position of two or more ribs is altered or disrupted.

In these cases, there is usually one rib that is responsible for causing the dysfunction. This rib is referred to as the **"key"** rib.

> *In inhalation dysfunctions the key rib is the lowest rib of the dysfunction. (see fig 3.3a)*
> *In exhalation dysfunctions the key rib is the uppermost rib of the dysfunction. (see fig 3.3b)*

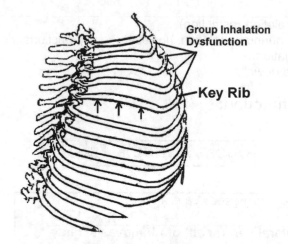

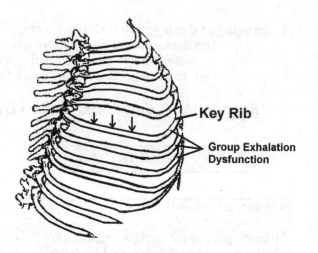

Fig 3.3a: Group inhalation dysfunction   Fig 3.3b Group exhalation dysfunction

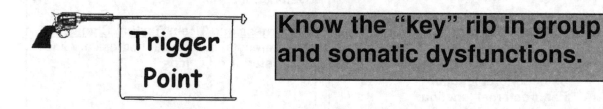

Trigger Point

Know the "key" rib in group and somatic dysfunctions.

Treating a Group Dysfunction

It is important to identify the key rib because, when treating a rib somatic dysfunction, treatment is directed at the key rib. For example, if a patient has a group exhalation dysfunction of ribs 2 - 5, osteopathic treatment would be directed at rib 2.

CHAPTER 3 REVIEW QUESTIONS

1. Using the "rule of three's", the transverse process of T5 can be located:
    A. Half way between the spinous process of T4 and T5.
    B. At the level of the spinous process of T5.
    C. Half way between the spinous process of T5 and T6.
    D. At the level of the spinous process of T6.
    E. At the level of the spinous process of T7.

2. The umbilicus is located in which dermatome?
    A. T4.
    B. T8.
    C. T10.
    D. T12.
    E. L1.

3. The main motion of the thoracic vertebrae is?
    A. Flexion/extension.
    B. Sidebending.
    C. Rotation.
    D. Sidebending and rotation.

4. All of the following are secondary muscles of respiration EXCEPT?
    A. Scalenes.
    B. Pectoralis minor.
    C. External intercostal.
    D. Quadratus lumborum.
    E. Latissimus dorsi.

5. Which of the following groups of ribs are considered false?
    A. Ribs 1-8.
    B. Ribs 7-10.
    C. Ribs 6-10.
    D. Ribs 8-10.
    E. Ribs 7-11.

6. Which of the following groups of ribs are considered atypical?
    A. Ribs 1,2,3,11,12.
    B. Ribs 1,2,3,12.
    C. Ribs 1,3,12.
    D. Ribs 1,2,11,12.
    E. Ribs 1,2,12.

7. A typical rib will have all of the following landmarks EXCEPT?
    A. Tubercle.
    B. Tuberosity.
    C. Head.
    D. Neck.
    E. Angle.

8. A 25 year old male comes to your office complaining of right sided thoracic pain. The pain started after a fall at work approximately one week ago. The severity of the pain has decreased throughout the week however it is still present, especially at maximum inhalation. Advil four times daily seems to decrease the pain. X-rays in your office reveal no fracture. EKG reveals normal sinus rhythm. On examination, you notice that ribs 6-9 on the right are restricted with inhalation, therefore you suspect a rib dysfunction. Which of the following statements correctly describes the diagnosis and treatment?
   A. Inhalation dysfunction and treatment should be directed at rib 9.
   B. Exhalation dysfunction and treatment should be directed at rib 9.
   C. Inhalation dysfunction and treatment should be directed at rib 6.
   D. Exhalation dysfunction and treatment should be directed at rib 6.

9. Which muscle would be used to correct this somatic dysfunction using muscle energy?
   A. Anterior scalene.
   B. Posterior scalene.
   C. Pectoralis minor
   D. Serratus anterior.
   E. Latissimus dorsi.

10. Which one of the following statements concerning ribs 6-9 is true?
   A. All of the ribs are considered typical.
   B. All of the ribs are considered typical except rib 9.
   C. All of the ribs are considered atypical.
   D. All of the ribs are considered typical except rib 6.

11. Which one of the following statements concerning the motion of ribs 6-9 is true?
   A. All of the ribs primarily move in a pump-handle motion.
   B. All of the ribs primarily move in a bucket-handle motion.
   C. All of the ribs primarily move in a caliper motion.
   D. All of the ribs primarily move in a pump-handle motion, except rib 9 which moves primarily in a bucket-handle motion.
   E. All of the ribs primarily move in a bucket-handle motion, except rib 6 which moves primarily in a pump-handle motion.

12. Which one of the following statements concerning the thoracic vertebral attachments of ribs 6-9 is true?
   A. Ribs 6-9 attach to T6-T10.
   B. Ribs 6-9 attach to T6-T9.
   C. Ribs 6-9 attach to T5- T9.
   D. Ribs 6-9 attach to T5-T10.

ANSWERS

1. A	7. B
2. C	8. D
3. C	9. D
4. C	10. A
5. D	11. B
6. D	12. C

CHAPTER 4

LUMBAR SPINE

I. Anatomy

A. Important clinical points

There are five lumbar vertebrae distinguishable by their large quadrangular spinous processes. The large cross-sectional area of the lumbar vertebral body is designed to sustain longitudinal loads. [1 p.582]

The posterior longitudinal ligament runs vertically along the posterior aspect of the vertebral body. This ligament begins to narrow at the lumbar region. At L4 and L5 the posterior longitudinal ligament is one-half the width of that at L1. This narrowing produces a weakness in the posteriolateral aspect of the intervertebral disc. This weakness makes the lumbar spine more susceptible to disc herniations.

In the thoracic and lumbar region a nerve root will exit the intervertebral foramen **below** its corresponding vertebrae (see fig 4.1). For example, the L4 nerve root will exit the spinal column between L4 and L5. The spinal cord usually terminates between L1 and L2. Therefore, the exiting nerve roots become longer as they approach the lower segments, causing the lumbar nerve roots to exit the superior aspect of their corresponding intervertebral foramina, just **above** the intervertebral disc. This information is important when considering disc herniations (discussed later).

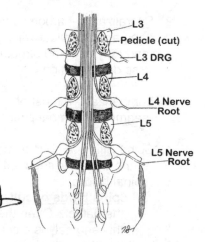

Fig 4.1: (DRG = Dorsal Root Ganglion) Lumbar nerve roots exit intervertebral foramen below the corresponding vertebrae, but above the intervertebral disc.

B. Muscles

Erector spinae group (spinalis, longissimus, iliocostalis)
Multifidus and rotatores
Quadratus lumborum
Iliopsoas - composed of the psoas major muscle and iliacus muscle.
   Origin - T12 - L5 vertebral bodies [3 p.385]
   Insertion - Lesser trochanter of femur
   Action - primary flexor of the hip
   Clinical importance - Somatic dysfunction of the iliopsoas muscle

> Memory Tool: [59 p.34]
> Erector spinae group = "SILO"
>
> S = Spinalis
> I = Iliocostalis
> LO = LOngissimus

is very common, and is usually precipitated from prolonged shortening of the muscle. *A pelvic side shift, a positive Thomas test, and somatic dysfunction of an upper lumbar segment is commonly seen with iliopsoas dysfunctions* (for further discussion see flexion contracture of the iliopsoas - Section IV C in this chapter). The iliopsoas also plays an important role in maintaining the lumbosacral angle.

C. Anatomical landmarks
        L4 - L5 intervertebral disc at the level of the iliac crest.
        T10 dermatome at the umbilicus, which is anterior to L3 and L4 intervertebral disc.

D. Anatomical variations
1. Facet (zygopophyseal) Trophism - An asymmetry of the facet joint angles. Normally facets in the lumbar spine are aligned in the sagittal plane (backwards and medial = BM). In facet tropism, lumbar facet joints are more closely aligned to the coronal plane.
        Clinical Importance - Considered the *most common anomaly in the lumbar spine.* [28 p.449] This may also predispose to early degenerative changes [30].

2. Sacralization- a bony deformity in which one or both of the transverse processes of L5 are long and articulate with the sacrum. Sacralization is present in 3.5% of individuals, [4 p.367] and may alter the structure-function relationship of the lumbosacral junction, leading to early disc degeneration.

3. Lumbarization- most often occurs from the failure of fusion of S1 with the other sacral segments. Lumbarization is much less common than sacralization.

4. Spina Bifida- a developmental anomaly in which there is a defect in the closure of the lamina of the vertebral segment. It usually occurs in the lumbar spine. There are three types of spinal bifida:
    a. **Spina bifida occulta** - No herniation through the defect. Often the only physical sign of this anomaly is a course patch of hair over the site. Rarely associated with neurological deficits.
    b. **Spina bifida meningocele** - A herniation of the meninges through the defect.
    c. **Spina bifida meningomyelocele** - A herniation of the meninges and the nerve roots through the defect. Associated with neruological deficits.

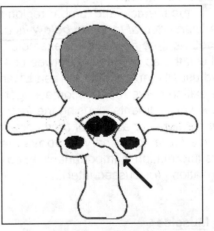

Fig 4.2: Spina bifida. Arrow demonstrates defect in lamina

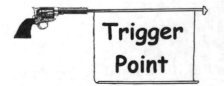

Trigger Point

Know the definition and different types of Spina Bifida.

II. Lumbar mechanics and Somatic dysfunction

Due to the alignment of the facets (backward and medial for the superior facets), *the major motion of the lumbar spine is flexion and extension.* There is a small degree of sidebending and a very limited amount of rotation. Motion of the lumbar spine will follow Fryette's laws. Somatic dysfunction may occur in any of the three planes of motion.

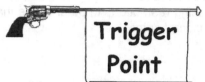

Trigger Point

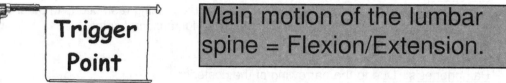

Main motion of the lumbar spine = Flexion/Extension.

A. Motion of L5 will influence the motion of the sacrum in two ways: [1 p.620]
  1. Sidebending of L5 will cause a sacral oblique axis to be engaged on the same side.
  2. Rotation of the L5 will cause the sacrum to rotate toward the opposite side.

For a further description of the influence of L5 on lumbosacral mechanics, see Chapter 6 Sacrum and Innominates.

III. Lumbosacral angle (Ferguson's angle) (see fig 4.3)

The lumbosacral angle is formed by the intersection of a horizontal line and the line of inclination of the sacrum. This angle is normally between 25° and 35°. [2 p.164] An increase in Ferguson's angle causes a shear stress placed on the lumbosacral joint, often causing low back pain.

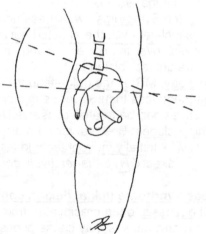

Fig 4.3: Ferguson's angle: The angle formed between the two dotted lines (normally 25° -35°).

IV. Problems that cause low back pain

Low back pain may be acute or chronic. Acute causes of low back pain may be due to fracture, recent strain or disc herniation, an infection, such as osteomyelitis or meningitis, or it may be referred pain. Chronic causes of low back pain are much more common. It is important as a physician to distinguish between congenital, metabolic, neoplastic, and degenerative cause of low back pain. Since there are several causes of low back pain, our discussion will be limited to the mechanical causes of low back pain. Although not very common, another important cause of low back pain is cauda equina syndrome, which will also be discussed.

A. Somatic dysfunctions of the lumbosacral spine (back strain/sprain)

Location of back pain: low back, buttock, posterior lateral thigh. [7 p.183]

Quality of pain: ache, muscle spasm. [7 p.183]

Signs and symptoms: increased pain with activity or prolonged standing or sitting, increased muscle tension.

Treatment: OMT consisting of counterstrain for tenderpoints, muscle energy or HVLA for restrictions. OMT should also be directed at decreasing restrictions in other areas that may alter the structure-function relationship of the lumbosacral spine.

B. Herniated nucleus pulposus

Pathogenesis: Due to the narrowing of the posterior longitudinal ligament, a posteriolateral herniation of the intervertebral disc is a common problem. Ninety-eight percent of herniations occur between L4 and L5, or between L5 and S1. [7 p.191] *A herniated disc in the lumbar region will exert pressure on the nerve root of the vertebrae below*. For example, a herniation between L3 and L4 will affect the nerve root of L4 (see fig 4.4).

Location of pain: lower back and lower leg.

Quality of pain: Numbness and/or tingling which may be accompanied by sharp, burning and/or shooting pain radiating down the leg, which worsens with flexion of the lumbar spine.

Signs and Symptoms: weakness and decreased reflexes associated with the affected nerve root. Sensory deficit over the corresponding dermatome. Positive straight leg raising test.

Radiology: MRI is the gold standard.

Treatment: less than 5% are surgical candidates. Most cases can be treated conservatively.

This includes: Bed rest for no more than 2 days. [31]

OMT - Initially indirect techniques, followed by gentle direct. HVLA is relatively contraindicated.

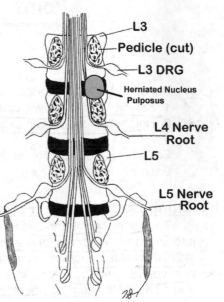

L3
Pedicle (cut)
L3 DRG
Herniated Nucleus Pulposus
L4 Nerve Root
L5
L5 Nerve Root

Fig 4.4: Herniated Nucleus Pulposus. Herniated disc at L3/L4 will likely exert pressure on L4 nerve root.

C. Psoas syndrome (a.k.a. flexion contracture of the iliopsoas)[56 p.747]

Pathogenesis: often precipitated from prolonged positions that shorten the psoas. [56 p.747] However organic causes may cause psoas spasm through viscero-somatic or somato-somatic reflexes. Organic causes must be ruled out before initiating treatment for mechanical causes.

Organic causes include: [56 p.747, 28 p.484]

1. Appendicitis
2. Sigmoid colon dysfunction
3. Ureteral calculi
4. Ureter dysfunction
5. Metastatic carcinoma of the prostate
6. Salpingitis

Location of pain: low back sometimes radiating to groin.

Quality of pain: ache, muscle spasm.

Signs and symptoms: increased pain when standing or walking, positive Thomas test, tender point medial to ASIS, nonneutral dysfunction of L1 or L2, positive pelvic shift test to the contralateral side, sacral dysfunction on an oblique axis and contralateral piriformis spasm.

Treatment:[1,489] An acute spasm may benefit from ice to decrease pain and edema. Do not initially use heat. Counterstrain to the anterior iliopsoas tenderpoint is very effective followed by muscle energy or HVLA to the high lumbar dysfunction. Stretching an acute psoas spasm may cause it to further spasm. Only stretch chronic psoas spasms. *Some authors[28] report that symptoms will not resolve until the high lumbar dysfunction is treated.*

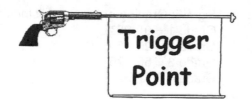

Trigger Point

A flexion contracture of the iliopsoas is often associated with a nonneutral dysfunction of L1 or L2.

D. **Spinal stenosis**

Definition: Narrowing of the spinal canal or intervertebral foramina usually due to degenerative changes, causing pressure on nerve roots (or rarely the cord). [32 p.540]

Pathogenesis: Degenerative changes in the lumbar spine can include:
1) Hypertrophy of the facet joints.
2) Calcium deposits within the ligamentum flavum and the posterior longitudinal ligament.
3) Loss of intervertebral disc height.

All of which can narrow the spinal canal and/or intervertebral foramina and result in nerve root compression.

Location of pain: low back to lower leg or legs.

Quality of pain: ache, shooting pain or paresthesias.

Signs and symptoms: Worsened by extension as when standing, walking or lying supine.

Radiology: osteophytes and decreased intervertebral disc space are usually present. *Foraminal narrowing may often be seen on oblique views.*

Treatment: OMT should be directed at decreasing any restrictions, improving range of motion. Additional conservative management includes: physical therapy, NSAID's or low dose tapering steroids. An epidural steroid injection may be used if conservative therapy is not effective. Surgical laminectomy with decompression is indicated if above fails.

E. **Spondylolisthesis** (see fig 4.7)

Definition: *anterior displacement* of one vertebrae in relation to the one below. [1 p.1138] Often occurs at L4 or L5, and is usually due to fatigue fractures in the pars interarticularis of the vertebrae.

Prevalence: 5% of the population. However, approximately half are asymptomatic. Patients who become symptomatic do so usually after the age of 20. [28p.366]

Location of pain: low back, buttock and/or posterior thigh. [29p.p.368]

Quality of pain: ache.

Signs and symptoms: Increased pain with extension-based activities. Tight hamstrings bilaterally. Stiffed-legged, short-stride, waddling type gait. [1p.1009, 28 p.367] Typically, there are no neurologic deficits. *Positive vertebral step-off sign (palpating the spinous processes there is an obvious forward displacement at the area of the listhesis).*

Radiology: forward displacement of one vertebrae on another seen on lateral films. Can be classified (grade 1 - 4) based on the degree of slippage (see figure 4.5)

Treatment: most patients (85 - 90%) can be managed with conservative management. The goals of manipulation is to reduce lumbar lordosis and somatic dysfunction [1 p.1011] *HVLA is contraindicated.* Additional conservative management includes, weight loss, avoiding high heels and avoiding flexion based exercises. [28 p.371-74] Heel lifts have been advocated to control postural mechanics. Lumbo-sacral orthotics can be considered for short term stability. [1p.1012]

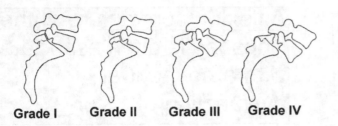

Fig 4.5: Grading of Spondylolisthesis.
Grade 1 = 0 - 25%
Grade 2 = 25 - 50%
Grade 3 = 50 - 75%
Grade 4 = >75%

Grade I   Grade II   Grade III   Grade IV

F. **Spondylolysis** (see figs 4.6 and 4.8) - a defect usually of the pars interarticularis **without** anterior displacement of the vertebral body. Symptoms and treatment are similar to spondylolisthesis. Since lateral lumbar x-rays will not reveal any slippage, **oblique views will identify the fracture of the pars interarticularis. It is often seen as a "collar" on the neck of the scotty dog.**

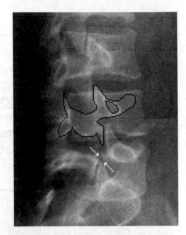

Fig 4.6: Oblique view of the lumbar spine. Black outline demonstrates the scotty dog. White arrows show lucency (a black collar around the neck of the scootty dog) in the pars interarticularis in the vertebrae below.

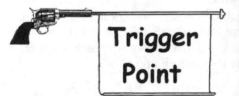

Trigger Point

Know the difference between spondylolisthesis, spondylolysis, and spondylosis

G. **Spondylosis** (see fig 4.9) - A radiographical term for degenerative changes within the intervertebral disc and ankylosing of adjacent vertebral bodies. [1] p.1138

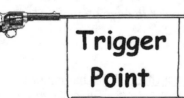

Trigger Point

Diagnose:
1) Spondylolisthesis with Lateral x-rays
2) Spondylolysis with Oblique x-rays

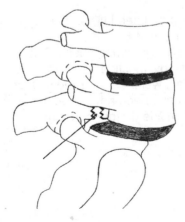 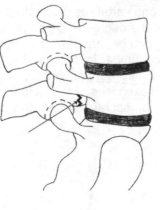

Fig 4.7 Spondylolisthesis (left): The arrow shows a fracture of the pars interarticularis with anterior displacement of L5 on the sacrum

Fig 4.8 Spondylolysis (right): The arrow shows a fracture of the pars interarticularis without anterior displacement.

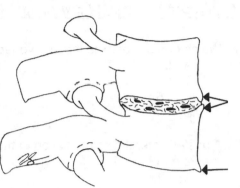

Fig 4.9 Spondylosis: Three arrows show the anterior lipping of the vertebral bodies. Note the associated degenerative changes within the intervertebral disc.

H. **Cauda Equina Syndrome**

Definition: pressure on the nerve roots of the cauda equina usually due to a massive central disc herniation.

Location of pain: low back.

Quality of pain: sharp.

Signs and symptoms: Saddle anesthesia, decreased deep tendon reflexes, decreased rectal sphincter tone, and loss of bowel and bladder control.

Treatment: Emergent surgical decompression of the cauda equina is imperative. If surgery is delayed too long, irreversible paralysis may result.

CHAPTER 4 REVIEW QUESTIONS

1. Which nerve root exits the intervertebral foramen between the L4 and L5 vertebrae?
   A. L3.
   B. L4.
   C. L5.
   D. S1.

2. A posteriolateral disc herniation of the intervertebral disc of L4/L5 is most likely to compress which nerve root?
   A. L3.
   B. L4.
   C. L5.
   D. S1.

3. All of the following may be seen in a patient with a right sided psoas syndrome EXCEPT?
   A. A positive Thomas test.
   B. Tenderpoint medial to the ASIS
   C. Pelvis shifted to the right
   D. A somatic dysfunction of the upper lumbar segments.

4. A posterior herniation of the meninges and the nerve roots through a defect in a lumbar vertebral body is called?
   A. Spina bifida occulta.
   B. Spina bifida meningocele.
   C. Spina bifida meningomyelocele
   D. Spondylolisthesis.
   E. Spondylosis.

5. The main motion of the lumbar spine is?
   A. Flexion/extension.
   B. Sidebending.
   C. Rotation.
   D. Sidebending and rotation.

6. A 55 year old male presents to your office with low back pain radiating to his lower extremities. He states that yesterday his feet felt numb and weak, and now this feeling has progressed into his thighs. Neurological examination of his lower extremities reveals: 0/4 deep tendon reflexes; 3/5 muscle strength in his ankle plantar flexors; 3/5 in ankle dorsiflexors; and 3/5 in knee flexors and extensors. You also notice a decreased rectal tone. Which one of the following statements describes the correct course of treatment?
   A. Immediate transportation by EMS to the hospital for neurosurgical evaluation.
   B. Indirect OMT techniques initially to decrease restrictions, followed by direct techniques such as muscle energy, one week later.
   C. Physical modalities, such as ultrasound and electrical stimulation to the low back.
   D. NSAIDS and referral to MRI clinic if pain not improved in one week.
   E. Referral to neurosurgical specialist for evaluation.

7. The anterior displacement of one vertebral body in relation to the one below is known as:
    A. Spondylosis.
    B. Spondylolysis.
    C. Spondylolisthesis.
    D. Spina bifida.
    E. Spinal stenosis.

8. Degenerative changes within the intervertebral disc and ankylosing of adjacent vertebral bodies is known as:
    A. Spondylosis.
    B. Spondylolysis.
    C. Spondylolisthesis.
    D. Spina bifida.
    E. Spinal stenosis.

9. All of the following concerning cauda equina syndrome is true EXCEPT:
    A. It can be due to a large central herniation on the cauda equina.
    B. It may result in a weakness in both legs.
    C. It is a surgical emergency.
    D. Paralysis may occur rapidly, but does not usually effect the bladder or rectum.
    E. A decreased sensation to the medial aspect of the thighs and groin, often called "saddle anesthesia" can occur.

10. All of the following may cause psoas syndrome EXCEPT:
    A. Ureter dysfunction
    B. Salpingitis
    C. Sigmoid colon dysfunction
    D. Appendicitis
    E. Cystitis

11. All of the following is true regarding spondylolisthesis EXCEPT:
    A. HVLA at the lumbosacral spine in contraindicated
    B. 30% of the vertebral displacement is considered a grade II spondylolisthesis
    C. Patients often walk stiffed-legged with a waddling type of gait
    D. Pain is relieved with extension based exercises
    E. The patient often has normal sensation in both lower extremities

ANSWERS

1. B	7. C
2. C	8. A
3. C	9. D
4. C	10. E
5. A	11. D
6. A	

A. Spondylosis
B. Scoliosis
C. Spondylolisthesis
D. Osteophyte
E. Disc stenosis

A. Supportive
B. Strong
C.
D.
E. Sphenoid base

A.
B.
C.
D.
E. Unsold

A.
B.
C.
D.

CHAPTER 5

SCOLIOSIS AND SHORT LEG SYNDROME

Scoliosis

I. **Definition** - an appreciable lateral deviation of the spine from the normally straight vertical line of the spine. [49] Due to Fryette's laws, any sidebending of the spine will automatically induce rotation. Therefore the term "rotoscoliosis" is thought to be more accurate.

    A. Epidemiology - 5% of school-age children develop scoliosis by age 15. [28 p.350] However, only 10% of those children have clinical symptoms related to their scoliotic curvatures. [28 p.350] Female: Male ratio = 4:1.

    B. Naming scoliosis -
        Curve that is sidebent left = scoliosis to the right = dextroscoliosis. (see fig 4.1a)
          Dextro - donoting a relationship to the right. [49]

        Curve that is sidebent right = scoliosis to the left = levoscoliosis. (see fig 4.1b)
          Levo - donoting a relationship to the left. [49]

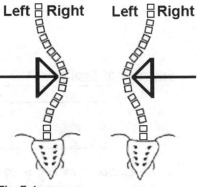

Fig 5.1a:
Dextroscoliosis

Fig 5.1b:
Levoscoliosis

> **Memory Tool:**
> The arrow points to the right in Dextroscoliosis
> The arrow points to the left in Levoscoliosis

II. **Classification of Scoliosis Curves**
    Two Types

        1) Structural Curve: [1 p.990, 25 p.433]
           A spinal curve that is relatively fixed and inflexible. A structural curve will not correct with sidebending in the opposite direction. It is associated with vertebral wedging and shortened ligaments and muscles on the concave side of the curve.

        2) Functional Curve: [1 p.990, 25 p.433]
           A spinal curve that is flexible and can be partially or completely corrected with sidebending to the opposite side. An uncorrected functional curve may eventually progress into a structural curve.

III. **Screening and Measuring Scoliosis**

A. **Screening**
It is generally recommended that children ages 10 - 15 years old be examined for scoliosis.

Procedure
1) Examine levelness of occiput, shoulders, iliac crests, PSIS's, and greater trochanters.
2) If any of the above are not level, have the patient bend forward at the waist. If a rib hump (a group of ribs that appear higher on one side as the patient bends forward) appears, the patient is likely to have scoliosis.
3) Screen for a lumbosacral somatic dysfunction that may give the appearance of a short leg (i.e. sacral shear). If present, treat the somatic dysfunction, recheck the scoliosis, and if it is still present then obtain standing x-rays.

B. **Measuring Scoliotic Curves**
Spinal curves are measured with x-rays using the Cobb method.

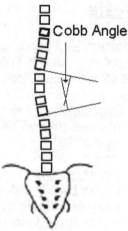

Cobb method: (fig 4.2)
1) Draw horizontal lines from the vertebral bodies of the extreme ends of the curve.
2) Draw perpendicular lines from these horizontal lines and measure the acute (Cobb) angle.

Fig 5.2: Cobb Angle shown measures the degree of scoliosis.

IV. **Severity of Scoliosis** [28 p. 351]

Severity	Cobb Angle
Mild	5^0 - 15^0
Moderate	20^0 - 45^0
Severe	$>50^0$

Respiratory function is compromised if the thoracic curvature is > 50^0.
Cardiovascular function is compromised if the thoracic curvature is >75^0.

V. **Causes of Scoliosis** [28 p.351, 32 p.643]

1) Idiopathic - Approximately 80% of all causes of scoliosis. Some patients may have a family history of scoliosis suggesting a genetic component.

2) Congenital - Often due to a malformation of the vertebrae. These cases are most often progressive.

3) Neuromuscular - Due to a muscular weakness or spasticity. [25 p. 434] Some examples include poliomyelitis, cerebral palsy, Duchenne's muscular dystrophy and meningomyelocele.

4) Acquired - Examples include tumor, infection, osteomalacia, sciatic irritability, psoas syndrome, and short leg syndrome.

VI. Treatment

5-15° (handwritten)

1) Mild Scoliosis - Conservative management will consist of physical therapy, Konstancin exercises and OMT. The goal of conservative treatment is to improve flexibility and strengthen trunk and abdominal musculature. OMT is not intended to completely straighten scoliotic curves. [1 p. 996] *Konstancin exercises is a series of specific exercises that has been proven to improve the patient with scoliotic postural decompensation.* [28 p.339]

20-45 (handwritten)

2) Moderate Scoliosis - In addition to the above, bracing with a spinal orthotic is often indicated.

>50° (handwritten)

3) Severe Scoliosis - Surgery is often indicated if there is respiratory compromise or if the scoliotic curve progresses quickly despite conservative management. *Resp > CV* (handwritten) *or curve incr Δ* (handwritten)

Short Leg Syndrome

I. Definition - Condition in which an anatomical or functional leg length discrepancy results in: [28 p.343]
1) Sacral base unleveling
2) Vertebral sidebending and rotation
3) Innominate rotation

II. Classifications
1) Anatomical leg length discrepancy - one leg anatomically shorter than the other.
   - *Most common cause is a hip replacement.*

2) Functional leg length discrepancy - one leg appears shorter than the other.

III. Signs and Symptoms
Although each person with short leg syndrome will compensate differently, certain structural findings will be present. They are: [28 p.344]

1) Sacral base unleveling - the sacral base will be lower on the side of the short leg.
2) Anterior innominate rotation on the side of the short leg.
3) Posterior innominate rotation on the side of the long leg.
4) Lumbar spine will sidebend away and rotate toward the side of the short leg.
5) Lumbosacral (Ferguson's) angle will increase $2°-3°$.
6) First the iliolumbar ligaments, then the SI ligaments may become stressed on the side of the short leg.

IV. Treatment [28 p. 346]

1) OMT directed at the spine and lower extremities done to remove or decrease as much somatic dysfunction as possible. If a leg length discrepancy is still present and short leg syndrome is still suspected then...
2) Obtain standing postural x-rays to quantify differences in the heights of the femoral head. If femoral head difference is > 5mm then consider a heel lift.

V. Heel Lift Guidelines [1 p.987, 28 p.346]
1) The heel lift should be applied to the side of the short leg.
2) The final lift height should be ½ - ¾ of the measured leg length discrepancy, unless there was a recent sudden cause of the discrepancy (i.e. hip fracture or hip prosthesis). In this case, lift the full amount that was lost.
3) The "fragile" (elderly, arthritic, osteoporotic, or having acute pain) patient should begin with a 1/16" (~1.5mm) heel lift and increase 1/16" every two weeks.

4) The "flexible" patient should begin with 1/8" (~3.2mm) heel lift and increase 1/8" every two weeks

5) A maximum of ¼" may be applied to the inside of the shoe. If > ¼" is needed then this must be applied to the outside of the shoe.

6) Maximum heel lift possible = ½". If more height is needed, an ipsilateral anterior sole lift extending from heel to toe should be used in order to keep the pelvis from rotating to the opposite side.

CHAPTER 5 REVIEW QUESTIONS

1. Which of the following is true regarding scoliosis?

   A) Approximately 50% of children with scoliosis develop clinical symptoms related to their scoliotic curves.
   B) Scoliosis is more common in males.
   C) Dextroscoliosis is a scoliotic curve that is sidebent to the left.
   D) A structural spinal curve is associated with a scoliosis greater than 15 degrees.

2. Which scoliotic curve typically results in respiratory compromise but not cardiovascular compromise?

   A) Scoliosis due to Duchenne's muscular dystophy
   B) Scoliosis due to osteomalacia
   C) A spinal curve with a Cobb angle measuring 52 degrees
   D) A spinal curve with a Cobb angle measureing 77 degrees

3. The most common cause of scoliosis is?
   A) Idiopathic
   B) Cerebral palsy
   C) Congenital malformation of the vertebrae
   D) Psoas syndrome
   E) Short leg syndrome

4. Surgery for scoliosis is likely to have favorable results in which of the following cases?
   A) In a patient with a spinal curve of 35 degees
   B) In a skeletally mature patient with a spinal curve of 50 degees.
   C) In a patient whose scoliosis pregressed 10 degrees in one year.
   D) In a patient with idiopathic scoliosis with a scoliotic curve measuring 30 degees
   E) In a patient whose scoliosis has progressed despite bracing, and is causing respiratory compromise.

5. All of the following signs and symptoms are typically seen in patient's with short leg syndrome EXCEPT?

   A) Anterior innominate rotation on the side of the short leg
   B) An increase in the lumbosacral angle of 2° - 3°
   C) Lumbar spine sidebent toward and rotated away from the side of the short leg.
   D) A sacral base that is lower on the side of the short leg

6. The most common cause of an anatomic leg length discrepancy is?

   A) Osteoarthritis at the hip
   B) Petrusio acetabulae due to rheumatod arthritis
   C) Total hip replacement
   D) Hip dislocation
   E) Scoliosis

7. A 75 year old female comes to your office with low back pain . On examination, she has a leg length discrepancy of 1.5cm. X-rays are without fracture but the right femoral head is 13mm cephalad when compared to the left. Which of the following choices explains the best course of action for this patient?

A) The patient should be perscribed a heel lift of 1.5 mm and increased 1.5mm every week until the pain has resolved

B) The patient should be perscribed a heel lift of 3.2 mm and increased 3.2mm every two weeks until the pain has resolved

C) The patient should be perscribed a lift of 1.5mm and increased 1.5mm every other week until a final height of 6 - 9 mm has been achieved.

D) The patient should be perscribed a shoe lift of 7.5 mm and follow-up in two weeks

E) A lift is not indicated in the above patient

ANSWERS

1. C	5. C
2. C	6. C
3. A	7. C
4. E	

CHAPTER 6
SACRUM & INNOMINATES

I. Anatomy

A. Bones and bony landmarks

1. <u>Innominate</u>: The innominate is composed of three fused bones. The ilium, the ischium and pubis bones are partially cartilaginous at birth and eventually fuse by age twenty. [1 p.601]

2. <u>Sacrum</u>: The sacrum is composed of <u>five fused</u> vertebrae. The anterior portion of the first segment (S1) is referred to as the *sacral promontory*. The *sacral base* is the top (most cephalad) part of the sacrum. In somatic dysfunctions, the sacral base can be recorded as shallow (or posterior) or deep (or anterior). The sacral apex is the bottom part of the sacrum, which articulates with the coccyx. The *sacral sulci* are located on the superior lateral part of the sacrum (see figure 6.1). They are recorded as posterior (or shallow) or anterior (or deep) in somatic dysfunctions. The *inferior lateral angles* (ILA's) of the sacrum are located at the inferior lateral part of the sacrum. They are recorded as shallow (or posterior), deep (or anterior), superior or inferior in somatic dysfunctions.

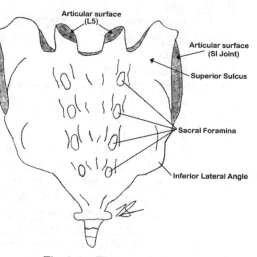

Fig 6.1: The sacrum

<u>NOTE:</u> In some osteopathic schools the right sacral sulcus is referred to as the right sacral base. The left sacral sulcus is referred to as the left sacral base. In somatic dysfunctions, the right (or left) sacral base could be anterior or posterior.

B. Articulations

The innominates articulate with the femur at the acetabulum, the sacrum at the SI joint, and the pubic bones articulate with each other at the pubic symphysis. The SI joint is an inverted "L" shaped joint with upper and lower arms converging anteriorly. These two arms join at S2. Somatic dysfunction may occur in one or both arms of the SI joint. [1 p. 619]

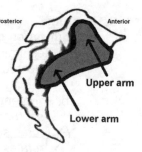

Fig 6.2: The SI joint is an inverted "L" joint with the 2 arms converging anteriorly.

C. Ligaments

Pelvic ligaments can be categorized into **true** and **accessory** pelvic ligaments. [28 p.406]

1. <u>True pelvic ligaments</u> (Sacroiliac ligaments)

   Anterior, posterior and *interosseous* sacroiliac ligaments surround and help stabilize the SI joint.

2. Accessory pelvic ligaments
   a. Sacrotuberous ligament - originates at the inferior lateral angle and attaches to the ischial tuberosity. Testing the tension of this ligament can help diagnose somatic dysfunction of the innominate or sacrum. [28 p.407]
   b. Sacrospinous ligament - originates at the sacrum and attaches to the ischial spines. This ligament divides the greater and lesser sciatic foramen.
   c. Iliolumbar ligament - originates from the transverse processes of L4 and L5 and attaches to the medial side of the iliac crest. It is often the first ligament to become painful in lumbosacral decompensation. [28 p.407]

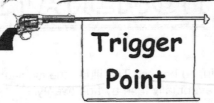

Trigger Point

The Sacrospinous ligament divides the greater and lesser sciatic foramen.

D. **Muscles**
   Pelvic muscles can be categorized into **primary and secondary** muscles. [28 p.408]
   1. Primary pelvic muscles - These muscles make up the *pelvic diaphragm*.
      a. Levator ani
      b. Coccygeus muscles
   2. Secondary pelvic muscles - These muscles have partial attachment to the true pelvis
      a. Iliopsoas - discussed in chapter 4
      b. Obturator internus
      c. Piriformis
         Origin - at the inferior anterior aspect of the sacrum.
         Insertion - the greater trochanter of the femur.
         Action - externally rotates, extends thigh and abducts thigh with hip flexed.
         Innervation - S1 & S2 nerve roots.
         Clinical importance - approximately 11% of the population will have either the entire or peroneal portion of the sciatic nerve running through the belly of the piriformis. Therefore, piriformis hypertonicity can cause buttock pain that radiates down the thigh, but not usually below the knee.

II. **Sacral and innominate mechanics**
   A. **Innominates** (see fig 6.3)
      Physiologically, the innominates rotate about an inferior transverse axis of the sacrum during the walking cycle (dotted line in figure 6.3). It is also the axis which an innominate anterior or innominate posterior somatic dysfunction occur.

   B. **Sacrum**
      1. **Four types of sacral motion** (see fig 6.3)
         a. Respiratory motion- *Motion occurs about the superior transverse axis of the sacrum.* It is located at approximately S2. [28 p.401] During inhalation, the sacral base will move posterior. During exhalation, the sacral base will move anterior. [1 p.607]
         b. Inherent (craniosacral) motion- *Motion occurs about the superior transverse axis of the sacrum* (same axis for respiratory motion). *During craniosacral flexion, the sacral base rotates posteriorly or* **counternutates**. *During craniosacral extension, the sacral base rotates anteriorly or* **nutates**. [1 p.607-8]
         c. Postural motion- *Motion occurs about the middle transverse axis of the sacrum.* As a person begins to bend forward, the sacral base moves anteriorly. At terminal flexion, the sacrotuberous ligaments become taut and the sacral base will move posteriorly. [1p.607, 28 p.176]

d. <u>Dynamic motion</u>- *Motion that occurs during ambulation*. As weight bearing shifts from one side to the other while walking, the sacrum engages two sacral oblique axes. *Weight bearing on the left leg (stepping forward with the right leg) will cause a left sacral axis to be engaged.* The opposite is true for weight bearing on the right leg. [1 p.608]

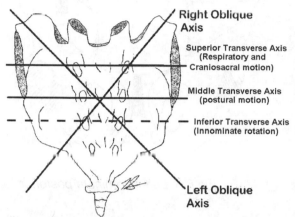

Right Oblique Axis

Superior Transverse Axis (Respiratory and Craniosacral motion)

Middle Transverse Axis (postural motion)

Inferior Transverse Axis (Innominate rotation)

Left Oblique Axis

Fig 6.3: Physiologic axes of the sacrum and innominate: Respiratory and craniosacral motions occurs about the superior transverse axis. Postural motion occurs about the middle transverse axis. Dynamic motion occurs about a left or right oblique axes. Innominate rotation occurs about an inferior transverse axis.

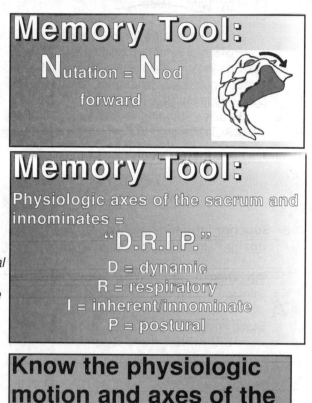

Memory Tool:

Nutation = Nod
forward

Memory Tool:

Physiologic axes of the sacrum and innominates =

"D.R.I.P."

D = dynamic
R = respiratory
I = inherent/innominate
P = postural

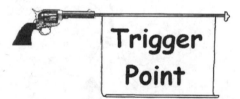

Trigger Point

Know the physiologic motion and axes of the sacrum.

III. Somatic dysfunctions of the innominates and sacrum

A. <u>Innominate dysfunction</u> (Remember, the side of the positive standing flexion test is the side of the dysfunction.)

1. **Anterior innominate rotation**
   One innominate will rotate anteriorly compared to the other. Rotation occurs about the inferior transverse axis of the sacrum.
   Etiology: tight quadriceps
   <u>Static findings:</u> [1 p.619, 33 p.219,]
   ASIS more inferior ipsilaterally.
   PSIS more superior ipsilaterally.
   Longer leg ipsilaterally. Unless it is compensatory for a anatomical short leg.
   <u>Dynamic findings:</u> [1 p.617, 33 p.219, 25 p.215]
   Positive standing flexion test ipsilaterally.
   Posterior innominate rotation is restricted ipsilaterally.
   ASIS restricted to compression ipsilaterally.

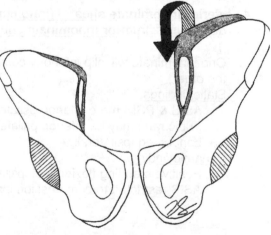

Fig 6.4: Left innominate anterior

2. **Posterior innominate rotation**
   One innominate will rotate posteriorly
   compared to the other. Rotation occurs about
   the inferior transverse axis of the sacrum.
   Etiology: tight hamstrings.
   Static findings: [1 p.617, 33 p.214]
   ASIS more superior ipsilaterally.
   PSIS more inferior ipsilaterally.
   Shorter leg ipsilaterally. Unless it is
   compensatory for a anatomical long leg.
   Dynamic findings: [33 p.214, 25 p.215]
   Positive standing flexion test ipsilaterally.
   ASIS restricted to compression ipsilaterally.

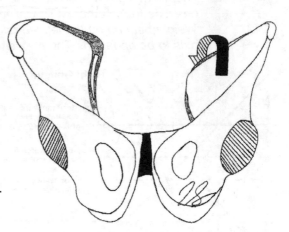

Fig 6.5: Left innominate posterior

3. **Superior innominate shear** [33] **(innominate
   upslip** [33]**, superior innominate subluxation** [1]**)**
   One innominate will slip superiorly compared to
   the other.
   Etiology: It can be due to a fall on the
   ipsilateral buttock or a mis-step
   Static findings: [1 p.617, 33 p.223, 25 p.215]
   ASIS & PSIS more superior ipsilaterally.
   Pubic rami may be superior ipsilaterally.
   Shorter leg ipsilaterally
   Dynamic findings: [33 p.223, 25 p.215]
   Positive standing flexion test ipsilaterally.
   ASIS restricted to compression ipsilaterally.

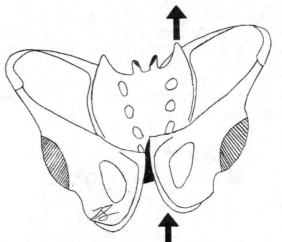

Fig 6.6: Left innominate upslip

4. **Inferior innominate shear** [33] **(innominate
   downslip** [33]**, inferior innominate subluxation**
   [1]**)**
   One innominate will slip inferiorly compared to
   the other.
   Static findings: [1 p.617, 25 p.215]
   ASIS & PSIS more inferior ipsilaterally.
   Pubic rami may be inferior ipsilaterally.
   Longer leg ipsilaterally
   Dynamic findings: [1 p.616, 25 p.215]
   Positive standing flexion test ipsilaterally.
   ASIS restricted to compression ipsilaterally.

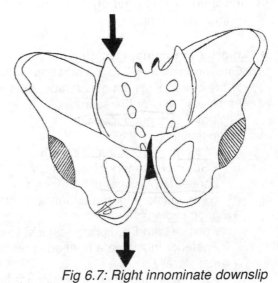

Fig 6.7: Right innominate downslip

5. **Superior pubic shear**

A condition where one pubic bone is displaced superiorly compared to the other.

Etiology: trauma or a tight rectus abdominus muscle.

Static findings: [1 p.618, 33 p.185]

ASIS's appear to be level.
PSIS's appear to be level.
Pubic bone superiorly ipsilaterally.

Dynamic findings: [33 p.185]

Positive standing flexion test ipsilaterally.
ASIS restricted to compression ipsilaterally.

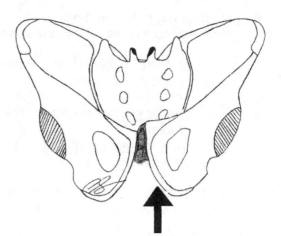

Fig 6.8: Left superior pubic shear

6. **Inferior pubic shear**

A condition where one pubic bone is displaced inferiorly compared to the other.

Etiology: trauma or tight adductors.

Static findings: [1 p.618, 33 p.187]

ASIS's appear to be level.
PSIS's appear to be level.
Pubic bone inferiorly ipsilaterally.

Dynamic findings: [33 p.187]

Positive standing flexion test ipsilaterally.
ASIS restricted to compression ipsilaterally.

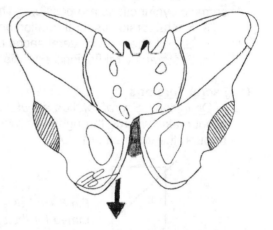

Fig 6.9: Right inferior pubic shear

7. **Innominate inflares**

A condition where the innominate will rotate medially.

Static findings: [33 p.224]

ASIS more medial ipsilaterally. Therefore the distance between the ASIS and umbilicus is less than the contralateral side.
Ischial tuberosity more lateral ipsilaterally.

Dynamic findings: [33 p.224]

Positive standing flexion test ipsilaterally.
ASIS restricted to compression ipsilaterally.

8. **Innominate outflare**

A condition where the innominate will rotate laterally.

Static findings: [33 p.224]

ASIS more lateral ipsilaterally. Therefore the distance between the ASIS and umbilicus is more than the contralateral side.
Ischial tuberosity more medial ipsilaterally.

Dynamic findings: [33 p.224]

Positive standing flexion test ipsilaterally.
ASIS restricted to compression ipsilaterally.

B. Sacral somatic dysfunction
There are two models to describe sacral dysfunction.

1. In 1938, Strachan described sacral movements in relation to the ilium. Strachan noted two sacral somatic dysfunctions.

    a. Anterior sacrum - the sacral base will rotate **forward** and sidebend to the opposite side of rotation.
    b. Posterior sacrum - the sacral base will rotate **backward** and sidebend to the opposite of the rotation.

NOTE: the two somatic dysfunctions listed above are older forms of describing sacral dysfunctions. Most osteopathic institutions do not teach this model, however in order to be complete, it was included here.

2. In 1958, Mitchell described sacral motion in relation to L5. According to Mitchell, three sacral somatic dysfunctions are possible. They are:
    a. Sacral torsions/sacral rotation on an oblique axis
    b. Sacral shears (unilateral sacral flexions/extensions)
    c. Bilateral sacral flexions/extensions

C. Sacral Torsions
1. Definition - *Sacral rotation about an oblique axis along with somatic dysfunction at L5.* The oblique axis will run through the superior sulcus ipsilaterally, diagonally across the sacrum, through the contralateral ILA.

Fig 6.10: Posterior view of the sacrum with a left oblique axis. The axis is named for the side of the superior pole it runs through.

2. Sacral Torsion Rules - Due to lumbosacral biomechanics, if a sacral torsion is present, certain reproducible L5 and seated flexion test findings are produced. These "Rules" can be summarized as follows:

Sacral Torsion Rules:
    a. **Rule #1**: *When L5 is sidebent, a sacral oblique axis is engaged on the same side as the sidebending.*
    b. **Rule #2**: *When L5 is rotated, the sacrum rotates the opposite way on an oblique axis.*
    c. **Rule #3**: *The seated flexion test is found on the opposite side of the oblique axis.*

Putting the rules together:
    If L5 is FR_RS_R:
        There will be a positive seated flexion test on the left.
        The sacrum will be rotated to the left on a right oblique axis or L on R.

    If L5 (or a group dysfunction of the lower lumbar region) is NS_LR_R:
        There will be a positive seated flexion test on the right.
        The sacrum will be rotated to the left on a left oblique axis or L on L.

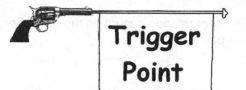

Trigger Point

Know the rules of L5 on the sacrum.

3. <u>Palpatory model for sacral torsions</u> [33]
   Springing over sacral landmarks in sacral torsions
      - *Springing (motion) present over the part of the sacrum that moved anterior.*
      - *Springing (motion) restricted over the part of the sacrum that moved posterior*
      - *Springing (motion) restricted over the poles that make up the oblique axis*
      - *Lumbosacral spring test is positive if the sacral base has moved posterior.*

Memory tool:
Torsion = twisting of two articulating structures (L5 and the Sacrum) in opposite directions.

In sacral torsions, L5 will always rotate in the opposite direction of the sacrum.

D. **Forward sacral torsion** (a.k.a. Anterior sacral torsion [56])
   In a forward sacral torsion, rotation is on the same side of the axis.
   Two dysfunctions are possible:

   1. <u>Left rotation on a left oblique axis (L on L)</u>: left rotation occurs as the right superior sulcus moves anterior while the left ILA moves posterior.

   <u>Static findings</u>: [1 p.620, 33 p.203]
      Right sulcus deeper.
      Left ILA posterior and slightly inferior
      Lumbar curve convex to the right.

   <u>Dynamic findings</u>: [25 p.218, 33 p.203]
      Positive seated flexion test on the RIGHT.
      Motion (springing) at the right base is present.
      Motion (springing) at the left ILA is restricted.
      Motion (springing) at the poles of the left oblique axis (left sulcus and right ILA) is restricted.
      Negative lumbosacral spring test
      L5 will be sidebent left rotated right ($NS_L R_R$).

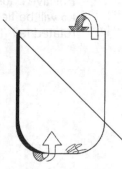

2. <u>Right rotation on a right oblique axis (R on R)</u>: right rotation occurs as the left superior sulcus moves anterior, while the right ILA moves posterior.

<u>Static findings</u>:[1 p.620, 33 p.203]
> Left sulcus deeper.
> Right ILA posterior and slightly inferior..
> Lumbar curve convex to the left.

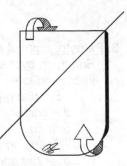

<u>Dynamic findings</u>: [25 p.219, 33 p.203]
> Positive seated flexion test on the LEFT.
> Motion (springing) at the left base is present.
> Motion (springing) at the right ILA is restricted.
> Motion (springing) at the poles of the right oblique axis
> (right sulcus and left ILA) is restricted.
> Negative lumbosacral spring test
> L5 will be sidebent right, rotated left (NS_RR_L).

E. **Backward sacral torsion** (posterior sacral torsion [56])
In a backward sacral torsion, rotation is on the opposite side of the axis.
Two dysfunctions are possible:

1. <u>Right rotation on a left oblique axis (R on L)</u>: right rotation occurs as the right superior sulcus moves posterior, and the left ILA moves anterior.

<u>Static findings</u>: [1 p.260, 33 p. 208]
> Right sulcus shallow.
> Left ILA anterior and slightly superior.
> Lumbar curve convex to the right.

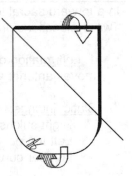

<u>Dynamic findings</u>: [1 p.615, 25 p.219, 33 p.203]
> Positive seated flexion test on the RIGHT.
> Motion (springing) at the right base is restricted.
> Motion (springing) at the left ILA is present.
> Motion (springing) at the poles of the left oblique axis
> (left sulcus and right ILA) is restricted.
> Positive lumbosacral spring test.
> Positive backward bending test.
> L5 will be flexed or extended (nonneutral), sidebent left,
> rotated left (NNR_LS_L).

50

2. <u>Left rotation on a right oblique axis (L on R)</u>: left rotation occurs as the left superior sulcus moves posterior, and the right ILA moves anterior.

<u>Static findings:</u>[1 p.260, 33 p. 208]
> Left sulcus shallow.
> Right ILA anterior and slightly superior.
> Lumbar curve convex to the left.

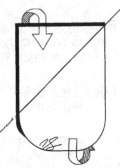

<u>Dynamic findings:</u> [1 p.615, 25 p.219, 33 p.203]
> Positive seated flexion test on the LEFT.
> Motion (springing) at the left base is restricted.
> Motion (springing) at the right ILA is present.
> Motion (springing) at the poles of the right oblique axis (right sulcus and left ILA) is restricted.
> Positive lumbosacral spring test.
> Positive backward bending test.
> L5 will be flexed or extended (nonneutral), sidebent right, rotated right (NNR_RS_R).

F. Sacral rotation on an oblique axis

Recently, the Educational Council on Osteopathic Principles has recognized another sacral somatic dysfunction, called **sacral rotation on an oblique axis**. This dysfunction is similar to sacral torsions, however **L5 is rotated to the same side as the sacrum.**

> <u>The possible dysfunctions include:</u>
> -Right sacral rotation on a right oblique axis
> -Right sacral rotation on a left oblique axis
> -Left sacral rotation on a right oblique axis
> -Left sacral rotation on a left oblique axis

Although there is no standardized treatment for a sacral rotation, it would stand to reason to first correct the lumbar dysfunction.

G. Bilateral sacral flexion and extension

1. <u>Bilateral sacral flexion (sacral base anterior)</u>
In this somatic dysfunction, the entire sacral base moves anterior about a middle transverse axis. [28 p.402]

<u>Static findings:</u> [1 p.620, 33 p.191]
> Right and left sulci deep.
> ILA's shallow bilaterally.
> Increased lumbar curve.

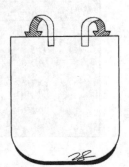

<u>Dynamic findings:</u> [1 p.615, 25 p.220, 33 p.191]
> FALSE negative seated flexion test.
> > <u>NOTE</u>: since both SI joints are restricted in this dysfunction, asymmetry cannot be appreciated, resulting in a false negative seated and standing flexion tests.
> Motion (springing) at both sulci (base) is present.
> Motion (springing) at both ILA's (apex) is restricted.
> Negative lumbosacral spring test.

51

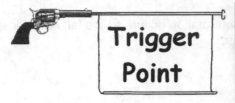

Trigger Point

Due to birth mechanics, bilateral sacral flexion is a common dysfunction in the post-partum patient. [1 p. 621]

2. Bilateral sacral extensions (sacral base posterior)
In this somatic dysfunction, the entire sacral base moves posterior about a middle transverse axis. [28 p.402]

Static findings: [1 p.620, 33 p.195]
Right and left sulci shallow.
ILA's deeper bilaterally.
Decreased lumbar curve.

Dynamic findings: [1 p.615, 25 p.220, 33 p.195]
FALSE negative seated flexion test.
NOTE: since both SI joints are restricted in this dysfunction, asymmetry cannot be appreciated. resulting in a false negative seated and standing flexion tests.
Motion (springing) at both sulci (base) is restricted.
Motion (springing) at both ILA's (apex) is present.
Positive lumbosacral spring test.

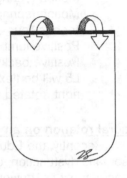

H. Sacral shears (unilateral sacral flexion/extension) (USF/USE) -
In this somatic dysfunction, the sacrum will shift anteriorly or posteriorly around a transverse axis. [1 p.621]

1. Unilateral sacral flexion on the right (USF$_R$) or left (USF$_L$).

Left unilateral sacral flexion	Right unilateral sacral flexion

Static findings: [33 p.211]
  Left sulcus deeper.
  Left ILA significantly inferior
  Left ILA slightly posterior.
Dynamic findings:
  Positive seated flexion test on the left.
  Motion (springing) at the left sulcus is present.
  Motion (springing) at the left ILA is restricted.
	Static findings: [33 p.211]
	  Right sulcus deeper.
	  Right ILA significantly inferior
	  Right ILA slightly posterior.
	Dynamic findings:
	  Positive seated flexion test on the right.
	  Motion (springing) at the right sulcus is present.
	  Motion (springing) at the right ILA is restricted.

2. Unilateral sacral extension on the right (USE$_R$) or left (USE$_L$).

Left unilateral sacral extension	Right unilateral sacral extension
Static findings: [33 p.213] Left sulcus shallow. Left ILA significantly superior. Left ILA slightly anterior. **Dynamic findings:** [1 p.615, 621, 33 p.213] Positive seated flexion test on the left. Motion (springing) at the left sulcus is restricted. Motion (springing) at the left ILA is present Positive lumbosacral spring test. Positive backward bending test.	**Static findings:** [33 p.213] Right sulcus shallow. Right ILA significantly superior. Right ILA slightly anterior. **Dynamic findings:** [1 p.615, 621, 33 p.213] Positive seated flexion test on the right. Motion (springing) at the right sulcus is restricted. Motion (springing) at the right ILA is present. Positive lumbosacral spring test. Positive backward bending test.

I. Sacral margin posterior

Some authors do not recognize this as a true somatic dysfunction, hence there is controversy on whether it exists. However, it is mentioned here because this dysfunction is taught at some osteopathic institutions. In a **sacral margin posterior,** the sacrum rotates posteriorly about a mid-vertical or parasagittal vertical axis. [33 p.198]

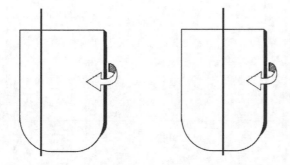

Figure 6.10: (left) Right sacral margin about a parasagittal vertical axis.

Figure 6.11: (right) Right sacral margin about a mid-vertical axis.

Right sacral margin *Vertical axis*	Right sacral margin *Parasagittal axis*
Static findings: Right sulci and right ILA shallow. Left sulci and left ILA deep Dynamic findings: Motion (springing) on the right sulcus and right ILA is restricted. Motion (springing) on the left sulcus and left ILA is present.	Static findings: Right sulci and right ILA shallow. Left sulci and left ILA normal Dynamic findings: Motion (springing) on the right sulcus and right ILA is restricted. Motion (springing) on the left sulcus and left ILA is present.

IV. Clinical pearls of innominate and sacral dysfunctions

As mentioned earlier, Mitchell described sacral motion in relation to L5. If a somatic dysfunction occurs in L5, a sacral somatic dysfunction is likely to be present. Therefore, if a physician uncovers a sacral somatic dysfunction, he/she should check L5 for restriction. If restriction is present then treatment should be directed toward L5 first. Most of the time the sacral dysfunction will spontaneously resolve with treatment of L5. [1 p. 622]

A psoas syndrome may cause L1 or L2 to be flexed, sidebent, and rotated to the same side of the iliopsoas contracture. For example, if a person has a flexion contracture of the iliopsoas on the right, L1 or L2 may be FR_RS_R. [1 p.597]

CHAPTER 6 REVIEW QUESTIONS

1. Which of the structure divides the greater and lesser sciatic foramen?
   A. Sacrotuberous ligament.
   B. Sacrospinous ligament.
   C. Sacroiliac ligament.
   D. Tendon of the obturator internus muscle.
   E. Tendon of the piriformis muscle.

2. Which of the following statements concerning sacral movement is true?
   A. During inhalation the sacral base will move anterior about a superior transverse axis.
   B. During postural flexion the sacral base will move anterior about a superior transverse axis.
   C. During swing phase of the right lower extremity the sacrum move about a left oblique axis.
   D. During craniosacral flexion the sacral base will move posterior about a middle transverse axis
   E. During exhalation the sacral base will move posterior about an inferior transverse axis

3. Which of the following movements will cause the sacral base to move anterior (sacral flexion)?
   A. Cranial extension.
   B. Counternutation.
   C. Inhalation.
   D. Weight bearing on the right leg..
   E. Weight bearing on the left leg.

4. Which of the following statements concerning sacral counternutation is true?
   A. It occurs during craniosacral flexion as the sacral base moves anterior.
   B. It occurs during craniosacral flexion as the sacral base moves posterior.
   C. It occurs during craniosacral extension as the sacral base moves anterior.
   D. It occurs during craniosacral extension as the sacral base moves posterior.

5. A 32 year old female presents to your office with sacroiliac pain. The pain started 2 days ago after picking up her 3 year old son. On examination you find a positive seated flexion test on the right, L5 $NS_L R_R$, her left ILA is shallow, right superior sulcus is deeper, and her lumbar curve is convex to the right. Based on these findings what is the most likely diagnosis?
   A. Right sacral rotation on a right oblique axis (R on R).
   B. Left sacral rotation on a left oblique axis (L on L).
   C. Right sacral rotation on a left oblique axis (R on L).
   D. Left sacral rotation on a right oblique axis (L on R).
   E. A unilateral sacral extension on the right (USE_R).

6. Which of the following L5 dysfunctions corresponds with right sacral rotation on a left oblique axis (R on L)?
   A. L5 $FR_L S_L$
   B. L5 $NS_L R_R$
   C. L5 $FR_R S_R$
   D. L5 $NS_R R_L$

7. A 21 year old male is complaining of gluteal pain for 2 days. He states that the pain started after biking several miles. He appears mildly obese and is not physically active. On examination, you notice that his sacral sulci appear shallow. There is a positive lumbosacral spring test. The seated and standing flexion tests are both negative. Based on the information given what is the most likely diagnosis?
    A. Unilateral sacral flexion on the right (USF$_R$).
    B. Bilateral sacral flexion (sacral base anterior).
    C. Unilateral sacral flexion on the left (USF$_L$).
    D. Bilateral sacral extension (sacral base posterior).
    E. Not enough information given to make a diagnosis.

8. A 25 year old medical student is complaining of right sided low back/sacroiliac pain. The pain started one week ago while studying for board exams. On examination, you notice tenderness over the right SI joint, a positive seated flexion test on the right, the sacral sulcus on the right is anterior, while the right ILA is inferior and shallow. Based on the information given what is the most likely diagnosis?
    A. Unilateral sacral extension on the left (USE$_L$).
    B. Unilateral sacral flexion on the left (USF$_L$).
    C. Unilateral sacral extension on the right (USE$_R$).
    D. Unilateral sacral flexion on the right (USF$_R$).
    E. Left sacral rotation on a left oblique axis (L on L).

9. A 30 year old male runner presents with left sided low back pain and left hip pain. The pain started yesterday after a five mile run. It is sharp but does not radiate into the lower extremities. On examination, you notice he has a positive standing flexion test on the left, his left ASIS is inferior, the left PSIS is superior, and his right leg is shorter. Based on the information given what is the most likely diagnosis?
    A. Right posterior innominate.
    B. Left anterior innominate.
    C. Left posterior innominate.
    D. Unilateral sacral flexion on the left (USF$_L$).
    E. Unilateral sacral extension on the left (USE$_L$).

10. All of the following can cause a positive seated flexion test on the right EXCEPT:
    A. Unilateral sacral extension on the right (USE$_R$).
    B. Unilateral sacral flexion on the right (USF$_R$).
    C. Left sacral rotation on a left oblique axis (L on L).
    D. Right sacral rotation on a right oblique axis (R on R).
    E. Sacral margin posterior on the right.

11. Which of the following will produce a deep sacral sulcus on the right?
    A. Unilateral sacral extension on the right (USE$_R$).
    B. Unilateral sacral flexion on the right (USF$_R$).
    C. Right sacral rotation on a left oblique axis (R on L).
    D. Right sacral rotation on a right oblique axis (R on R).
    E. Unilateral sacral flexion on the left (USF$_L$).

12. Which of the following findings is present in a left innominate anterior rotation?
    A. PSIS inferior on the left.
    B. PSIS superior on the right.
    C. PSIS superior on the left.
    D. ASIS superior on the left.
    E. PSIS and ASIS posterior on the left.

ANSWERS

1. B	7. D
2. C	8. D
3. A	9. B
4. B	10. D
5. B	11. B
6. A	12. C

CHAPTER 7
UPPER EXTREMITIES

Shoulder
I. Anatomy
  A. Bones
-Clavicle - acts as a strut for upper limb to allow maximum freedom of motion, as well as transmit forces from the upper extremity to the axial skeleton. It is the only bone connecting the upper extremity and the axial spine.
-Scapula
-Humerus

  B. Joints
-Scapulothoracic (pseudo-joint)
-Acromioclavicular
-Sternoclavicular
-Glenohumeral

  C. Muscles
1. Rotator cuff - is the name for the group of 4 muscles that serve to protect the shoulder joint and give it stability by holding the head of the humerus in the glenoid fossa. [3 p.537]

mnemonic: SITS
    S= supraspinatus - abduction of the arm.
    I= infraspinatus - external rotation of arm.
    T= teres minor - external rotation of arm.
    S= subscapularis - internal rotation of arm.

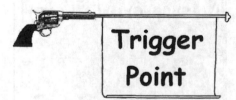

Trigger Point

Know the rotator cuff muscles.

2. Other muscles of the shoulder Table 7.1 [1 p.549]

Action	Muscle
Primary flexor	Deltoid (anterior portion)
Primary abductor	Deltoid (middle portion)
Primary extensors	Latissimus dorsi, Teres major and Deltoid (posterior portion)
Primary adductors	Pectoralis major, Latissimus dorsi
Primary external rotators	Infraspinatus, Teres minor
Primary internal rotator	Subscapularis

D. Arterial supply

-The subclavian artery passes between the anterior and middle scalenes. The subclavian vein passes anterior to the anterior scalene. Therefore, contracture of the anterior and middle scalenes may compromise arterial supply to the arm, but not affect venous drainage.

-The subclavian artery becomes the axillary artery at the lateral border of the first rib.

-The axillary artery becomes the brachial artery at the inferior border of the teres minor muscle.

-The profunda brachial artery is the first major branch of the brachial artery. It accompanies the radial nerve in its posterior course of the radial groove. [3 p.547]

-The brachial artery divides into the ulnar and radial arteries under the bicipital aponeurosis.

-The radial artery courses the lateral aspect of the forearm supplying blood to the elbow, wrist, dorsal aspect of the hand, and eventually forming most of *the deep palmar arterial arch*.

-The ulnar artery courses the medial aspect of the forearm supplying blood to the elbow, wrist, dorsal aspect of the hand and eventually forming most of *the superficial palmar arterial arch*.

E. Lymphatic drainage of the upper extremities

Right upper extremity drains into the right (minor) duct.

Left upper extremity drains into the left (main) duct.

For a more detailed description of the lymphatic system see Chapter 13 "Lymphatics"

Treatment to relieve lymph congestion of the upper extremity [28 p. 604]

      1. Open the thoracic inlet.

      2. Redome the thoraco-abdominal diaphragm.

      3. Posterior axillary fold technique.

F. Nerves

The brachial plexus (fig 7.1) is responsible for supplying the nerves to the upper extremity. It is composed of nerves from roots C5-C8 and T1. A thorough neurological examination of the upper extremity demands that every physician have a good understanding of the brachial plexus.

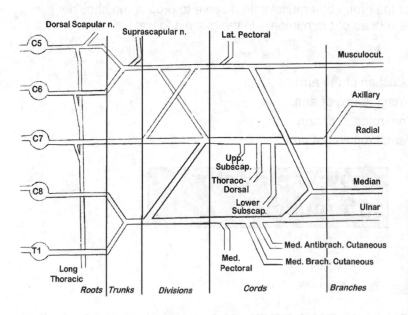

Fig 7.1: The brachial plexus:

Roots exit the spinal cord to form

Trunks which form

Divisions which form

Cords which form

Branches.

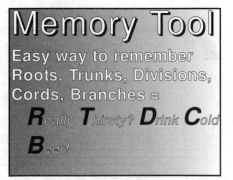

Memory Tool

Easy way to remember Roots, Trunks, Divisions, Cords, Branches =

Really **T**hirsty? **D**rink **C**old **B**eer!

II. Motion and somatic dysfunction of the shoulder

A. Motion of the shoulder

Normally, the arm can abduct to 180^0 with active motion, 120^0 is due to glenohumeral motion and 60^0 is due to scapulothoracic motion. *Therefore, for every 3^0 of abduction, the glenohumeral joint moves 2^0 and the scapulothoracic joint moves 1^0.* [1 p.548] A careful history and examination will reveal to the physician which joint has a restriction.

A good screening examination for gross range of motion of the shoulder is Apley's Scratch test (see Chapter 18 Special Tests). The Spencer techniques can more accurately test individual motions of the shoulder (see Chapter 17 Articulatory Techniques). This modality can be expanded to include treatment as well.

B. Somatic dysfunction of the shoulder

-The most common somatic dysfunction of the shoulder is restriction in internal and external rotation. [28 p.607]
-The second most common somatic dysfunction of the shoulder is restriction in abduction. [28 p.607]
-The least common somatic dysfunction of the shoulder is restriction in extension. [28 p.607]

C. Motion at the clavicle [28 p.163]

-Each end of the clavicle can glide:
  -Anterior or Posterior   **OR**   Superior or Inferior
  -Motions at either end of the clavicle are in opposite directions.
    -For example, if the lateral end of the clavicle has moved superior (e.g shoulder shrug) the medial end would move inferior.
    -Example #2, if the lateral end of the clavicle has moved posterior, the medial end would move anterior.
  -The clavicle can also rotate around a transverse axis (with internal or external rotation of the arm).

1. Sternoclavicular joint
   -Most common somatic dysfunction = Clavicle, anterior and superior on the sternum. [28 p. 596]
     -Findings: [33 p.229]
        - Clavicle will resist posterior and inferior glide at the sternum.
        - Superior glide present with shoulder depression.
        - Inferior glide restricted with shoulder elevation.
        - Anterior glide present with shoulder retraction.
        - Posterior glide restricted with shoulder protraction.
        - Decreased motion of clavicle around transverse axis.

2. Acromioclavicular joint
   - Stabilized by
        - Acromioclavicular ligament
        - Coracoacromial ligament
        - Coracoclavicular ligament
   - The most common somatic dysfunction = Clavicle, superior and lateral on the acromion. [28 p.597]
        - Findings [33 p.231]
           - "Step-off" seen at the AC joint
           - Clavicle will resist inferior glide at the AC joint.
           - Tenderness over the AC joint

61

III. Common problems of the shoulder

A. Thoracic outlet syndrome

Pathogenesis: Compression of the neurovascular bundle (subclavian artery and vein, and the brachial plexus) as it exits the thoracic outlet.

Compression can occur in three places: [28, p.528-9, 56 p.704]
1. *Between the anterior and middle scalenes.*
2. *Between the clavicle and the first rib.*
3. *Between pectoralis minor and the upper ribs.*

Compression may be due to:
1. a cervical rib
2. excessive tension of the anterior or middle scalenes
3. somatic dysfunction of the clavicle or upper ribs
4. abnormal insertion of pectoralis minor

Location of pain: Neck pain or pain radiating to arm.

Quality of pain: Ache or paresthesias.

Signs and Symptoms: On examination, the scalenes, a cervical rib, or the clavicle may be tender. Pulses in the upper extremity may be normal or diminished. *Often there is a positive Adson's test (if compression between scalenes), Military posture test (if compression between clavicle and rib 1) or Hyperextension test (if compression occurs between under pectoralis minor) (see Chapter 18 Special Tests).*

Treatment: OMT should be directed at C2-C7, T1, rib 1, thoracic inlet, clavicle, and scalenes if somatic dysfunction is present. [1 p.561, 28 p.528] Exercises to strengthen trapezius and levator scapula. [4 p.463]

B. Supraspinatus Tendinitis

Pathogenesis: Continuous impingement of the greater tuberosity against the acromion as the arm is flexed and internally rotated.

Location of pain: Tenderness, especially at the tip of the acromion.

Signs and symptoms: It is usually a gradual onset and may be preceded by a strain. The pain is usually exacerbated by abduction, especially from $60°-120°$. This is commonly referred to as the *"painful arc"*.

Clinical manifestations: Chronic tendinitis may lead to calcification of the supraspinatus tendon.

Treatment: Rest, ice and NSAIDS for the acute stages. For severe cases, a sling and injection with lidocaine or steriods may provide relief. OMT should be directed at the shoulder complex, upper thoracic and ribs to free up motion and loosen the fascia of the shoulder girdle to expedite the healing process.

C. Bicipital tenosynovitis

Pathogenesis: An inflammation of the tendon and its sheath of the long head of the biceps. It is usually due to overuse, combined with physiological wear and tear, leading to adhesions that bind the tendon to the bicipital groove. It also may result from a subluxation of the bicepital tendon out of the bicipital groove. [1 p.559]

Location of pain: Anterior portion of the shoulder which may radiate to the biceps.

Signs and symptoms: Tenderness is usually present over the bicipital groove. Pain is usually aggravated by resisted flexion or supination of the forearm. [8 p. 1366]

Treatment: Rest and ice for acute injury. For severe cases, an injection with lidocaine or steriods may provide relief. OMT should include freeing up any restrictions in the glenohumeral area, and myofascial release.

D. __Rotator cuff tear__
   Definition: A tear at the insertion of one of the rotator cuff tendons, usually the supraspinatus. Minor tears of the cuff are common. However, a complete tear can occur resulting in retraction of the affected muscle, and sharp shoulder pain.
   Etiology: Often associated with trauma.
   Location of pain: Tenderness just below the tip of the acromion.
   Quality of pain: A transient sharp pain in the shoulder followed by a steady ache that may last for days. [4 p.470]
   Signs and symptoms: In supraspinatus tears, a weakness in active abduction is often present along with a *positive drop arm test* (see Chapter 18 Special Tests). Atrophy is a common sign. Often the patient will experience pain for months especially at night.
   Treatment: For minor tears, rest, ice and NSAIDS in the acute stages. OMT should be directed at freeing up any restrictions in the glenohumeral area as well as treating the clavicle, upper thoracic, and ribs for somatic dysfunction. Surgery is often required for complete avulsion.

E. __Adhesive capsulitis/ Frozen shoulder syndrome__
   Definition: A common condition characterized by pain and restriction of shoulder motion that increasingly gets worse over the course of one year.
   Signs and symptoms: Decreased range of motion, with active and passive movements. Abduction, internal and external range of motion is often effected. Extension is typically preserved. Pain is often present at the end of the range of motion. [32 p.98]
   Epidemiology: It is most often seen in patients over 40 years of age. [4 p.469]
   Etiology: *It is typically caused by prolonged immobility of the shoulder.*
   Location of pain: Tenderness is usually at the anterior portion of the shoulder.
   Treatment: The main goal is prevention. Early mobilization following shoulder injury is essential. Injection of corticosteriods and NSAIDS may help. OMT, especially Spencer techniques, should be directed at improving motion and lysing adhesions. Treatment of the glenohumeral joint and upper thoracic often provide relief.

F. __Shoulder dislocation__
   Common in athletes and usually occurs as a result of trauma. *Humeral dislocation usually occurs anteriorly and inferiorly.* Recurrent shoulder dislocations are common and require less force. Injury to the axillary nerve can occur with shoulder dislocation.

G. __Winging of the scapula__
   Usually a weakness of the anterior serratus muscle due to a long thoracic nerve injury. This condition is evident if the scapula protrudes posteriorly while the patient is pushing on a wall.

H. __Brachial plexus injuries__
   The nerves of the brachial plexus are susceptible to traction injury especially during childbirth. *Erb-Duchenne's palsy is by far the most common form of brachial plexus injury. It is an upper arm paralysis caused by injury to C5 and C6 nerve roots usually during childbirth.* It can result in paralysis of the deltoid, external rotators, biceps, brachioradialis, and supinator muscles. Klumpke's palsy is much less common, and is due to injury to C8 and T1. Paralysis usually occurs in the intrinsic muscles of the hand.

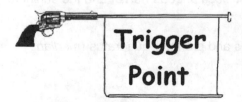
Trigger Point

Most common type of brachial plexus injury is Erb-Duchenne's palsy.

I. Radial nerve injury

The radial nerve is the most common nerve injured in the upper extremity due to direct trauma. It may be injured in the axilla by direct pressure, such as **crutch palsy**, caused by improper use of crutches. More commonly, it is injured as it travels within the spinal groove in **humeral fractures**. **Saturday night palsy** is caused by compression of the nerve against the humerus, as the arm is draped over the back of a chair during intoxication or deep sleep. These injuries typically will result in wrist drop, and possibly triceps weakness depending on the location of the nerve injury.

Elbow, Wrist and Hand

I. Anatomy

A. Bones

Radius
Ulna
Eight carpal bones

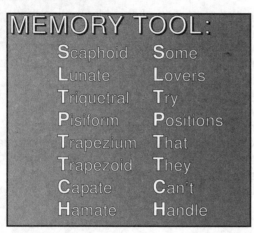

MEMORY TOOL:

Scaphoid	**S**ome
Lunate	**L**overs
Triquetral	**T**ry
Pisiform	**P**ositions
Trapezium	**T**hat
Trapezoid	**T**hey
Capate	**C**an't
Hamate	**H**andle

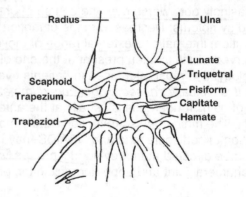

Fig 7.2: The carpal bones

Five metacarpals
Fourteen phalanges

B. Joints

Elbow (ulna and humerus)
Ulna and Radial (distal and proximal)
Intercarpals, Carpometacarpals, Metacarpophalangeal (MCP), Interphalangeal (PIP & DIP).

C. Muscles and innervations [1] p.550

Primary **flexors of the wrist and hand** originate on or near the medial epicondyle of the humerus. Most of which are *innervated by the median nerve* (except for flexor carpi ulnaris - ulnar nerve).

Primary **extensors of the wrist and hand** originate at the lateral epicondyle of the humerus. All of which are *innervated by the radial nerve*.

Primary **supinators** of the forearm are the biceps (*musculocutaneous nerve*) and the supinator (*radial nerve*).

Primary **pronators** of the forearm are the pronator teres and pronator quadratus (*median nerve*).

64

D. Muscles of the hand

Muscles in the thenar eminence are innervated by the *median nerve* (except for adductor pollicis brevis - ulnar nerve).

Muscles in the hypothenar eminence and interossi are innervated by the *ulnar nerve.*

Lumbricals (4)

First and Second lumbricals innervated by the *median nerve.*

Third and Fourth lumbricals innervated by the *ulnar nerve.*

NOTE: Remember that the flexor digitorum profundus attaches to the distal interphalengeal joint (DIP). The flexor digitorum superficialis attaches to the proximal interphalangeal joint (PIP).

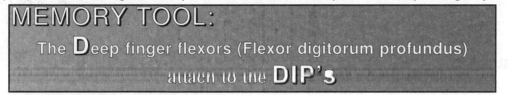

MEMORY TOOL:

The **D**eep finger flexors (Flexor digitorum profundus)

attach to the **DIP's**

II. Motion of the Elbow and Forearm

A. Carrying angle (fig 7.3)

-Formed by the intersection of two lines. The first line is the longitudinal axis of the humerus. The second line starts at the distal radial-ulna joint, and passes through the proximal radial ulna joint.

-The normal carrying angle in men is 5°.

-The normal carrying angle in women is 10°-12°.

-A carrying angle > 15° is called cubitus valgus or **abduction of the ulna** if somatic dysfunction is present.

-A carrying angle < 3° is called cubitis varus or **adduction of the ulna** if somatic dysfunction is present.

Carrying Angle

Fig 7.3: The angle formed between the two dotted lines represents the carrying angle.

-The carrying angle has a direct influence on the position of the wrist.

-Due to a parallelogram effect, **an increase in the carrying angle (abduction of the ulna) will cause an adduction of the wrist.**

Conversely, **a decrease in the carrying angle (adduction of the ulna) will cause an abduction of the wrist**. [1] p.554

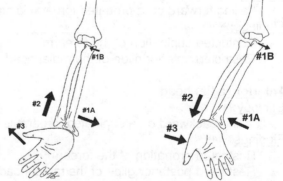

Fig 7.4 (left): Adduction of the ulna (arrow #1A) and lateral glide of the olecranon (proximal ulna) (arrow #1B) will cause the radius to be pulled proximally (arrow #2). This will result in abduction of the wrist (arrow #3).-

Fig 7.5 (right): Abduction of the ulna (arrow #1A) and medial glide of the olecranon (proximal ulna) (arrow #1B) will cause the radius to be pushed distally (arrow #2). This will result in adduction of the wrist (arrow #3).

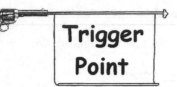

Trigger Point

Table 7.5

Carrying Angle	Ulna Movement	Wrist Movement
Increased	Abduction	Adduction
Decreased	Adduction	Abduction

B. Radial head motion

The radial head will glide anteriorly and posteriorly with supination and pronation respectively of the forearm.

When the forearm is pronated, the radial head will glide posteriorly.
When the forearm is supinated, the radial head will glide anteriorly.

SAPP

III. Somatic dysfunction of the forearm

A. Abduction of the ulna (See figure 7.5)

Findings: [33 p.239]

-Carrying angle increased (olecranon deviated medially and distal ulna deviated laterally).
-Olecranon process restricted in lateral glide.
-Radial head may be compressed against the lateral humeral condyle.
-Distal ulna resticted in medial glide.
-The wrist/hand will be adducted and restricted in abduction.

B. Adduction of the ulna (See figure 7.4)

Findings: [33 p.240]

-Carrying angle decreased (olecranon deviated laterally and distal ulna deviated medially).
-Olecranon process restricted in medial glide.
-Radial head may be distracted from the lateral humeral condyle.
-Distal ulna resticted in lateral glide.
-The wrist/hand will be abducted and restricted in adduction.

C. Posterior radial head

Etiology:
-Falling forward on a pronated forearm is often a common cause. [1 p.556]
Findings: [33 p.242]
-Restricted supination of the forearm.
-Restricted anterior glide of the radial head.

Food?

D. Anterior radial head

Etiology:
Falling backward on a supinated forearm is often a common cause. [1 p.556]
Findings: [33 p.244]
-Restricted pronation of the forearm.
-Restricted posterior glide of the radial head.

FBoosh

IV. Common complaints of the wrist and elbow

A. Carpal tunnel syndrome

Definition: Entrapment of the median nerve at the wrist. [32 p.192]
Quality and location of pain: *The patient usually complains of paresthesias on the thumb and the first 2 ½ digits.*
Signs and symptoms: Weakness and atrophy usually appear late. On examination, symptoms are reproduced with *Tinel's, Phalen, and prayer tests.*
Diagnosis: Nerve conduction studies/electromyography remain the gold standard.

66

Treatment: Treatment usually consists of splints, NSAIDS, and steroid injections. Surgery is indicated if medical treatment has failed.

Osteopathic treatment for carpal tunnel syndrome: [1 p.560]

1. Treating rib and upper thoracic somatic dysfunctions to decrease sympathetic tone in the upper extremity.
2. Treating cervical somatic dysfunctions and myofascial restrictions to enhance brachial plexus function and remove potential sites of additional compression.
3. Treating the carpal tunnel with direct release techniques to increase the space in the carpal tunnel.

B. Lateral epicondylitis (tennis elbow)

Definition: A strain of the extensor muscles of the forearm near the lateral epicondyle.

Pathogenesis: Commonly develops as a result of overuse of the forearm extensors and supinators. Aggravating activities includes hitting a ball in racquet sports with improper techniques and turning a screwdriver. [?? p.139]

Location of pain: The patient usually complains of pain over the lateral epicondyle that worsens with wrist extension against resistance.

Quality of pain: Pain may radiate to the lateral aspect of the arm and forearm.

Signs and symptoms: Tenderness at the lateral epicondyle or just distal to it. Pain often worsens with activity.

Treatment: NSAIDS, rest, and ice. To prevent reoccurrences, a tennis elbow strap worn just below the elbow often helps. [32 p.141] OMT should be directed toward correcting cervical or upper thoracic dysfunctions, counterstrain to affected muscles (usually extensors), and myofascial release to decrease fascial restrictions.

C. Medial epicondylitis (golfer's elbow)

Definition: A strain of the flexor muscles of the forearm near the medial epicondyle.

Pathogenesis: Commonly develops as a result of overuse of the forearm flexors and pronators. [32 p.139]

Location/quality of pain, signs/symptoms, treatment: Same for tennis elbow but directed at the medial epicondyle.

V. Contractures and deformities of the wrist and hand

A. Swan-neck deformity (fig 7.6)
-Flexion contracture of the MCP and DIP.
-Extension contracture of the PIP.
-Results from a contracture of the intrinsic muscles of the hand and is often associated with *rheumatoid arthritis*.

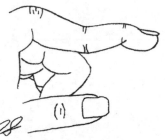

Fig 7.6: Swan neck deformity

B. Boutonniere deformity (fig 7.7)
-Extension contracture of the MCP and DIP.
-Flexion contracture of the PIP.
-Results from a rupture of the hood of the extensor tendon at the PIP. It is often associated with *rheumatoid arthritis*.

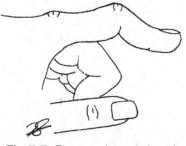

Fig 7.7: Boutonniere deformity

C. <u>Claw hand</u>
   Extension of the MCP.
   Flexion of the PIP and DIP.
   Results from median and ulnar injury (loss of intrinsic muscles and overactivity of the extensor
      muscles).

D. <u>Ape hand</u>
   Similar to the claw hand, but in addition, there is a wasting of the thenar eminence, and the
      thumb is adducted.
   Results from median nerve damage.

E. <u>Bishops deformity</u>
   Contracture of the last two digits with atrophy of the hypothenar eminence due to *ulnar nerve
      damage.*

F. <u>Dupuytren's contracture</u>
   Flexion contracture of the MCP and PIP usually seen with contracture of the last two digits.
      However, unlike Bishops contracture, *this is due to a contracture of the palmar fascia.*

G. <u>Drop-wrist deformity</u>
   Radial nerve damage results in paralysis of the extensor muscles.

CHAPTER 7 REVIEW QUESTIONS

1. All of the following muscles make up the rotator cuff EXCEPT:
    A. Supraspinatus.
    B. Infraspinatus.
    C. Teres major.
    D. Teres minor.
    E. Subscapularis.

2. Which one of the following muscles is the primary internal rotator of the humerus?
    A. Teres minor.
    B. Subscapularis.
    C. Infraspinatus.
    D. Pectoralis minor.
    E. Deltoid.

3. Which one of the following statements is true concerning the radial artery?
    A. It branches directly from the profunda (deep) brachial artery and accompanies the radial nerve in the posterior course of the radial groove.
    B. It branches directly from the axillary artery to supply the lateral aspect of the forearm.
    C. It branches directly from the axillary artery to supply the medial aspect of the forearm.
    D. It forms most of the deep palmar arch of the hand.

4. What is the correct sequence of nerve divisions leaving the spinal cord to form the brachial plexus?
    A. Roots, trunks, branches, cords, divisions.
    B. Roots, divisions, trunks, cords, branches.
    C. Roots, trunks, cords, branches, divisions.
    D. Roots, cords, trunks, branches, divisions.
    E. Roots, trunks, divisions, cords, branches.

5. Which of the following nerves only carries fibers from the C5 nerve root?
    A. Musculocutaneous
    B. Lateral Pectoral
    C. Suprascapular
    D. Long Thoracic
    E. Dorsal scapular

6. Upper arm paralysis caused by an injury to the C5 and C6 nerve roots usually during childbirth is also known as?
    A. Klumpke's palsy.
    B. Erb-Duchenne's palsy.
    C. Stick palsy.
    D. Long thoracic nerve palsy.
    E. Bell's palsy.

7. Which of the following findings is most likely to be present in a patient that suffers from a lower motor neuron injury affecting the C5 and C6 nerve roots?
    A. A decreased biceps reflex.
    B. An increased triceps reflex.
    C. Weak finger flexors.
    D. Decreased sensation over the ring and little fingers.
    E. Decreased sensation over the medial epicondyle.

8. A 31 year old female presents to your office with neck pain following a motor vehicle accident two days ago. She states that her pain is a dull ache on the right side of her neck that radiates into her arm. On examination, you notice a right anterior scalene tenderpoint and positive Adson's test. Neurological exam reveals no sensory deficits, 5/5 muscle strength, and normal deep tendon reflexes. Your most likely diagnosis is?
    A. Bicipital tenosynovitis.
    B. A rotator cuff tear.
    C. Thoracic outlet syndrome.
    D. Supraspinatus tendonitis.
    E. Herniated nucleus propulsis of the cervical spine.

9. Thoracic outlet syndrome is due to compression of the neurovascular bundle (subclavian artery and vein and brachial plexus). This compression can occur in all of the following locations EXCEPT:
    A. Between the anterior and middle scalene muscles.
    B. Between joint of Luschka and facet joint.
    C. Between the pectoralis minor and the upper ribs.
    D. Between the clavicle and the first rib.

10. Humeral dislocation is most likely to occur in which position?
    A. Inferior and posterior.
    B. Anterior and inferior.
    C. Superior and anterior.
    D. Superior.
    E. Posterior.

11. A 21 year old right-handed minor league pitcher presents to your office with right shoulder pain. The pain has increased gradually over the past month, and worsens with pitching. Ice and ibuprofen seem to decrease the pain. On examination, you notice tenderness at the tip of the acromion. He has full range of motion of the right shoulder, but has pain with abduction, especially from 60° - 120°. He has a positive drop arm test. Neurological examination of the upper extremity is within normal limits. The most likely cause of his pain is?
    A. Bicipital tenosynovitis.
    B. Adhesive capsulitis.
    C. Supraspinatus tendonitis.
    D. Complete rupture of the supraspinatus tendon.
    E. A cervical rib.

12. Winging of the scapula can be caused by damage to which nerve?
    A. Axillary.
    B. Long thoracic.
    C. Suprascapular.
    D. Lower subscapular.
    E. Thoracodorsal.

13. Which of the following carpal bones is located most medially?
    A. Scaphoid
    B. Trapezoid
    C. Trapezium
    D. Capitate
    E. Hamate

14. Pronators of the forearm are primarily innervated by which one of the following nerves?
    A. Median.
    B. Ulnar.
    C. Radial.
    D. Musculocutaneous.

15. A 15 year old female presents to your office with left wrist and elbow pain. The pain started one week ago. On examination, you notice tenderpoints at the elbow and wrist, she has an increased carrying angle on her left side. Her wrist appears to be restricted in abduction. And X-rays show no evidence of any fractures. Assuming she has somatic dysfunction at her left elbow, which choice is the most likely diagnosis?
    A. Posterior radial head.
    B. Anterior radial head.
    C. Adduction of the ulna.
    D. Abduction of the ulna.

16. Which of the following movements will cause the radial head to glide anterior?
    A. Pronation of the forearm.
    B. Supination of the forearm.
    C. Flexion of the wrist.
    D. Extension of the wrist.
    E. Extension of the elbow.

17. A 35 year old female presents with numbness and tingling over the palmar surface of her right thumb. She states symptoms often radiates into her first and middle fingers. It started six months ago and has gotten increasingly worse. Tylenol and Advil seem to alleviate the symptoms somewhat. On examination, you notice a decreased sensation at the pads of the first and middle fingers, and decreased grip strength of the right hand. Tinel's test at the wrist is positive. The most likely cause of her pain is?
    A. Thoracic outlet syndrome.
    B. Syphilis.
    C. A scaphoid fracture.
    D. Carpal tunnel syndrome.

18. Which nerve is most likely to be effected in the above question?
    A. Median nerve.
    B. Ulnar nerve.
    C. Radial nerve.
    D. Musculocutaneous nerve.

19. Tennis elbow is often associated with tenderness at which anatomical landmark?
    A. The olecrenon.
    B. The bicipital aponeurosis.
    C. The lateral epicondyle.
    D. The medial epicondyle.
    E. The humeral condyles

20. Wrist drop deformity is associated with damage to which one of the following structures?
    A. Median nerve.
    B. Wrist flexor muscles.
    C. Flexor retinaculum.
    D. Ulnar nerve.
    E. Radial nerve.

21. The origin of the brachial artery is located at:
    A. The superior border of pectoralis minor.
    B. The lateral border of the first rib.
    C. The superior border of teres minor.
    D. The inferior border of teres minor.
    E. The inferior/lateral border of the clavicle.

22. All of the following is associated with abduction of the ulna somatic dysfunction EXCEPT:
    A. Cubitis valgus.
    B. An increased carrying angle.
    C. Adduction of the wrist.
    D. Lateral glide of the olecranon.

ANSWERS

1.	C	12.	B
2.	B	13.	E
3.	D	14.	A
4.	E	15.	D
5.	E	16.	B
6.	B	17.	D
7.	A	18.	A
8.	C	19.	C
9.	B	20.	E
10.	B	21.	D
11.	C	22.	D

CHAPTER 8

LOWER EXTREMITIES

Hip and Knee

I. Anatomy

A. Bones and bony landmarks

1. <u>Femur</u> - proximally articulates with the acetabulum; distally articulates with the medial and lateral menisci that are situated on the tibial plateau.
2. <u>Patella</u> - a sesamoid bone that attaches to the quadriceps tendon superiorly, and the patella tendon inferiorly.
3. <u>Tibia</u>
4. <u>Fibula</u>

B. Muscle of the hip and knee

1. <u>Hip</u>

Primary extensor:	Gluteus maximus
Primary flexor:	Iliopsoas

2. <u>Knee</u>

Primary extensor:	Quadriceps (rectus femoris, vastus lateralis, medialis and intermedius)
Primary flexors:	Semimembranosus and semitendinosus (hamstrings)

C. Ligaments and joints

1. <u>Hip</u>

a. <u>Femoroacetabular joint (hip joint)</u> - a ball and socket joint that is held in place by the surrounding musculature and four ligaments.

<u>Iliofemoral ligament</u>
<u>Ischiofemoral ligament</u>
<u>Pubofemoral ligament</u>
<u>Capitis femoris</u> - the ligament at the head of the femur attaching to the acetabular fossa.

b. <u>Hip motion and somatic dysfunction</u>
1) <u>Major motions</u>
   - Flexion/Extension
   - Abduction/Adduction
   - Internal rotation/External rotation
2) <u>Minor motions</u>
   - Anterior Glide
     The head of the femur will glide anteriorly with external rotation of the hip. [28 p.663]
   --Posterior Glide
     The head of the femur will glide posteriorly with internal rotation of the hip. [28 p.664]

3) <u>Somatic dysfunction of the hip</u>

| <u>External rotation somatic dysfunction:</u>
<u>Findings:</u>
    Hip restricted in internal rotation
<u>Etiology:</u>
    Piriformis or iliopsoas spasm | <u>Internal rotation somatic dysfunction:</u>
<u>Findings:</u>
    Hip restricted in external rotation
<u>Etiology:</u>
    Spasm of internal rotators (gluteus minimus, semimembranosus, semitendinosus, TFL, adductor magnus, adductor longus.) [3] |

2. <u>Knee</u>

The knee is composed of three joints and four major ligaments.

a. <u>Tibiofemoral joint</u> - the largest joint in the body. [5 p.372]   The articular surfaces of the tibia and femur are separated by two "C" shaped menisci. [5 p.372]   The medial and lateral menisci act as shock absorbers and also aid in nutrition and lubrication of the joint. Between the two menisci are two ligaments that help stabilize the knee.

   1) <u>The anterior cruciate ligament (ACL)</u> - originates at the posterior aspect of the femur, and attaches to the anterior aspect of the tibia. It *prevents anterior translation of the tibia on the femur.*

   2) <u>The posterior cruciate ligament (PCL)</u> - originates on the anterior aspect of the femur and inserts on the posterior aspect of the tibia. It *prevents posterior translation of the tibia on the femur.*

b. <u>Lateral stabilizers of the knee</u>

   1) <u>Medial collateral ligament</u> (tibial collateral ligament) - originates at the femur and inserts on the tibia. This ligament also articulates with the medial meniscus.

   2) <u>Lateral collateral ligament</u> (fibular collateral ligament) - originates at the femur and inserts on the fibula.

c. <u>Patellofemoral joint</u>

d. <u>Tibiofibular joint</u> - a synovial joint composed of the lateral aspect of the proximal tibia and the proximal fibular head. Movement at this joint occurs with pronation and supination of the foot.

   -The fibular head will *glide anteriorly with pronation of the foot.* (fig 8.1)
      Pronation (dorsiflexion, eversion and abduction) of the foot causes the talus to push the distal fibula posteriorly, and reciprocally the proximal fibular will move anterior.

   -The fibular head will *glide posteriorly with supination of the foot.* (fig 8.2)
      Supination (plantarflexion, inversion and adduction) of the foot causes the anterior talofibular ligament to pull the distal fibula anteriorly, and reciprocally the proximal fibular will move posterior. [28 p. 686]

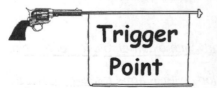

Trigger Point

| 1. *Dorsiflexion, eversion, and abduction =* <u>*PRONATION*</u> *of the ankle.* [1 p.636]
2. *Plantarflexion, inversion, and adduction =* <u>*SUPINATION*</u> *of the ankle.* [1 p.636] |

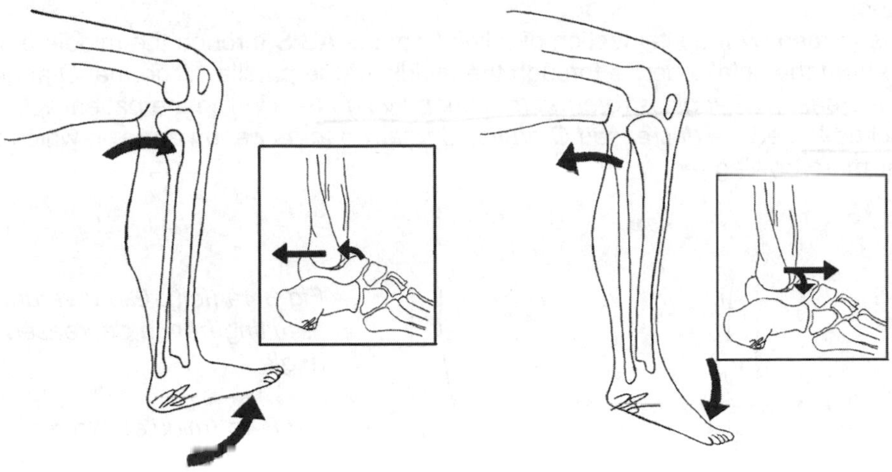

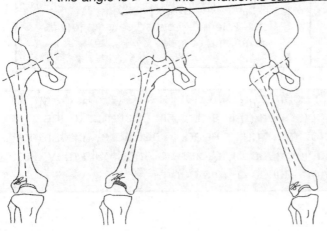

Fibular head movement:

Fig 8.1: (left) Fibular head movement. Pronation at the ankle will cause the fibular head to glide anteriorly.

Fig 8.2: (right) Supination at the ankle will cause the fibular head to glide posteriorly.

I. Nerves

A. Femoral nerve - (L2-L4) [6, 27]

Motor - innervates quadriceps, iliacus, sartorius and pectineus.

Sensory - anterior thigh and medial leg.

B. Sciatic nerve - (L4-S3) [6, 27] Courses through the greater sciatic foramen. In 85% of the population the sciatic nerve will be inferior to the piriformis muscle.

Two divisions:

1. Tibial
   a. Motor - Hamstrings except short head of the biceps femoris, most plantar flexors, and toe flexors.
   b. Sensory - Lower leg and plantar aspect of foot.

2. Peroneal
   a. Motor - Short head of biceps femoris, evertors and dorsiflexors of the foot, and most extensors of the toes.
   b. Sensory - Lower leg and dorsum of foot.

III. Anatomical variations of the femur and Q angle (quadriceps angle)

A. Angulation of the head of the femur (figs 8.3 a-c)

The normal angle between the neck and shaft of the femur is 120° -135°.
If this angle is < 120° this condition is called **coxa vara.**.
If this angle is > 135° this condition is called **coxa valga**.

Fig 8.3a (left): Normal angle between the neck and shaft of the femur is approximately 120°-135°.

Fig 8.3b (middle): Coxa valga; the angle between the neck and the shaft of the femur is >135°.

Fig 8.3c (right): Coxa vara; the angle between the neck and the shaft of the femur is <120°.

B. Q angle (figs 8.4a-c)

N = 10-12

↑ Q = Valgu

↓ Q = Varus

The Q angle is formed by the intersection of a line from the ASIS through the middle of the patella, and a line from the tibial tubercle through the middle of the patella. A normal Q angle is 10°-12°. [1 p.627] *An increased Q angle is referred to as genu valgum*, in which the patient will appear more knocked-kneed. *A decreased Q angle is referred to as genu varum*, in which the patient will appear more bowlegged. [1 p.627]

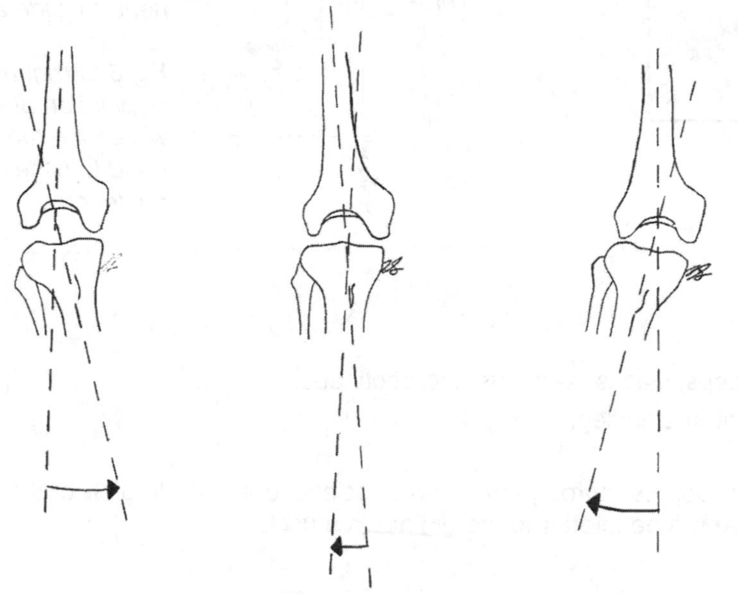

Fig 8.4a (left): Genu varum, resulting from a decreased Q angle.

Fig 8.4b (middle): Normal Q angle approximately 10°-12°.

Fig 8.4c (right): Genu valgum, resulting from an increased Q angle.

IV. Somatic dysfunction of the fibular head

A. Fibular head dysfunction

Like all synovial joints in the body, the tibiofibular joint may develop restrictions. This may result in knee pain with activity because the fibula can bear up to 1/6 of the body weight. [5 p 374] For fibular head movement see figures 8.1 and 8.2.

Two somatic dysfunctions are possible with fibular head movement:

Posterior fibular head	Anterior fibular head
Findings [33 p.292]	Findings [33 p.295]
Proximal fibular head resists anterior spring.	Proximal fibular head resists posterior spring.
Distal fibula may be anterior and resists posterior springing.	Distal fibula may be posterior.
Talus internally rotated causing foot to invert and plantarflex.	Talus externally rotated causing foot to evert and dorsiflex.

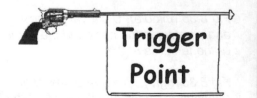

Trigger Point

The common peroneal nerve (a.k.a. common fibular nerve) lies directly posterior to the proximal fibular head. Therefore, a posterior fibular head or fracture of the fibula may disturb the function of this nerve. [28 p. 686-7]

V. Clinical considerations of the hip and knee

A. Patello-femoral syndrome (a.k.a lateral patello-femoral tracking syndrome)

Pathophysiology: An imbalance of the musculature of the quadriceps (strong vastus lateralis and weak vastus medialis). This imbalance will cause the patella to deviate laterally, and eventually lead to irregular or accelerated wearing on the posterior surface of the patella. The quadriceps imbalance is generally thought to be due to biomechanics related to a larger Q angle [1 pp.627-8]

Signs and Symptoms: Deep knee pain is present, especially when climbing stairs. The physician may notice atrophy in the vastus medialis, and often the patient will have patella crepitus.

Prevalence - Mostly in women. A wider pelvis often results in a larger Q angle.

Treatment - Strengthen the vastus medialis muscle.

B. Ligamentous injury

Three grades of sprains. [1 p.623-624]

    a. First degree: no tear resulting in good tensile strength and no laxity.

    b. Second degree: partial tear resulting in a decreased tensile strength with mild to moderate laxity

    c. Third degree: complete tear resulting in no tensile strength and severe laxity.

NOTE: In most cases, third degree sprains may require surgery, while first and second degree sprains generally can be treated conservatively.

C. Compartment syndrome

Usually results from trauma or vigorous overuse leading to an increase in intracompartmental pressure. This will compromise circulation within that compartment.

The lower leg can be divided into four compartments:

    1. Anterior
    2. Lateral
    3. Deep posterior
    4. Superficial posterior

The anterior compartment is most often affected. [32 p.9] This often results in severe unrelenting pain after and during exercise. The anterior tibilais muscle is hard and tender to palpation, pulses are present and stretching the muscle causes extreme pain. [32 p.10] Treatment usually consists of ice and myofascial release, to increase venous and lymph return. Since muscle necrosis can develop within 4 to 8 hours, if intracompartmental remains elevated a surgical fasciotomy is indicated. [1 p.655]

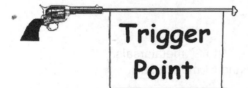

Trigger Point

O'Donahue's triad (terrible triad): a common knee injury resulting in the injury to the ACL, MCL and medial meniscus.

Ankle and foot

I. Anatomy

This region consists of 26 bones, 55 articulations, 30 synovial joints, and supported by over 100 ligaments and 30 muscles.

A. Bones (flg 8.5)
Talus
Calcaneus
Navicular
Cuboid
3 Cuneiforms
5 Metatarsals
14 Phalanges

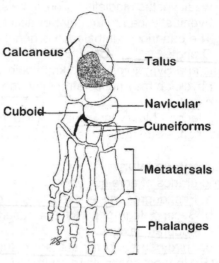

Fig 8.5: Bones of the foot: Note the gray area of the talus, (trochlea of the talus - this portion of the talus articulates with the ankle mortise); it is wider anteriorly, making the foot more stable in dorsiflexion.

B. Joints

1. Talocrural joint (tibiotalar joint): a hinge joint located between the talus and the medial malleolus of the tibia, and the lateral malleolus of the fibula. [5] *p.448*

   Main motions = plantar flexion and dorsiflexion.
   Minor motions = anterior glide of the talus (with plantar flexion) and posterior glide of the talus (with dorsiflexion).
   Due to the configuration of the talus and the ankle mortise, the ankle is more stable in dorsiflexion than plantar flexion (see fig. 8.5). This is the reason why 80% of ankle sprains occur in plantar flexion.

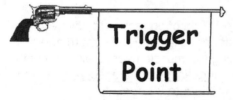

Trigger Point

The ankle is more stable in dorsiflexion.

2. Subtalar joint (talocalcaneal joint): acts mostly as a shock absorber, and also allows internal and external rotation of the leg while the foot is fixed.

C. Arches

1. Longitudinal arches:
   a. Medial longitudinal arch: talus, navicular, cuneiforms, 1st to 3rd metatarsals. [1] *p.639*
   b. Lateral longitudinal arch: calcaneus, cuboid, and 4th and 5th metatarsals. [1] *p.639*

2. Transverse arch: navicular, cuneiforms, and cuboid.

3. **Somatic dysfunction of the arches**
   Somatic dysfunctions usually occur within the transverse arch. The navicular, cuboid or cuneiforms may displace, causing pain. This is often seen in long distance runners.

Three somatic dysfunctions of the transverse arch: (fig 8.6)
  a. Cuboid: the medial edge will glide toward the plantar surface.
  b. Navicular: the lateral edge will glide toward the plantar surface.
  c. Cuneiforms: usually caused by the second cuneiform gliding
      directly downward, toward the plantar surface.

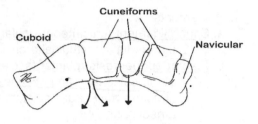

Fig 8.6: Transverse arch of the foot. It is composed of the cuboid, cuneiforms, and the navicular. Arrows show three possible somatic dysfunctions.

D. Ligaments

Since there are over one hundred ligaments in the foot and ankle, we are going to limit our discussion to the major stabilizing ligaments.

1. Lateral stabilizers of the ankle: These ligaments prevent excessive supination.

  a. Anterior talofibular ligament
  b. Calcaneofibular ligament
  c. Posterior talofibular ligament

Fig 8.7: Lateral stabilizers of the ankle

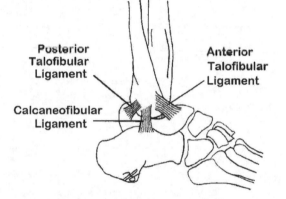

Important note: Due to the less stable supination position of the ankle, sprains often cause damage to these ligaments. *The most common injured ligament is the anterior talofibular ligament.* [10] Sprains associated with the supination position are classified into 3 types depending on the extent of ligamentous injury.[1 p.637]

Type I: involves the anterior talofibular ligament.
Type II: involves the anterior talofibular ligament and the calcaneofibular ligament.
Type III: involves the anterior talofibular ligament, calcaneofibular ligament and the posterior talofibular ligament.

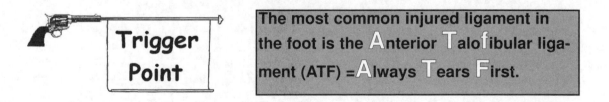

Trigger Point

The most common injured ligament in the foot is the Anterior Talofibular ligament (ATF) = Always Tears First.

2. <u>Medial stabilizer of the ankle</u>: This ligament prevents excessive pronation.
    a. <u>Deltoid ligament</u>: Since the ankle is more stable in the pronation position and the deltoid ligament is very strong, pronation sprains are very uncommon. Excessive pronation usually results in a fracture of the medial malleolus rather than pure ligamentous injury.

3. <u>Plantar ligaments</u>
    a. <u>Spring ligament (calcaneonavicular ligament)</u>: This ligament strengthens and supports the medial longitudinal arch.
    b. <u>Plantar aponeurosis (plantar fascia)</u>: Strong, dense, connective tissue that originates at the calcaneus and attaches to the phalanges. Chronic irritation to this structure may cause calcium to be laid down along the lines of stress, leading to a heel spur. [1] p.639

CHAPTER 8 REVIEW QUESTIONS

1. Which muscle is considered to be the primary flexor of the hip?
    A. Gluteus medius.
    B. Gluteus maximus.
    C. Iliopsoas.
    D. Quadriceps.
    E. Hamstrings.

2. Which structure prevents hyperextension of the knee?
    A. The posterior cruciate ligament.
    B. The anterior cruciate ligament.
    C. The medial meniscus.
    D. The medial collateral ligament,
    E. The lateral collateral ligament.

3. An insult to the knee often referred to as "O'Donahue's triad", "the terrible triad", or "the unhappy triad" results in injury to which of the following structures?
    A. The medial meniscus, the anterior cruciate ligament and the lateral collateral ligament.
    B. The lateral meniscus, the anterior cruciate ligament and the medial collateral ligament.
    C. The medial meniscus, the anterior cruciate ligament and the lateral meniscus.
    D. The medial meniscus, the anterior cruciate ligament and the medial collateral ligament.
    E. The medial meniscus, the posterior cruciate ligament and the lateral collateral ligament.

4. All of the following is true regarding a posterior fibular head dysfunction EXCEPT:
    A. It often occurs following a supination ankle sprain.
    B. The talus will be externally rotated on the affected side.
    C. The distal fibular head may be anterior.
    D. Dorsiflexion of the ankle will be restricted on the affected side.

5. The condition in which there is a decrease in the angle between the neck and the shaft of the femur is called:
    A. Coxa valga.
    B. Coxa vara.
    C. Genu varum.
    D. Genu valgum.
    E. A decreased Q angle.

6. A decreased Q angle is associated with which one of the following conditions?
    A. Genu valgum.
    B. Patello-femoral syndrome.
    C. A bow-legged appearance.
    D. Coxa vara.

7. All of the following is true concerning lateral femoral patella tracking EXCEPT:
    A. It is associated with accelerated wearing on the posterior surface of the patella.
    B. It occurs most often in women.
    C. It is associated with a positive Lachman's test.
    D. The patient may complain of deep knee pain that worsens when climbing stairs.

8. The treatment for lateral femoral patella tracking is focused on strengthening which muscle(s)?
    A. Rectus femoris.
    B. Vastus lateralis.
    C. Vastus medialis.
    D. The hamstrings.
    E. Gastrocnemius.

9. An injury to a ligament, in which a portion of the fiber is disrupted, is referred to as which of the following types of sprains?
    A. First degree sprain.
    B. Second degree sprain.
    C. Third degree sprain.
    D. Fourth degree sprain.

10. Which compartment of the lower leg is most often effected in "compartment syndrome"?
    A. The lateral compartment.
    B. The anterior compartment.
    C. The deep posterior compartment.
    D. The superficial posterior compartment.

11. All of the following are lateral stabilizers of the ankle (ligaments that prevent excessive supination) EXCEPT:
    A. The anterior talofibular ligament.
    B. The calcaneonavicular ligament.
    C. The calcaneofibular ligament.
    D. The posterior talofibular ligament.

12. The ligament most often injured in supination ankle sprains is:
    A. The anterior talofibular ligament.
    B. The calcaneonavicular ligament.
    C. The calcaneofibular ligament.
    D. The posterior talofibular ligament.

13. The ankle is most stable in which one of the following positions?
    A. Supination.
    B. Inversion.
    C. Plantar flexion
    D. Dorsiflexion.

14. A type II supination ankle sprain implies that there is injury to which of the following ligaments?
    A. The anterior talofibular ligament.
    B. The anterior talofibular and the calcaneofibular ligament.
    C. The anterior talofibular the calcaneofibular, and the posterior talofibular ligament.
    D. The posterior talofibular and the calcaneofibular ligament.
    E. The deltoid ligament.

15. A fracture of the proximal fibular head is most likely to effect which nerve?
    A. Sciatic nerve.
    B. Common fibular nerve.
    C. Tibial nerve.
    D. Sural nerve.
    E. Femoral nerve.

16. All of the following are components of the lateral longitudinal arch EXCEPT:
    A. Navicular.
    B. Cuboid.
    C. Fourth metatarsal.
    D. Fifth metatarsal.
    E. Calcaneus.

ANSWERS

1. C	9. B
2. B	10. B
3. D	11. B
4. B	12. A
5. B	13. D
6. C	14. B
7. C	15. B
8. C	16. A

CHAPTER 9

CRANIOSACRAL MOTION

I. Introduction

The cranial field was established by William Garner Sutherland D.O., D.Sc (Hon) (1873-1954). Sutherland, who graduated from the American School of Osteopathy, was an early student of A.T. Still. As a student, Sutherland noticed that the articular surfaces of the cranial bones had a unique design. After years of research and careful observations he noticed that the CNS, CSF, dural membranes, cranial bones and sacrum functioned as a unit. He named this unit the primary respiratory mechanism (PRM). [56 p.987]

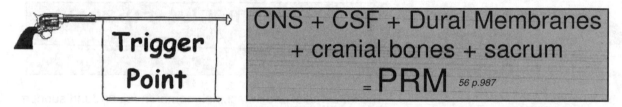

Trigger Point

CNS + CSF + Dural Membranes + cranial bones + sacrum = PRM [56 p.987]

The CNS, CSF, dural membranes, cranial bones and sacrum (PRM) function together as a physiological unit to control and regulate pulmonary respiration (which Sutherland termed *secondary respiration*), circulation, digestion. and elimination.

The PRM is composed of five anatomical-physiological elements.
1. The inherent motility of the brain and spinal cord.
2. Fluctuation of CSF.
3. The movement of the intracranial and intraspinal membranes. Dur
4. The articular mobility of the cranial bones.
5. The involuntary mobility of the sacrum between the ilia.

A. The inherent motility of the brain and spinal cord

The brain and spinal cord have a subtle inherent slow pulse-wavelike motion. [56 p.986] The brain and spinal cord lengthens and thins during the exhalation phase and shortens and thickens during the inhalation phase of the primary respiratory mechanism. [11]

B. The fluctuation of the cerebral spinal fluid (CSF)

Since direct observation of the CSF would change the hydrodynamic condition under which it normally exists, experimentation is difficult. However, several authors agree that the CSF circulates with a pulsating rhythm. Hyden and others demonstrated that glial cells grown in tissue culture pulsate continuously. [11 p.24]

Sutherland discovered rhythmic impulses could be palpated on a human skull. Later this was called the **"Cranial Rhythmic Impulse"** or the **C.R.I.** [11 p.24] The C.R.I. is commonly reported to be 10 - 14 cycles per minute in most major osteopathic texts[1 p.904, 11 p.25, 14 p.165, 35 p.140 , 36 p.122], however 8 - 12 cycles per minute has also been reported. Two other "tidal" motions have been reported, one occurring 2.5 times a minute and another "large tide" occurring six times every ten minutes. However, for the board exams, just remember the rate of the C.R.I. to be 10-14 cycles per minute.

Factors that will DECREASE the rate and quality of the C.R.I.	Factors that will INCREASE the rate and quality of the C.R.I.
1. Stress (emotional, physical) 2. Depression 3. Chronic fatigue 4. Chronic infections	1. Vigorous physical exercise 2. Systemic fever 3. Following OMT to the craniosacral mechanism

C. Movement of the Intracranial and intraspinal membranes

The intracranial and intraspinal membranes (i.e. meninges), surround, support, and partition the CNS. The meninges have three membranes:

1. Dura mater

The dura mater is the outermost membrane. It is thick, inelastic and forms the *falx cerebri and tentorium cerebelli. The dura projects caudally down the spinal canal, with firm attachments at foramen magnum, C2, C3, and S2.*

2. Arachnoid mater
3. Pia mater

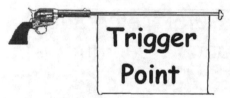

Trigger Point

Dural attachments: Foramen magnum, C2, C3 and S2.

The intracranial and intraspinal membranes surround support and partition the CNS. The inherent motility of the brain and spinal cord, and the fluctuation of the CSF will cause these membranes to move. Since the dura is inelastic and is attached to the cranial bones, any motion of the dura will influence the cranial bones. Therefore, the meninges will act as an inelastic rope causing the cranial bones to move in response to the motility of the brain and spinal cord, and fluctuation of the CSF. Sutherland called this "inelastic rope" the **Reciprocal Tension Membrane (RTM)**. The RTM has been described as an automatic, shifting, suspension fulcrum.

D. Articular mobility of the cranial bones

While Sutherland was still in medical school, he became intrigued with the articulations of the cranial sutures. The beveled surface of the sphenoid bone, and the squamous portions of the temporal bones, led Sutherland to think that articular mobility was possible. After 30 years of research on himself, and careful observation of his patients, he was convinced that the cranial bones moved in a very specific and a rhythmic type of pattern. More recently, Heisey and T. Adams demonstrated quantitatively in animal models, that cranial bones move in relation to each other. [1] p.903

E. Involuntary mobility of the sacrum between the ilia

The inherent motility of the brain and spinal cord, and the fluctuation of CSF will cause the RTM to move. Since a portion of the RTM (the dura) *attaches to the posterior superior aspect of the second sacral segment*, any motion of the RTM will cause the sacrum to move. Research has shown that a slight rocking motion of the sacrum occurs about a *transverse axis that runs though the superior transverse axis of the sacrum.*

II. Physiologic motion of the primary respiratory mechanism

The *sphenobasilar synchondrosis* (SBS) is the articulation of the sphenoid with the occiput. It is the keystone of all cranial movement. The SBS is moved through a biphasic cycle (*flexion and extension*), in response to the pull of the dural membranes that are influenced by the coiling and uncoiling of the CNS, and the fluctuation of the CSF. [1] p.904

A. _There are two motions that can occur at the SBS_:
 1. **_Flexion_**

   - _During flexion, the midline bones of the cranium (sphenoid, occiput, ethmoid, vomer) move through a flexion phase. The paired bones of the cranium will move through an external rotation phase._ An easy way to remember this relationship is:

   During "fl **ex** ion" of midline bones,

   external rotation of paired bones occur.

   - _Flexion at the SBS will cause the dura to be pulled cephalad, moving the sacral base posterior through the superior transverse axis of the sacrum. This movement at the sacral base (originally termed sacral extension) is called **counternutation** (Fig 9.1)._

   - _Flexion will widen the head slightly and decrease its anterioposterior diameter (Fig 9.2)._

Fig 9.1 (right): Flexion of the SBS will cause the dura to be pulled cephalad, resulting in counternutation of the sacrum.
Fig 9.2 (left): Craniosacral flexion (dotted lines) will widen the head slightly and decrease the AP diameter.

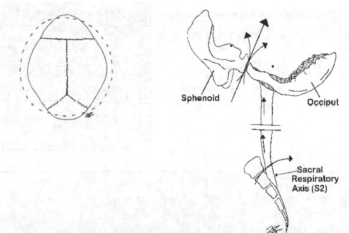

Sphenoid   Occiput

Sacral Respiratory Axis (S2)

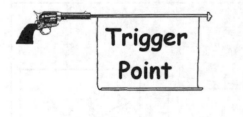

Trigger Point

Craniosacral Flexion:
1. Flexion of the midline bones.
2. Sacral base posterior (counternutation).
3. Decreased AP diameter of the cranium.
4. External rotation of paired bones.

 2. **_Extension_**
   - _During extension, the midline bones of the cranium (sphenoid, occiput, ethmoid, vomer) move through a extension phase. The paired bones of the cranium will move through an internal rotation phase._

   - _Extension at the SBS will cause the dura to fall caudad, moving the sacral base anterior through the superior transverse axis of the sacrum. This movement at the sacral base (originally termed sacral flexion) is called **nutation** (Fig 9.3)._

   - _Extension will narrow the head slightly and increase its anterioposterior diameter (Fig 9.4)._

Fig 9.3 (right): Extension of the SBS will cause the dura to fall caudad, resulting in nutation of the sacrum.

Fig 9.4 (left): Craniosacral extension (dotted lines) will narrow the head slightly and increase the AP diameter.

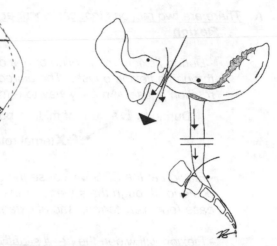

Trigger Point

Craniosacral Extension:

1. Extension of the midline bones.
2. Sacral base anterior (nutation).
3. Increased AP diameter of the cranium.
4. Internal rotation of the paired bones.

Memory Tool:

An easy way to distinguish craniosacral flexion from extension is to identify the movement of the sphenoid.

-In craniosacral flexion, the sphenoid looks like it is flexing forward.

-In craniosacral extension, the sphenoid looks like it is extending.

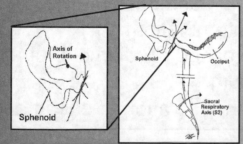

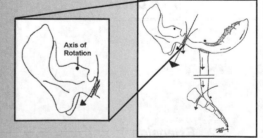

-Therefore one could say that you name craniosacral flexion and extension in the direction of sphenoid movement.

In addition, MOST (not all) craniosacral strains are also named for which direction the sphenoid has moved. See specific strains for details.

III. Strains of the sphenobasilar synchondrosis

From before birth until death, the body is subject to strains and stresses. Childbirth, traumatic brain injury, musculoskeletal dysfunction, surgery, and even everyday emotional stress are all examples of strains and stresses that may cause the PRM to be compromised. There are six types of strains that can occur at the SBS. They are: [12 p.36]

1. Flexion and extension
2. Torsion
3. Sidebending and rotation
4. Vertical strain
5. Lateral strain
6. Compression

A. Torsion

A torsion is a type of strain that occurs when there is a twisting at the SBS. *The sphenoid and other related structures of the anterior cranium rotate in one direction about an anterioposterior axis, while the occiput and the posterior cranium rotate in the opposite direction.*[1 p.906] *The torsion is named for the greater wing of the sphenoid that is more superior.* For example, if the sphenoid is rotated, so that the greater wing of the sphenoid is more superior on the right, this is called a right torsion.

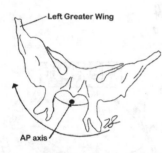 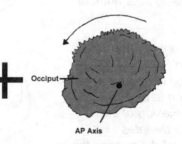

| Fig 9.5a: Posterior view of sphenoid rotating clockwise, such that the left greater wing is superior. | Fig 9.5b: Posterior view of occiput rotating counterclockwise. | Fig 9.5c: Putting together figures a & b produces a left cranial torsion. |

B. Sidebending/Rotation

This type of strain has two distinct motions that occur simultaneously about three separate axes. Rotation occurs about an AP axis through the SBS (same axis as a torsion strain) (Fig 9.6b). However, unlike a torsion, in this type of strain the sphenoid and the occiput rotate in the same direction. Both bones will either rotate clockwise or counterclockwise. Sidebending occurs about two parallel vertical axes - one axis passes through foramen magnum and the other through the center of the sphenoid (Fig 9.6a). Motion will occur about these two axes so that the SBS will deviate to the right or to the left. Due to the upward convexity of the SBS, sidebending to the left (deviation of the SBS to the left) will cause the sphenoid and occiput to rotate so that they are inferior on the left. This is denoted as SBR$_L$.

NOTE: the above strains (Right torsion, Left torsion, SBR$_L$, SBR$_R$) are all considered physiologic if their presence does not interfere with the flexion or extension components of the mechanism. [1 p.906]

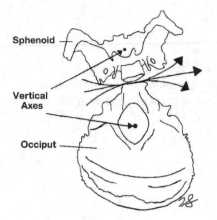

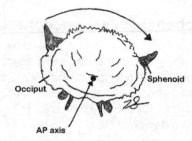

Fig 9.6a (left): Right sidebending of the SBS about two vertical axes will cause the SBS to deviate to the right.
Fig 9.6b (above): Right rotation of the SBS about an AP axis.

C. Flexion/Extension

As mentioned earlier, flexion and extension are natural physiologic components of cranial movement. A strain pattern occurs when the mechanism does not move through flexion and extension equally. *An extension lesion occurs when the SBS deviates caudad, decreasing the amount of flexion at the SBS. (Fig 9.7a). Conversely, a flexion lesion occurs when the SBS is deviates cephalad, decreasing the amount of extension at the SBS (Fig 9.7b).*

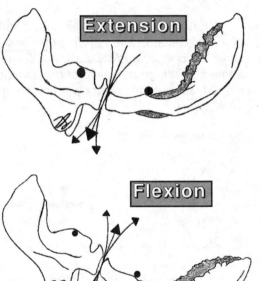

> *Fig 9.7a (above right): Extension of the SBS. The SBS deviates caudad (arrows) decreasing the amount of flexion at the SBS.*
> *Fig 9.7b (right): Flexion of the SBS:. The SBS deviates cephalad (arrows) decreasing the amount of extension at the SBS.*

D. Vertical strain

A vertical strain of the SBS is present when the sphenoid deviates cephalad (superior vertical strain) or caudad (inferior vertical strain) in relation to the occiput. Rotation will occur about <u>two transverse axes</u>. One through the center of the sphenoid, the other superior to the occiput.

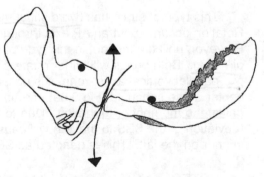

> *Fig 9.8: Superior vertical strain. The sphenoid deviates cephalad in relation to the occiput.*

E. Lateral strain

A lateral strain of the SBS is present when the sphenoid deviates laterally in relation to the occiput. If the sphenoid deviates to the left, it is termed a left lateral strain. If the sphenoid deviates to the right, it is termed a right lateral strain. Rotation will occur about two vertical axes, one through the center of the sphenoid, the other through foramen magnum. Palpation of a lateral strain will feel as if the cranium is shaped like a parallelogram.

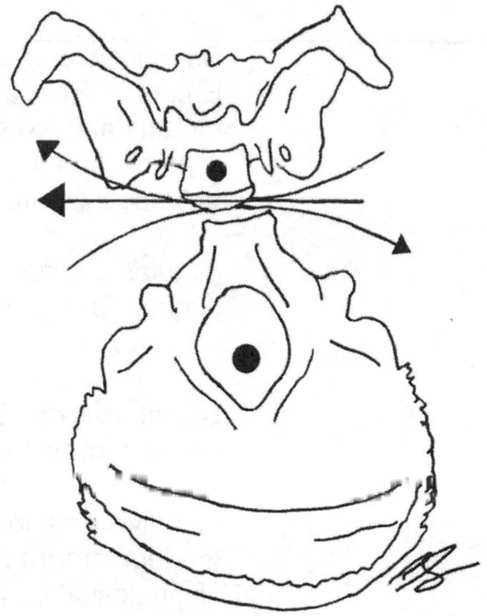

Fig 9.9: Left lateral strain. The sphenoid deviates laterally in relation to the oooiput.

NOTE: Vertical and lateral strains may be superimposed on other strains.

F. Compression

This type of strain occurs when the sphenoid and occiput have been pushed together. As a result there will be a decrease in the amplitude of the flexion and extension components of the CRI. If the compression is severe enough the CRI can be almost completely obliterated. [11 p.135] It can be due to trauma to the back of the head. [56 p.993]

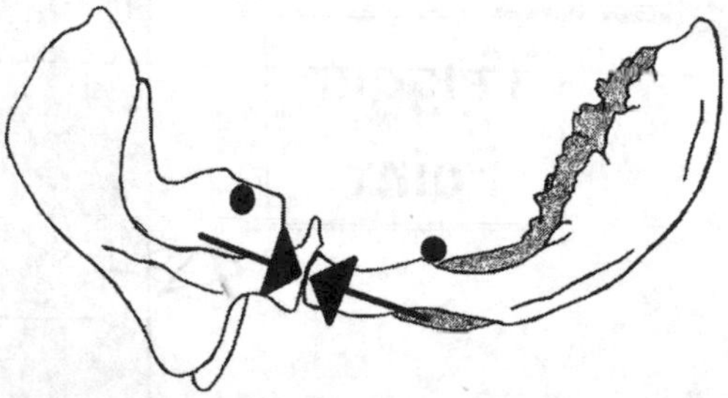

Fig 9.10: SBS compression

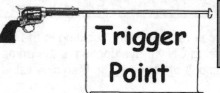

Trigger Point

> **Compression strain of the SBS can result in severely decreased C.R.I. It is usually due to trauma, especially to the back of the head.** [56 p.993]

IV. Cranial nerves

Table 9.1 Summary of the cranial nerves [1. p. 524-30]

Nerve		Exits the cranium	Somatic Dysfunction	Symptoms associated with the Dysfunction
CN I		Cribiform plate	3 Sphenoid, frontal, ethmoid	Altered sense of smell
CN II		Optic canal	2 Sphenoid, occiput	Visual changes
CN III		Superior orbital fissure	2 Sphenoid, temporal	Diplopia, ptosis or accomodation problems
CN IV		Superior orbital fissure	2 Sphenoid, temporal	Diplopia
CN V	V₁	Superior orbital fissure	2 Sphenoid, temporal	Decreased sensation to the eyelid and scalp
	V₂	Foramen rotundum	4 Sphenoid, temporal, maxillae, mandible	Tic Douloureux
	V₃	Foramen ovale	1 Sphenoid	Decr. sensation to the mandible

91

Nerve	Exits the cranium	Somatic Dysfunction	Symptoms associated with the Dysfunction
CNVI	Superior orbital fissure *2*	Sphenoid, temporal	Diplopia, esotropia
CNVII	Enters internal acoustic *3* meatus and exits the stylomastoid foramen.	Sphenoid, temporal, occiput	Bell's palsy
CNVIII	Int'l acoustic meatus *3*	Sphenoid, temporal, occiput	Tinnitus, vertigo or hearing loss
CN IX	Jugular foramen *2*	Temporal, occiput	
CN X	Jugular foramen *5*	Temporal, occiput, OA, AA, C2	Headaches, arrhythmias, GI upset, respiratory problems
CNXI	Spinal division (C1-C6) *2* enters foramen magnum joins with the cranial division and exits the jugular foramen	Temporal, occiput	Tenderness in the SCM or trapezius
CN XII	Hypoglossal canal *1*	Occiput	Dysphagia

Trigger Point

1. Vagal somatic dysfunction can be due to OA, AA and/or C2 dysfunction.
2. Dysfunction of CN VIII can cause tinnitus, vertigo or hearing loss.
3. [Occipital] Condylar compression (CN XII) can result in poor suckling in the newborn. Dysfunctions of CN IX and X at the jugular foramen can also cause suckling dysfunctions in the newborn.

NOTE: Some authors report that dysfunctions of CN's IX and X can result in poor suckling in the newborn, [35 p.7] other authors state that condylar compression causing CN XII dysfunction is the primary cause of poor suckling. [11 p. 234] The most recent edition of Foundations of Osteopathic Medicine list all three nerves as a possible cause. [56 p.674]

V. Craniosacral treatment

The goal of craniosacral treatment is to reduce venous congestion, mobilize articular restrictions, balance the SBS and enhance the rate and amplitude of the C.R.I. [14 p.171] Although treatment varies from practitioner to practitioner, there are some general techniques that every osteopathic physician should be familiar with in order to treat the patient successfully. All of the following techniques ultimately depend upon the inherent motility of the brain and spinal cord to reestablish normal mobility. For a full description of the craniosacral techniques see Greenman's Principles of Manual Medicine, Chapter 12, pages 169-170.

A. Venous sinus technique

The venous sinuses drain approximately 85 - 95% of the blood from the cranium. The remaining 5% of venous blood drains via the facial veins and external jugular. [35 p.6, 25 p.390]
Purpose - To increase venous flow through the venous sinuses so that blood may exit the skull through the jugular foramen. [14 p.169]
Procedure - The operator gently, but directly spreads apart the sutures of the cranium that overly the occipital, transverse and sagittal sinuses.

92

B. CV4: Bulb decompression

Purpose - To enhance the amplitude of the C.R.I. This is done by first resisting the flexion phase and encouraging the extension phase of the C.R.I. until a "still point" is reached, then allowing restoration of normal flexion and extension to occur. [14 p.169-70] The CV4 technique has also been reported to be helpful in fluid homeostasis [35 p.61] and help induce uterine contraction in post-date gravid women. [35 p.157]

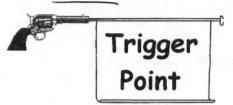

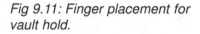
The CV4 will increase the amplitude of the C.R.I.

C. Vault hold

Purpose - To address the strains at the SBS. The operator can use either a direct or indirect method of treatment. Most commonly, an indirect method is used to balance membranous tension. [14 p.170]

    Finger placement for the vault hold is as follows: [1 p.539, 25 p.410]
        Index finger - greater wing of the sphenoid
        Middle finger - temporal bone in front of the ear
        Ring finger - mastoid region of temporal bone
        Little finger - squamous portion of the occiput

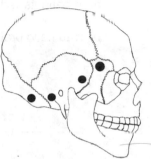

Fig 9.11: Finger placement for vault hold.

D. V spread

Purpose - To separate restricted or impacted sutures. The principle can be applied to any suture. [14 p.170]

E. Lift technique

Purpose - Frontal and parietal lifts are commonly used to aid in the balance of membranous tension. [14 p.170]

VI. Indications for craniosacral treatment

Craniosacral treatment can be used for common strain patterns caused by any stresses that disturb the PRM. Craniosacral treatment can also be used in the following scenarios:

1. After the birth of a child
    Trauma to the cranial bones often and dural membranes occur during delivery. Craniosacral treatment within the first few days of life facilitates bony remodeling of the skull. If no treatment is given and sutures continue to overlap, the cranial bones will grow together, forming a synostosis. [1 p.909]

2. Trauma to the PRM
    This can occur from mild forces, such as orthodontics or severe forces such as a car accident. Regardless of the cause, the PRM will remain compromised. Craniosacral treatment should be directed at normalizing the rate and amplitude of the C.R.I.

3. Dentistry
    Extraction of teeth, the filling of cavities, or improperly fitted dentures can compromise the PRM. Headaches, vertigo or TMJ dysfunction may result from improperly directed forces associated with dentistry. [1 p.911]

93

VII. Complications and Contraindications to craniosacral treatment

A. Complications

Although uncommon, headaches, tinnitus, or dizziness has been reported following some treatments. SBS strain treatment may cause an alteration in heart rate, blood pressure, respiration, and gastrointestinal irritability. [14 p.171]

B. Contraindications

1. Absolute contraindications
   a. Acute intracranial bleed or increased intracranial pressure
   b. Skull fracture

2. Relative contraindications
   a. In patients with known seizure history or dystonia, great care must be used in order not exacerbate any neurological symptoms.
   b. Traumatic brain injury

CHAPTER 9 REVIEW QUESTIONS

1. All of the following are components of the primary respiratory mechanism EXCEPT:
   A. The CNS.
   B. The CSF.
   C. The dural membranes.
   D. The ilium.

2. All of the following are anatomical - physiological elements that make up the PRM EXCEPT:
   A. The inherent motility of the brain and spinal cord.
   B. The fluctuation of the CSF.
   C. Mobility of the intracranial and intraspinal membranes.
   D. The immobility of the sphenobasilar synchondrosis.
   E. The involuntary mobility of the cranial bones.

3. The dura mater has firm attachments to all of the following structures EXCEPT:
   A. Foramen magnum.
   B. C2.
   C. C3.
   D. C7.
   E. S2.

4. All of the following are considered midline bones EXCEPT:
   A. Sphenoid.
   B. Occiput.
   C. Frontal.
   D. Vomer.
   E. Ethmoid.

5. Flexion of the midline bones will cause:
   A. Internal rotation of the paired bones and a decrease in the anterio-posterior diameter of the cranium.
   B. External rotation of the paired bones and a decrease in the anterio-posterior diameter of the cranium.
   C. Internal rotation of the paired bones and an increase in the anterio-posterior diameter of the cranium.
   D. External rotation of the paired bones and an increase in the anterio-posterior diameter of the cranium.

6. All of the following is associated with craniosacral flexion EXCEPT:
   A. Deviation of the SBS caudad.
   B. Counternutation.
   C. Sacral extension about a superior transverse axis.
   D. An increased width of the cranium.
   E. External rotation of the temporal bones.

7. While palpating a patient's cranium you notice that the greater wing of the sphenoid feels more superior on the right than the left. You also notice that the occiput is rotated in the opposite direction. This best describes which type of strain pattern?
   A. A right torsion.
   B. A left torsion.
   C. A left lateral strain.
   D. Sidebending and rotation to the left.
   E. Sidebending and rotation to the right.

8. Which of the following strains can be considered physiologic if it does not interfere with the flexion/extension components of the mechanism?
   A. A vertical strain.
   B. A lateral strain.
   C. Compression at the SBS.
   D. A torsion.

9. Which of the following strains is associated with a virtually absent C.R.I.?
   A. A vertical strain.
   B. A lateral strain.
   C. Compression at the SBS.
   D. A torsion.
   E. Sidebending and rotation strain.

10. Which of the following cranial somatic dysfunctions may result in tinnitus?
    A. Sphenoid restriction interfering with CN X.
    B. Temporal restriction interfering with CN VIII.
    C. Ethmoid restriction interfering with CN I.
    D. Temporal restriction interfering with CN VII.

11. Somatic dysfunction in all of the following may cause diplopia EXCEPT:
    A. The sphenoid.
    B. The temporal.
    C. The occiput.
    D. CN III.
    E. CN VI.

12. Dysfunction of which cranial nerve can cause symptoms similar to Tic Douloureux?
    A. CN V V_1.
    B. CN V V_2.
    C. CN V V_3.
    D. CN III.
    E. CN VII.

13. Which one of the following cranial nerves exit the foramen rotundum?
    A. CN V V_1.
    B. CN V V_2.
    C. CN V V_3.
    D. CN III.
    E. CN VII.

14. All of the following cranial nerves exit the jugular foramen EXCEPT:
    A. CN IX.
    B. CN X.
    C. CN XI.
    D. CN XII.

15. Somatic dysfunction of C2 may alter the function of which cranial nerve?
    A. CN IX.
    B. CN X.
    C. CN XI.
    D. CN XII.

16. All of the following are relative or absolute contraindications to craniosacral therapy EXCEPT:
    A. An acute intracranial bleed.
    B. A skull fracture.
    C. Traumatic brain injury.
    D. A migraine headache.
    E. A history of seizure disorder.

MATCHING
    A. Venous sinus technique.
    B. CV4 technique.
    C. Vault hold.
    D. Temporal rocking.
    E. V spread.

17. Enhances venous blood flow through the venous sinuses.
18. Separates restricted or impacted sutures.
19. A valuable technique to help TMJ dysfunction.
20. Diagnose strains at the SBS.
21. Enhances the amplitude of the C.R.I.

ANSWERS

1. D	12. B
2. D	13. B
3. D	14. D
4. C	15. B
5. B	16. D
6. A	17. A
7. A	18. E
8. D	19. D
9. C	20. C
10. B	21. B
11. C	

CHAPTER 10 FACILITATION

I. Facilitation

Definition - the maintenance of a pool of neurons (e.g., premotor neurons, motoneurons of preganglionic sympathetic neurons in one or more segments of the spinal cord) in a state of partial or sub-threshold excitation. In this state, less afferent stimulation is required to trigger the discharge of impulses. Facilitation may be due to a sustained increase in afferent input, or changes within the affected neurons themselves, or their chemical environment. Once established, facilitation can be sustained by normal CNS activity. [1] p.1130

A. Neurophysiologic mechanism of facilitation

If facilitation occurs at an individual spinal level it is termed segmental facilitation. In order to closely examine segmental facilitation we must first look at the spinal reflex. A spinal reflex is thought to have three simple parts: [15] p.65

1. An afferent limb (sensory input)
2. A central limb (spinal pathway)
3. An efferent limb (motor pathway)

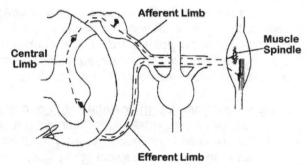

Fig 10.1: Simplification of a spinal reflex: Sensory input is transmitted by a afferent limb, processed by the central limb (interneurons) then a motor response is transmitted by the efferent limb.

Unfortunately, this is an oversimplification. In actuality, sensory input originates from many places causing a variety of effects throughout the spinal cord. Within the spinal cord, ascending/descending, branching, and crossing interneurons process (and further complicate) the sensory information. Output at the spinal segment could be to lower motor neurons (dorsal/ventral rami) to muscle or to viscera via the autonomic nervous system. Thus, a spinal reflex is actually part of a vast ever-changing network of neurons that is finely tuned to regulate the activity of the body. [15] p.65

B. How does a segment become (and stay) facilitated? (Figs 10.2 a,b)
A spinal cord segment can receive input from three areas:
1. From higher centers (brain).
2. From viscera via sympathetic or parasympathetic visceral afferents.
3. From somatic afferents (muscle spindles, Golgi tendons, nociceptors, etc.).

Any abnormal and steady sensory stimulus from one of these three areas can cause the interneurons at a spinal cord level to become sensitive to the stimulus. These "sensitized" interneurons will have an increased or exaggerated output to the initiating site as well as other areas (neighboring muscles, or organs via autonomic efferents). Once the sensitized state is established, the segment is then considered to be facilitated. Any continuous sensitizing input or the presence of normal input through sensitized interneurons, will maintain the process allowing the abnormal situation to continue.

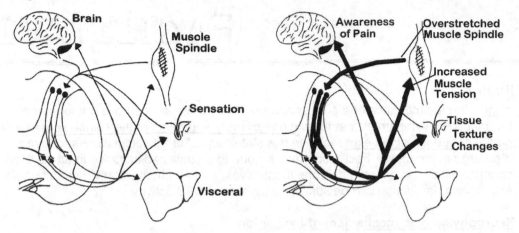

Fig 10.2a (above left): Normal afferent and efferent circuit. Fig 10.2b (above right): Facilitated segment: An abnormal sensory stimulus from an overstretched muscle spindle sensitizes two interneurons in the spinal cord. This will result in an increased or exaggerated output to the initiating site (resulting in increased muscle tension), as well as the brain (resulting in an awareness of pain), and local cutaneous tissue (resulting in tissue texture changes).

C. How does facilitation correlate with somatic dysfunction?

Let us investigate what might occur when a patient strains his deltoid muscle.

1. Abnormal and continuous sensory input from the overstretched muscle spindle sensitizes the interneurons in the spinal cord at C5.
2. A reflex occurs so that muscle tension is produced at the deltoid muscle. This will result in a **restricted** range of motion of the deltoid and **tenderness** upon palpation.
3. Prolonged muscle tension causes continuation of the sensitizing input, and the maintenance of the facilitated segment.
4. Muscle tension at the initiation site (deltoid) causes nociceptor activation in the neighboring areas, and a release of bradykinins, serotonin, histamines, potassium, prostaglandins, substance P, and leukotrienes. [1] [p.917] These substances will cause local vasodilatation and **tissue texture changes.**
5. The abnormal and continuous sensory input into C5 may also cause a paraspinal muscle spasm. The facilitated interneurons may cause an exaggerated motor output through the dorsal rami at C5 causing increased muscle tension in the deep paraspinal muscles. The resulting increase in muscle tension will cause C5, to rotate or sidebend so that **asymmetry** is present.
6. Therefore, a facilitated segment can lead to:
    1. **T**issue texture change.
    2. **A**symmetry.
    3. **R**estriction.
    4. **T**enderness.

TART = the diagnostic criteria for somatic dysfunction.

D. Reflexes

    1. **Viscero-somatic reflex** (Fig 10.3)

        According to the Glossary of Osteopathic Terminology, a viscero-somatic reflex occurs when localized visceral stimuli produce patterns of reflex response, in segmentally related somatic structures. For example, acute cholecystitis often refers pain to the mid-thoracic region at the tip of the right scapula.

    2. **Somato-visceral reflex**

        Somatic stimuli may produce patterns of reflex response in segmentally related visceral structures. For example, a triggerpoint located in the right pectoralis major muscle, between the fifth and sixth ribs and just medial to the nipple line, has been known to cause supraventricular tachyarrhythmias.[1 p.931]

Although viscero-somatic and somato-visceral reflexes are probably the most common, other reflexes are also possible. They include: somato-somatic, viscero-visceral, psycho-somatic, and psycho-visceral reflexes.

E. How does facilitation correlate with these reflexes?

    Lets investigate how acute cholecystitis can cause referred pain to the mid-thoracic region at the tip of the right scapula, and somatic dysfunction of T5 - T9 (a common viscero-somatic reflex).

    1. Continued gallbladder dysfunction, most often caused by gallstones,[8 p.926] will transmit an abnormal sensory input (from visceral receptors) into the spinal cord. This will result in segmental facilitation of T5 - T9.

    2. Normal sensory input from general afferents (e.g., muscle spindle) at T5 - T9 will become amplified at the sensitized interneurons, resulting in an exaggerated motor response. This will cause an increase in tension in the paraspinal musculature of T5 - T9. Tenderness and pain can then be elicited at this region.

    3. In addition, the increased muscle tension in the paraspinal muscles, will cause T5 - T9 to rotate and sidebend so that somatic dysfunction is present.

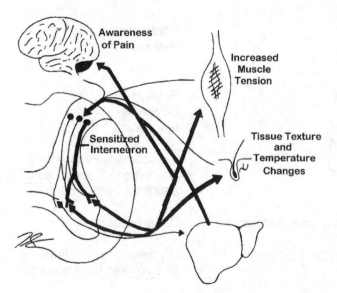

Fig 10.3: Viscero-somatic reflex: Continued visceral dysfunction will transmit abnormal sensory input into the spinal cord, resulting in facilitation of the interneurons. This will result in an exaggerated efferent response to somatic structures and the brain.

NOTE: Another common viscero-somatic reflex is T1-T5 somatic dysfunction, and pain radiating into the jaw and left arm, associated with cardiac dysfunction.

II. **Autonomic innervation**

Since visceral dysfunction transmits information to the spinal cord via autonomic afferents, it is essential for the osteopathic physician to understand the somatic areas likely to show effects of underlying visceral pathologic conditions through viscero-somatic reflexes. [1 p.572] Table 10.1 demonstrates the effects of the autonomic nervous system on various organ systems. Fig 10.4 on the following page details the visceral innervation of the parasympathetic nervous system. Table 10.2 shows the visceral innervation of the sympathetic nervous system.

Table 10.1 [13 p.275, 16 p.250, 17 p.672, 35 pp. 38, 126, 127,188]

Structure	Parasympathetic Function	Sympathetic Function
Eye		
pupil	Constricts (miosis)	Dilates (mydriasis)
lens	Contracts for near vision	Slight relaxation for far vision
Glands		
nasal, lacrimal, parotid, submandibular, gastric and pancreatic	Stimulates copious secretion	Vasoconstriction for slight secretion.
Sweat Glands	Sweating on palms of hands	Copious sweating (cholinergic)
Heart	Decreases contractility and conduction velocity	Increases contractility and conduction velocity
Lungs		
Bronchiolar smooth muscle	Contracts	Relaxes
Respiratory epithelium	Decreases # of goblet cells to enhance thin secretions	Increases # of goblet cells to produce thick secretions
GI tract		
Smooth muscle		
lumen	Contracts	Relaxes
sphincters	Relaxes	Contracts
Secretion and Motility	Increases	Decreases
Systemic arterioles		
skin and visceral vessels	None	Contracts
skeletal muscle	None	Relaxes
Genitourinary		
bladder wall (detrusor)	Contracts	Relaxes
bladder sphincter (trigone)	Relaxes	Contracts
penis	Erection	Ejaculation
Kidneys	Unknown	Vasoconstriction of afferent arterioloe=> Decreased GFR => decreased urine volume
Ureters	Maintains normal peristalsis	Ureterospasm
Liver	Slight glycogen synthesis	Glycogenolysis (release of glucose into bloodstream)
Uterus		
body (fundus)	Relaxation	Constricts
cervix	Constricts	Relaxes

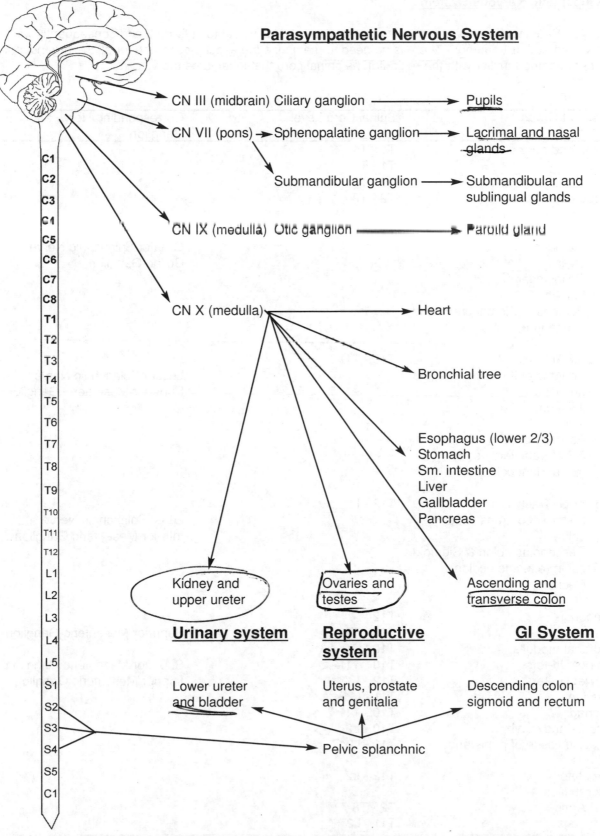

Parasympathetic Nervous System

CN III (midbrain) Ciliary ganglion ⟶ Pupils

CN VII (pons) ⟶ Sphenopalatine ganglion ⟶ Lacrimal and nasal glands

Submandibular ganglion ⟶ Submandibular and sublingual glands

CN IX (medulla) Otic ganglion ⟶ Parotid gland

CN X (medulla) ⟶ Heart

Bronchial tree

Esophagus (lower 2/3)
Stomach
Sm. intestine
Liver
Gallbladder
Pancreas

Kidney and upper ureter

Ovaries and testes

Ascending and transverse colon

Urinary system

Reproductive system

GI System

Lower ureter and bladder

Uterus, prostate and genitalia

Descending colon sigmoid and rectum

Pelvic splanchnic

Figure 10.4: Visceral innervation of the Parasympathetic Nervous System

Sympathetic Nervous System

NOTE: Segmental sympathetic innervation varies from individual to individual and consequently will vary from author to author. There is no need to memorize the exact innervation for all the organs, but rather become familiar with the region of the spinal cord that innervates the viscera.

Table 10.2 [1 p.56, 18 p.459, 35 pp. 125, 192-3]

Visceral Organ	Spinal Cord Level	Corresponding Nerve and Ganglion
Head and neck	T1 - T4	
Heart	T1 - T5	
Respiratory System	T2 - T7	
Esophagus	T2 - T8	
Upper GI Tract	T5 - T9	
Stomach		Greater Splanchnic Nerve
Liver		Celiac Ganglion
Gallbladder		
Spleen		
Portions of the pancreas and duodenum		
Middle GI tract	T10 - T11	
Portions of the pancreas and duodenum		Lesser Splanchnic Nerve
Jejunum		Superior Mesenteric Ganglion
Ilium		
Ascending Colon & proximal 2/3 of transverse colon (a.k.a. right colon)		
Lower GI Tract	T12 - L2	
Distal 1/3 of transverse colon		Least Splanchnic Nerve
Descending colon & Sigmoid colon (a.k.a. left colon)		Inferior Mesenteric Ganglion
Rectum		
Appendix	T12	
Kidneys	T10 - T11	Superior Mesenteric Ganglion
Adrenal medulla	T10	
Upper Ureters	T10 - T11	Superior Mesenteric Ganglion
Lower Ureters	T12 - L1	Inferior Mesenteric Ganglion
Bladder	T11 - L2	
Gonads	T10 - T11	
Uterus and cervix	T10 - L2	
Erectile tissue of penis and clitoris	T11 - L2	
Prostate	T12 - L2	
Extremities		
Arms	T2 - T8 [35 p.192]	
Legs	T11 - L2 [35 p.192]	

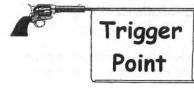

It is essential for anyone taking the COMLEX boards to understand the segmental innervation to each visceral organ. Approximately 20% of the OMT boards questions will stem from Fig 10.4 and Table 10.2.

A. Key points concerning autonomic innervations

   1. **Parasympathetic**

      Most COMLEX questions will test on which structures receive innervation from the vagus vs. the pelvic splanchnic.

      Here's an easy way to distinguish the difference:
        - All viscera above the diaphragm = Vagus nerve
        - Below the diaphragm there are three main organ systems:

      1) GI system:
        - Entire small intestine = vagus
        - Large intestine: There are four sections of the large intestine. Ascending, transverse, descending and recto-sigmoid. Divide the large intestine in half:

          Proximal half = Ascending and transverse = Vagus
     Distal half = Descending and recto-sigmoid = Pelvic splanchnic

      2) GU system: There are three major structures. The kidneys, ureters and bladder (leave the urethra out of this it is not considered a major structure).
        Proximal half = Kidneys and upper ureter = Vagus
     Distal half = Lower ureter and bladder = Pelvic splanchnic

      3) Reproductive system: The ovaries and testes descend from a higher region in the posterior abdominal wall. [3 p.145] therefore their innervations are from the vagus. All other reproductive structures are innervated by the pelvic splanchnic.

   2. **Sympathetic**
      a. T1-T4 = Head and neck
      b. T1-T5 = Heart
      c. T2 - T7 = Lungs
      d. T5-L2 = Entire GI tract.

              An easy way to divide the GI tract
      Remember two landmarks
      1) **Ligament of Treitz** - (divides the duodenum and jejunum)
      2) **Splenic flexure of the large intestine** (divides the transverse and descending colon)

        Anything before the ligament of Treitz = T5 - T9
        Anything between these two landmarks is innervated by T10 - T11.
        Anything after the Splenic flexure = T12 - L2

      e. T2-T8 = Upper Extremities [35 p.192]
      f. L3-L5 = **NOTHING**!!

III. Osteopathic manipulation directed at the autonomic nervous system

A. Autonomic nervous system
Irvin Korr PhD. (osteopathic researcher) established that there is hypersympathetic activity in disease processes. [28 p.73] Therefore, it is important to curb sympathetic activity (or enhance parasympathetic activity) when treating disease states.

B. Sympathetic nervous system

1. Rib raising
   Purpose #1: *Normalize (decrease) sympathetic activity.*
   Since the thoracic sympathetic ganglia lie anterior to their corresponding rib, gentle anterior pressure on these ganglia will initially produce a short-lived increase in sympathetic activity, but this is followed by long lasting sympathetic inhibition. [28 p.57]
   Examples:
   1. Hypersympathetic activity to mucus membranes of the sinuses and the bronchial tree promotes the proliferation of goblet cells and produces thick, sticky, tenacious secretions. Rib raising to T2 - T7 will thin mucous secretions thus enhance expectoration. [28.p.65]
   2. Rib raising and paraspinal inhibition reduced the incidence of an ileus in post-surgical patients to 0.3% from 7.6%. [28 p.76]

   Purpose #2: *Improve lymphatic return*
   Example:
   Since there is sympathetic innervation to the larger lymphatic vessels, rib raising should improve lymphatic return, in addition it will create pressure gradients directly affecting lymph return. [28 p.66]

   Purpose #3: Encourages maximum inhalation and provokes a more effective negative intrathoracic pressure. [35 p.195]

   Indications: [35 p.228]
   - Visceral dysfunction
   - Decreased rib excursion
   - Lymphatic congestion
   - Fever
   - Paraspinal muscle spasm

   Contraindications: [35 p.228]
   - Spinal or rib fracture
   - Recent spinal surgery

2. Soft tissue paraspinal inhibition [35 p.198]
   Purpose: *Normalize (decrease) sympathetic activity (Ileus prevention)*
   The upper lumbar (L1 and L2) sympathetic ganglia is continuous with that of the thoracic paraspinal ganglia. However, due to the absence of ribs, direct paraspinal pressure on the erector spinae mass produces the same autonomic effects as rib raising. [28 p.57]

3. Celiac ganglion, Superior mesenteric, Inferior mesenteric releases
   Purpose: *Normalize (decrease) sympathetic activity*
   Midline abdominal pressure over the celiac, superior mesenteric, and/or inferior mesenteric ganglia will reduce hypersympathetic activity. Pressure is applied until a fascial release is palpable. [28 p.76]

106

Indications: [35 p.227]
- GI dysfunction
- Pelvic dysfunction

Contraindications: [35 p.227]
- Aortic aneurysm
- Open surgical wound

4. Treatment of Chapman's reflexes
    Purpose: *Decrease sympathetic tone to associated visceral tissues*
        Diagnose and treat Chapman's reflexes for visceral dysfunction. Chapman's points are treated using soft, circular manipulation over the point itself. Posterior Chapman's points feel rubbery, similar to a classic viscerosomatic reflex.

5. Treatment of cervical paraspinal sympathetic ganglia
        Treatment techniques adjacent to the superior (C1 - C3), middle (C6 - C7), and inferior (C7 - T1) ganglia may influence sympathetic tone to the head and neck structures. [28 p.58]

C. **Parasympathetic nervous system**

1. Cranial manipulation
    Purpose: Aids in dural strains and improves parasympathetic function in head structures innervated by CN III, VII, IX and X. [35 p.224]

2. Sphenopalatine ganglion technique
    Purpose: Enhancing parasympathetic activity will encourage thin watery secretions through short intermittently manual finger pressure intraorally to the sphenopalatine ganglion. [28 p.65]

    Indications: [35 p.231]
    - Thick nasal secretions

3. Condylar decompression
    Purpose: This technique will help free parasympathetic responses to structures innervated by cranial nerves IX and X by freeing the passage through the jugular foramen (i.e. occipito-mastoid suture). [28 p.79]
    NOTE: Some authors report that condylar compression causes dysfunction of CN's IX and X, [35 p.7] other authors state that CN XII is primarily involved. [11 p.234]
    Example: Condylar compression as a result of childbirth may cause suckling difficulties for the newborn and thus failure to thrive. [35 p.7] Treat this problem with condylar decompression.

4. Treatment through vagus nerve influence
    Purpose: Balance parasympathetic influence to the viscera. Manipulation of the OA, AA or C2 joints will influence parasympathetic tone via the vagus nerve. [28 p.79, 35 p.224]

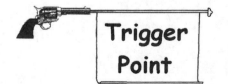

Trigger Point

Condylar compression may cause suckling difficulties for the newborn.

5. <u>Treatment of sacral somatic dysfunctions</u>
   <u>Sacral inhibition</u>
   <u>Purpose:</u> [35 p.231]
       1 *Normalize hyperparasympathetic activity in the left colon, and pelvic structures.*
       2 *Reduce labor pain caused by cervical dilation.*

   <u>Indications:</u>
       - <u>Dysmenorrhea</u>
       - <u>Labor pain from cervical dilation</u>
       - <u>Constipation</u>

   <u>Contraindications:</u>
       - <u>Local infections or incisions</u>

Chapter 10 Review Questions

1. All of the following are true concerning stimulation of sympathetic chain ganglia at T3 EXCEPT:
    A. It will cause dilation of the pupil.
    B. It will cause an increase in heart rate.
    C. It will cause bronchodilation.
    D. It will stimulate lacrimal secretion.

2. Which of the following vertebral segments will have the least effect on cardiac function?
    A. T3.
    B. T7.
    C. T4.
    D. OA.
    E. AA.

3. All of the following are true concerning vagus nerve stimulation EXCEPT:
    A. It will cause a decrease in contractility of the heart.
    B. It will cause pupillary constriction.
    C. It will cause an increase in gastric motility.
    D. It will cause urinary retention

4. All of the following are true concerning a facilitated segment EXCEPT:
    A. Less afferent stimulation is required to trigger a discharge of efferent neurons.
    B. Once established, it can be sustained by normal CNS activity.
    C. It has an increased efferent output.
    D. Usually caused by an increase in afferent input.
    E. It has a high threshold of excitation.

5. A 15 year old male presents to your office with an acute asthmatic exacerbation. Viscero-somatic changes associated with asthma can be seen at which spinal levels?
    A. C2-C7.
    B. T2-T6.
    C. T5-T10.
    D. T9-T11.
    E. T12-L2.

6. Treatment of the occiput and atlas may effect all of the following visceral structures EXCEPT:
    A. Prostate.
    B. Kidney.
    C. Ureter.
    D. Transverse colon.
    E. Ovaries.

7. Which of the following will result from hypersympathetonia?
    A. Increase in gastric motility.
    B. glycogen synthesis.
    C. Increase in respiratory rate.
    D. Lacrimation.
    E. Miosis.

8. A 42 year old obese female presents to your office with right upper quadrant pain. Pain radiates to the tip of the right scapula. On examination, you notice a positive Murphy's sign. You suspect acute cholecystitis. At which vertebral levels would you expect to find somatic changes?
   A. T1-T4.
   B. T6-T9.
   C. T9-T11.
   D. T11-L2.

9. Obstruction of a ureter from a calcium oxalate stone resulting in hydronephrosis and acute pyelonephritis will have the least effect on which of the following structures?
   A. Vagus.
   B. Pelvic splanchnic.
   C. Sympathetic chain ganglia of T12-L1.
   D. Sympathetic chain ganglia of T8-T9
   E. Sympathetic chain ganglia of T10-T11.

10. A viscero-somatic reflex resulting from a right colon cancer would be associated with somatic changes at which spinal segment?
    A. T5
    B. T8
    C. T11
    D. L2

11. Stimulation of sympathetic chain ganglia may cause all of the following EXCEPT:
    A. Digestion.
    B. Ejaculation.
    C. Vasodilation of blood vessels supplying skeletal muscle.
    D. Diaphoresis.
    E. Increased heart rate.

12. Which of the following spinal segments may alter the parasympathetic innervation to the appendix?
    A. AA.
    B. C7.
    C. T9-T12.
    D. T12-L1.
    E. S2-S4.

13. Sympathetic innervation to the liver courses through which one of the following ganglia?
    A. Otic
    B. Celiac..
    C. Superior mesenteric.
    D. Inferior mesenteric.
    E. Pelvic mesenteric.

14. A 75 year old male presents to your office with difficulty urinating. You suspect a prostate problem. Treatment to which one of the following spinal segments may calm the sympathetic influence on the prostate?
    A. T5.
    B. T8.
    C. T11.
    D. L1.
    E. S2.

15. Restriction of the occipitomastoid suture at the jugular foramen may cause all of the following visceral dysfunctions EXCEPT:
    A. Gastritis.
    B. Diarrhea.
    C. Bradycardia.
    D. Stress incontinence.
    E. Irritable bowel syndrome.

16. An increase in the sympathetic tone to the abdominal cavity will result in all of the following EXCEPT:
    A. An increase in gluconeogenesis.
    B. An increase in pancreatic secretion.
    C. A decrease in gastric motility.
    D. A decrease in GI absorption.
    E. Hypertension

17. Which of the following will influence the parasympathetic supply to the ovaries?
    A. The vagus nerve.
    B. The lesser splanchnic nerve
    C. The least splanchnic nerve
    D. The pelvic splanchnic nerve

18. A 25 year old female presents to your office with dysmenorrhea. Viscero-somatic reflex changes associated with uterine dysfunction may be at which spinal level?
    A. AA.
    B. C7.
    C. T12.
    D. L4.

19. A 45 year old male with paroxysmal hypertension secondary to an adrenal pheochromocytoma may have somatic changes at which spinal level?
    A. OA.
    B. T8.
    C. T10.
    D. T12.
    E. L2.

20. Parasympathetic stimulation may cause all of the following EXCEPT:
    A. Lacrimation.
    B. Bradycardia.
    C. Miosis.
    D. Thick bronchial secretions

21. Sympathetic stimulation of segments T10-L2 may cause which one of the following reactions?
    A. Ejaculation.
    B. Erection.
    C. Bradycardia.
    D. Increased lymphatic drainage of the lower extremities.
    E. Pancreatic secretion.

ANSWERS

1. D	12. A
2. B	13. B
3. D	14. D
4. E	15. D
5. B	16. B
6. A	17. A
7. C	18. C
8. B	19. C
9. D	20. D
10. C	21. A
11. A	

CHAPTER 11
CHAPMAN'S POINTS AND TRIGGER POINTS

I. Chapman's Points
Definition:

Starting in the 1920's, Frank Chapman D.O. discovered that specific "gangliform contractions" were associated with visceral dysfunction. [19] These "gangliform contractions" were later called Chapman's reflex points or simply Chapman's points. Anteriorly, these reflexes are *smooth, firm, discretely palpable nodules, approximately 2-3 mm in diameter, located within the deep fascia or on the periosteum of a bone.* Posteriorly, most are located between the spinous and transverse processes of vertebrae and have been described as rubbery, similar to tissue texture changes associated with the classic viscero-somatic reflex. Gentle pressure at a Chapman's point will usually elicit a sharp, nonradiating, and exquisitely distressing pain. [p.936]

Chapman's reflexes, in current clinical practice, are used more for diagnosis than for treatment. *They are thought to represent viscero-somatic reflexes.* **Therefore, a Chapman's point represents the somatic manifestation of a visceral dysfunction.** Palpating for a Chapman's reflex point can often provide the physician with clinical evidence of the presence or absence of visceral disease.

A. Important Chapman's reflex points
Table 11.1

Reflex point	Location
1. **Appendix**	**Anteriorly - At the tip of the right 12th rib.** Posteriorly - At the transverse process of T11 vertebrae. **The presence of this particular reflex point helps to direct the differential diagnosis more toward acute appendicitis.
2. Adrenals	Anteriorly - 2" superior and 1" lateral to the umbilicus Posteriorly - Between the spinous and transverse processes of T11 and T12.
3. Kidneys	Anteriorly - 1" superior and 1" lateral to the umbilicus Posteriorly - Between the spinous and transverse processes of T12 and L1.
4. Bladder	Periumbilical region
5. Colon	On the lateral thigh within the iliotibial band from the greater trochanter to just above the knee). (see fig 11.1)

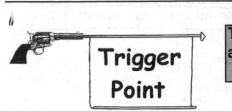 Trigger Point

The appendix Chapman's point is located at the tip of the right 12th rib.

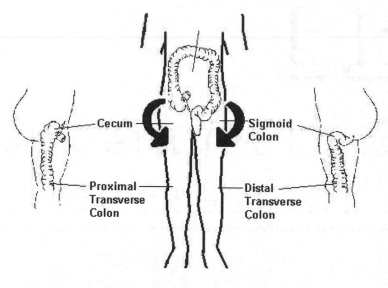

Fig 11.1: Anterior Chapman's reflexes for the colon.

To determine what portion of the colon corresponds to the Chapman's reflex, split the colon in the middle of the transverse colon, flip each side on to the corresponding iliotibial band.

The cecum point is located at the right proximal femur, the proximal transverse colon at the hepatic flexure is located at the right distal femur.

The sigmoid colon is located at the left proxima femur, the distal transverse colon at the splenic flexure is located at the left distal femur.

II. <u>Travell's Myofascial Trigger Points</u>

A trigger point is a hypersensitive focus, usually within a taut band of skeletal muscle or in the muscle fascia. It is painful upon compression and can give rise to a characteristic referred pain, tenderness, and autonomic phenomena. [20 p. 3]

A. <u>Diagnostic characteristics</u>

The patient may complain of tightness or soreness in a particular muscle that may or may not have followed an injury. On examination, the physician can palpate a taut band within the muscle. Upon compression of the band, the patient will experience pain at the site *and pain referring to an area of the body.* This referred pain is reproducible and specific for certain muscles. For example, trigger points located within the sternocleidomastoid will refer pain to occipital and temporal regions ipsilaterally. [20]

B. <u>Pathophysiology</u>

The spinal cord plays an important role in the establishment and maintenance of trigger points. Direct stimuli, such as a muscular strain, overwork fatigue, or postural imbalance, can initiate trigger points. [1 p.916] This concept is very similar to facilitation. For example, if a person were to strain his deltoid, abnormal and continuous sensory input from the overstretched muscle spindle will sensitize the interneurons at C5. A reflex occurs so that muscle tension is produced within the deltoid at the initiating site, resulting in a taut band. If this taut band refers pain when compressed, then it is considered a trigger point.

Other stimuli, such as visceral dysfunction, may also facilitate the spinal cord (viscero-somatic reflex). For example, sixty-one percent of patients with cardiac disease were reported to have chest muscle trigger points. [20 p.586] Conversely, trigger points may facilitate the spinal cord and cause visceral dysfunction (somato-visceral reflex). [1 p.917] *For example, a trigger point located in the right pectoralis muscle between the fifth and sixth ribs (intercostal space) near the sternum has been associated with supraventricular tachyarrhythmias.* [21 p.577] **Therefore, a trigger point represents the somatic manifestation of a viscero-somatic, somato-visceral or somato-somatic reflex.**

C. Treatment

   Myofascial trigger points can be treated in many ways. All techniques are directed toward eliminating the trigger point using a neurological or vascular method. The following procedures have been successful in eliminating trigger points: [21] p.9-10

   Spray and stretch using vapocoolant spray
   Injection with local anesthetic or dry needling
   Muscle energy techniques
   Myofascial release
   Ultrasound, reciprocal inhibition, or ischemic compression

D. Trigger point vs. tenderpoint

   Tenderpoints were first introduced by Lawerence Jones, D.O. Tenderpoints are small, hypersensitive points in the myofascial tissues of the body used as diagnostic criteria, and as a treatment monitor for counterstrain (Glossary of Osteopathic Terminology). Tenderpoints are similar to trigger points in that they are taut myofascial bands that are painful upon compression. *However, tenderpoints do not refer pain beyond the location compressed.* Some authors note a significant overlap in the location between trigger points and tenderpoints, [22] while some authors state that their distinction is somewhat arbitrary. [23]

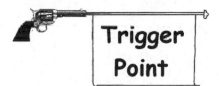

	Trigger Point

Trigger points may refer pain when pressed.
Tenderpoints DO NOT refer pain when pressed.

Travell = Referred pain on palpation

CHAPTER 11 REVIEW QUESTIONS

1. All of the following are true concerning Chapman's reflex points EXCEPT:
    A. They are thought to represent viscero-somatic reflexes.
    B. They are discretely palpable nodules 2-3 mm in diameter.
    C. Upon compression they can give rise to a characteristic referred pain, tenderness or autonomic phenomena.
    D. They are used more for diagnosis than treatment in current clinical practice.

2. Which one of the following Chapman's reflex points is associated with appendicitis?
    A. The tip of the eleventh right rib.
    B. The tip of the twelfth right rib.
    C. The spinous process of L1.
    D. The spinous process of L2.
    E. The spinous process of T12.

3. All of the following statements are true concerning tenderpoints EXCEPT:
    A. They are hypersensitive points in myofascial tissue.
    B. They act a treatment monitor for counterstrain.
    C. They often refer pain when compressed.
    D. They are painful when compressed.

ANSWERS

1. C
2. B
3. C

CHAPTER 12

MYOFASCIAL RELEASE

I. Myofascial Release

Myofascial Release is a form of manual medicine that combines several types of OMT In order to stretch and release muscle (myo) and fascia (fascial) restrictions. Counterstrain, facilitated positional release, unwinding, balanced ligamentous release, functional indirect release, direct fascial release, cranial osteopathy, and visceral manipulation are all forms of myofascial release. [25] [p.380] Since counterstrain and facilitated positional release have unique features, they are discussed separately in chapter 14.

Myofascial release treatment can be direct or indirect, active or passive (see Chapter 1, The Basics, for a further explanation of these types of treatment). It also can be performed anywhere from head to toe, because fascia surrounds and compartmentalizes all structures throughout the body. For this reason, there are several hundred different types of myofascial release techniques. It is not in the scope of this text to describe all of these treatments, but rather, a typical myofascial release procedure will be outlined, along with two very common myofascial release techniques.

A. Typical Myofascial Release Treatment

1. The physician must first palpate a restriction.
   -A restriction may present itself as muscle tension, tenderness or decreased movement of an articulation.

2. Once a restriction is palpated, the physician must then decide the type of treatment.
   -In a direct treatment, the physician will move myofascial tissues toward a restrictive barrier. This can be accomplished by using a limb as a lever and monitoring tissue tension at the restriction, or it can be accomplished by directly applying a **traction** along the long axis of the muscle.
   -In an indirect treatment, the physician will move myofascial structures away from the restrictive barrier. Again, this can be accomplished by using a limb as a lever, or by applying a **compression** along the long axis of the muscle.

3. Then the physician will add other forces to "fine tune" the treatment.
   -**Twisting** the myofascial structures (clockwise or counter-clockwise)or applying **transverse forces** perpendicular to the long axis of the muscle are added in a direct or indirect fashion. Also, passive movement of a limb may aid in the fine tuning of the myofascial treatment.

4. After the physician has correctly addressed the myofascial structures, the patient is asked to use "enhancers" to help induce a release.
   Enhancers include active movement of the patient (respiration, eye movement or muscle contraction). Again, these movements are added in a direct or indirect fashion.

5. The physician then awaits a release. A release may come in many forms, a change in temperature, a tightness may "melt" or "give way". The release may occur at different levels of the fascia or in several directions. The release phenomena is subtle and can only be appreciated by the skilled practitioner. Therefore, it may take several attempts before the osteopathic student can experience the release phenomenon.

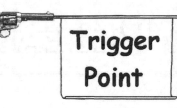

Myofascial release procedure
1. **Palpate restriction**
2. **Apply compression (indirect) or traction (direct)**
3. **Add twisting or transverse forces**
4. **Use enhancers**
5. **Await release**

B. Goal of Myofascial Release
1. Restore functional balance to all integrative tissues in the musculoskeletal system.
2. **Improve lymphatic flow** by removing myofascial restrictions.

C. Indications and Contraindications
    Myofascial release techniques are typically gentle and can be performed on acutely ill hospitalized patients and elderly patients who cannot tolerate more aggressive therapy. Since these techniques can be done in multiple positions, they also can be done on those patients who cannot tolerate much movement.
    Since myofascial release is a form of manual medicine that combines several types of OMT and has many applications, it is difficult to list specific indications and contraindications. It is important to remember that a goal of myofascial release is to improve lymphatic flow. Therefore, several of the indications and contraindications of lymphatic treatments can be applied to myofascial release techniques. For a list of indications and contraindications of specific myofascial release techniques, please see Appendix A.

D. Physiologic diaphragms
There are four diaphragms in the human body. All play a role in lymphatic return (the most important being the abdominal diaphragm).
    The four diaphragms are:
        Tentorium cerebelli
        Thoracic inlet
        Abdominal diaphragm
        Pelvic diaphragm

E. Diaphragm Release Techniques

1) **Thoracic Inlet Release** (a.k.a. thoracic outlet release)
    Purpose - To relax soft tissue restrictions and enhance lymphatic drainage from the head and neck.

    Procedure: (Direct technique) [1 p.949]
    1. Patient supine with arm abducted to 90°.
    2. Physician seated at the side of the patient.
    3. With one hand, place your fingers in the patient's supraclavicular fossa and apply traction towards the patient's wrist.
    4. With the other hand, move the patient's wrist superiorly until tension develops in the supraclavicular fossa. Hold this until some relaxation is noted.

118

5. Repeat this procedure two to three times.

2) Thoracoabdominal Diaphragm Release

Purpose - To increase pressure gradients within the thoracic and abdominal cavities, thereby increasing lymphatic return. [1 p.951] There are several different types of thoracoabdominal release, the following is example of an indirect myofascial release.

Procedure:
1. Patient seated.
2. Physician standing behind patient.
3. Pass your hands around the thoracic cage (under the patient's arms) and introduce your fingers underneath the costal margin.
4. Test for motion by gently rotating the thoracic tissues.
5. Treatment phase: With your fingers still underneath the costal margin, hold the thoracic tissues in the direction which it moves more freely. Allow the fascia to unwind, until it settles into a rhythmic vertical motion.

II. Fascial Patterns (Common Compensatory Patterns)

Many authors have noted that the musculoskeletal system in most individuals is asymmetric. These authors postulate that fascias of the body have a tendency to rotate in a certain direction. The fascia at one area will rotate one way, and the fascia in another area will rotate the opposite direction to compensate. J. Gordon Zink, D.O. was the first to provide documented material about these fascial preferences. Zink states that there are four compensatory curves throughout the spine. [1 p.946]

They are located at:
1. Occipitoatlantal junction
2. Cervicothoracic junction
3. Thoracolumbar junction
4. Lumbosacral junction

Rotatory testing of these segments reveal that in approximately 80% of **healthy individuals** the OA is rotated left, the cervicothoracic rotated right, the thoracolumbar rotated left and the lumbosacral rotated right. *Zink called this the Common Compensatory Pattern.* The remainder of **healthy individuals** (20%) had the opposite pattern. *Zink called this the Uncommon Compensatory Pattern.* He also noticed that unhealthy individuals, such as hospitalized patients, or those patients that recently experienced a traumatic event or stress, did not show this type of alternating pattern. In other words, their fascial preference did not alternate in direction from one reference area to the next. [28 p.46]

Table 12.1

Junction	Common Compensatory Pattern (80%) Rotation	Uncommon Compensatory Pattern (20%) Rotation
Occipitoatlantal	Left	Right
Cervicothoracic	Right	Left
Thoracolumbar	Left	Right
Lumbosacral	Right	Left

CHAPTER 12 REVIEW QUESTIONS

1. When performing indirect myofascial release, which barrier is engaged?
    A. Pathologic
    B. Restrictive
    C. Anatomic
    D. Physiologic
    E. Both A and B

2. Which of the following is **NOT** an appropriate endpoint of myofascial release treatment?
    A. A warming of the region treated
    B. Restoration of symmetry
    C. "Melting" of the restrictive barrier
    D. A sufficient amount of time has passed and no release was felt
    E. All are appropriate

3. Which of the following is an indication for treatment utilizing myofascial release?
    A. Febrile bacterial infection
    B. Peripheral edema
    C. Osseous fracture
    D. Advanced stage cancer
    E. Traumatic disruption of internal organs

4. Which of the following structures is considered to be a physiologic diaphragm?
    A. Hard and soft pallate
    B. Tentorium cerebelli
    C. Greater omentum
    D. Broad ligament of the uterus
    E. Mediastinum

5. Which of the following is **INCORRECTLY** matched according to the common compensatory pattern described by Zink?
    A. Occipito-atlantal fascia rotated left
    B. Cervicothoracic junction rotated right
    C. Lumbosacral junction rotated right
    D. All are correctly matched
    E. None are correctly matched

ANSWERS

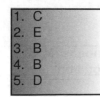

1. C
2. E
3. B
4. B
5. D

CHAPTER 13 LYMPHATICS

"We strike at the source of life and death when we go to the lymphatics." [45 p.68]
                                                                    - A.T. Still, M.D.

"What we meet with in all diseases is dead blood, stagnant lymph, and albumen in a semi-vital or dead and decomposing condition all through the lymphatics and other parts of the body, brain, lungs, kidneys, liver and fascia." [46 p.71]
                                                                    - A.T. Still, M.D.

Note: Primary information for this chapter is derived from: Wallace, et al, Foundations for Osteopathic Medicine; Kuchera and Kuchera, Osteopathic Considerations in Systemic Dysfunction; Dowling, An Osteopathic Approach to Diagnosis and Treatment; and Willard, et al, Foundations for Osteopathic Medicine. Proceeds from this chapter will be given to the Undergraduate American Academy of Osteopathy, (UAAO).

JOHN D. CAPOBIANCO, D.O., F.A.A.O.

I. Overview:

The right upper extremity, the right hemicranium (including the head and face), and the heart and the lobes of the lung (except the left upper lobe) drain into the right (minor) lymphatic duct. [1 p.943] Lymph from the remainder of the body empties into the left (major) duct. The thoracic duct traverses Sibson's fascia of the thoracic-inlet up to the level of C7 before turning around and emptying into the left (major) duct. The right (minor) duct only traverses the thoracic inlet once. [35 p.86, 210]

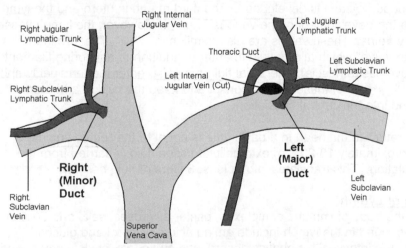

Fig 13.2 (above): The right (minor) duct drains into the right brachiocephalic vein. The left (major) duct drains the junction of the left internal jugular and subclavian veins.

Fig 13.1 (above):The right upper extremity, the right hemicranium, and the heart and the lobes of the lung (except left upper lobe) drain into the right (minor) duct. Lymph from remainder of the body empties into the left (major) duct.

The lymphatic drainage of the right (minor) duct is variable; it usually drains into the right brachiocephalic vein or the junction of the right internal jugular and subclavian veins.

The lymphatic drainage of the left (major) duct is more consistent: it drains into the junction of the left internal jugular and subclavian veins.

Therefore, lymphatic drainage from an infection of the right first toe would drain into the left (major) lymphatic duct via the thoracic duct. A right maxillary sinus infection would drain into the right (minor) duct, as would extracellular fluid resulting from lymphedema of the right upper extremity.

II. Anatomicophysiologic Relationships

Lymphatics are tubes lined with endothelial cells, which drain the interstitium and viscera in general. [47] [p.1605] Lymphoid tissues are aggregates of lymphocytes and other immune cells. [47 p.1605] Not all lymphoid tissues (for example, lymph nodes) are connected to lymphatic capillaries. Not all lymphatics are connected to the lymphoid tissue. The thyroid, esophagus and the coronary and triangular ligaments of the liver bypass lymphoid tissue and drain directly into the thoracic duct. [47 p.1605] Traditionally, the superficial skin, deep portions of the peripheral nerves, the endomysium of muscles, and bones were thought not to have lymphatic vessels. However, they have prelymphatics, the Haversian canals being an example. Two-thirds of the lymphatic fluid is produced by the liver and intestines. [17 p.180] Also, the cerebrospinal fluid is the de facto lymph of the central nervous system.

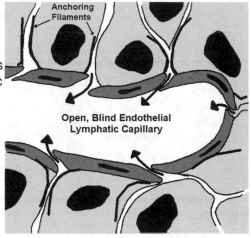

Fig 13.3: Lymphatic fluid draining into a lymphatic capillary terminal.

The thoracic duct extends approximately 18 inches from the cisterna chyli below the diaphragm (at the level of L2), through the aortic hiatus (at the level of T12) into the neck for about 3 centimeters before draining into the left (major) duct. [35 p.86]

Embryologically, the lymphatic system is developed by the third month in utero and the lymph vessels are closely related to the development of the venous system. However, the lymph vessels have more valves than do the veins. These valves are also semilunar. [47 p.1605] The terminal lymphatic capillary has a "flap valve" which allows fluid to enter in addition to anchoring filaments into the surrounding connective tissue (fascia). Interstitial fluid may also enter the terminal lymphatic vessel via micropinocytosis. [47 p.1605] All of these factors conspire to keep the fluid in and propel it proximally to lymph nodes and into the central circulation.

Ordinarily, the lymphatic return to the heart in a day's time is equal to the "entire volume of serum of the body". [35 p.39] Approximately 10-20% of extracellular tissue fluid is carried from the interstitium to the blood circulation. This translates into at least 3 liters of fluid per day. [1 p.944, 47 p.1605]

III. Composition and Function of Lymph

The lymphatics cleanse the body of immune complexes, bacteria, viruses, salts and 50% of the plasma proteins. Substances found in the lymph include amino acids, glycerol and glucose [25 p.256] Vital to one's nutritional state, the intestinal lymphatics absorb long chain fats, chylomicrons, and cholesterol. [1 p.944-45] Lymph also contains clotting factors. The main cells found in lymph are lymphocytes. Hence, the lymph is essential for bringing particulate matter to both immune cells (for example, lymphocytes) and lymphoid tissue (for example, nodes). [1 pp.943-44]

IV. Innervation of Lymphatic System

It is important to realize that the lymphatic capillary is under the same sympathetic influences as are other vasculature. The sympathetics constrict the lymphatic capillaries. Initially, this will lead to an increase in peristalsis of the lymph vessel. However, sustained inappropriate hypersympathetic tone may decrease the overall movement of lymphatic fluids. Although there are cholinergic fibers in the lymphatics, little is known of the parasympathetic influence upon the lymph movement. The sympathetic control to the lymphatic duct is topographically innervated by the intercostal nerves. The cisterna chyli is innervated by T11. [1 p.120]

V. Factors Influencing Lymphatic Fluid Movement:

The lymphatics relieve the body's excess fluids and wastes by both intrinsic and extrinsic forces.

Extrinsic forces include:
- Osteopathic manipulative treatment
- Exercise
- Contraction of muscles [47 p.1606]
- Pulsation of adjacent arteries [47 p.1606]
- Respiratory movement to increase negative intrathoracic pressure [47 p.1606]

Intrinsic forces include:
- Smooth muscle contraction [47 p.1606]
- Interstitial fluid pressure

Interstitial fluid pressure is normally -6.3mmHg and flows at a rate of 120cc/hr. Any increase of interstitial fluid pressure will increase the absorption of lymph into lymph capillaries. An increase to 0mmHg will increase lymph flow twenty-fold. [1 p.945] However at levels above 0mmHg interstitial fluid pressure becomes so great that it causes the lymphatic capillaries to collapse. As a result, there is a decrease in lymphatic drainage.

Factors allowing extracellular fluid to enter the lymphatic capillary:
According to Guyton: [17 p.182]

1. Increased arterial capillary pressure.
2. Decreased plasma colloidal osmotic pressure.
3. Increased protein in the interstitium.
4. Increased capillary permeability.

In addition, from an osteopathic standpoint other factors include:
5. Connective tissue movement.
6. Fluid fluctuations.

Factors increasing interstitial pressure above 0mmHg that correlate to numbers 1-4 above:
According to Wallace, et al.: [1 p.945]

1. Systemic hypertension.
2. Cirrhosis (decreased plasma protein synthesis).
3. Hypoalbuminemia associated with starvation.
4. Toxins such as rattlesnake poisoning.

VI. Osteopathic Diagnosis for Lymphatic Dysfunction: [35 p.206]

According to Drs. Kuchera this includes but is not limited to the following:

1. Supraclavicular fullness and bogginess resulting from lymphatic congestion of the head and neck. Eg., sinusitis.
2. Posterior axillary fold fullness and bogginess resulting from lymphatic congestion of the arm. Eg., post-mastectomy lymphedema.
3. Epigastric area fullness and bogginess resulting from organ congestion of the chest or abdomen. Eg., cirrhosis.
4. Inguinal area fullness and bogginess resulting from lymphatic congestion of the lower extremity. Eg., infection.
5. Popliteal area fullness and bogginess resulting from lymphatic congestion of the leg. Eg., thrombophlebitis.
6. Achilles tendon fullness and bogginess resulting from lymphatic congestion of the ankle or foot. Eg., sprained anterior talofibular ligament.

Additionally, many other areas of dysfunction may lead to lymphatic congestion. Some of these include:

7. Tense pelvic diaphragm (levator ani and coccygeus muscles).
8. Restricted thoracic cage motion [25 p.258]
9. Viscerosomatic tissue texture changes (Chapman's reflexes) from lymphatic congestion of any organ.
10. Paravertebral muscle spasm causing an increased lumbar lordosis with resultant flattened diaphragm.
11. Torsioned thoracic-inlet.
12. Cranial base strain, particularly along the attachments of the tentorium cerebelli (occiput, parietals, temporals, sphenoid or ethmoid).

VII. Osteopathic Treatment for Lymphatic Dysfunction

This includes but is not limited to the following:

1. Chapman's reflexes

Lymphatic congestion of the bronchus, upper or lower lung may involve a gangliform contraction of the third or fourth intercostal space along the parasternal border respectively anteriorly or a rubbery nodule (it feels like a classic viscerosomatic reflex) between the spinous and transverse processes of T2, T3 or T4 respectively. There are about 100 recorded Chapman's reflexes in the body.

2. Thoracic pump (of Miller)

This facilitates increased rib cage motion in addition to mobilizing total lymphatic fluid movement.

3. Pedal pump (of Dalrymple)

Again, this encourages total body lymphatic movement and is particularly useful for the pediatric patient.

4. Osteopathy in the cranial field

This will decrease dural strains of what is considered the uppermost diaphragm of the body, the tentorium cerebelli and the reciprocal tension membrane in general. This will also increase venous return from the head by undoing strains at the occipital and temporal regions, which make up the jugular foramen. In addition, the CSF not only is considered the lymphatic fluid of the brain but also drains directly into the facial and spinal lymphatics.

5. Muscle energy or any treatment to the thoracic-inlet

Remember Sibson's fascia is made up of the connective tissues of the scalenes and longus colli muscle and is traversed by both right and left lymphatic ducts.

6. Rib raising

This will increase thoracic motion by lessened somatic dysfunction of the spine, ribs and sternomanubrial-clavicular complex. Also, normalization of the parathoracic sympathetic ganglia are achieved by rib raising.

7. Splenic/Liver pump

This facilitates bringing toxins and other antigens into close contact with the macrophages of the liver (Kupffer cells) and allows the spleen to screen and remove damaged cells form the circulation [1 p.957, 25 p.258]

8. Facial sinus pressure/Galbreath technique

This includes direct "stroking" of the frontal, nasal, maxillary and zygomatic bones and/or TMJ in order to facilitate lymph movement toward the jugulodigastric node (just anterior to the TMJ) and eventually distally to the right and left lymphatic ducts. This is useful in sinus congestion or otitis media.

9. Anterior cervical mobilization

Basically, gentle translatory (right to left, vice versa) motion of the hyoid, thyroid, cricoid and trachea will also encourage lymphatic drainage of the head, neck and throat.

10. Extremity pump (of Wales)

Involves effleurage wave-like motions of the arms and legs in order to move lymph proximally to the axillae and groin respectively before terminating into the right and left lymphatic ducts.

VIII. Types of Lymphatic Treatments [56 p.1062]

Lymphatic treatments can be divided into two catagories. Those that improve restrictions and those that augment lymphatic flow. Treatment protocols should include techniques from both catagories. First starting with techniques that remove restriction, then appling techniques that augment flow. A basic sequence for lymphatic treatment program should include:

1. Treat any thoracic inlet somatic dysfunction

Since the thoracic duct and right lymphatic duct traverse Sibson's fascia in the thoracic inlet, somatic dysfunction here can cause decreased lymphatic drainage from anywhere in the body

2. Rib raising or paraspinal inhibition

This will mobilize the ribs for improved respiration, and normalize any hypersympathetic activity

3. Redome the thoracoabdominal diaphragm

This will optimize thoracoabdominal pressure gradients to maximize lymph return.

4. Apply lymphatic pump techniques

Once the diaphragms are free of restriction and sympathetic tone is normalized. Lymphatic pumps will help return lymph through open channels.

IX. Indications for lymphatic treatment
According to Wallace, et al, this list includes but is not limited to the following:

1. Upper respiratory infections such as sinusitis, otitis, pharyngitis.
2. Bronchitis, pneumonia, asthma, COPD, atelectasis.
3. Post myocardial infarction, congestive heart failure, and infections of the heart.
4. Mastitis, lymphedema.
5. Gastrointestinal disorders such as hiatal hernia, Crohn's or colitis.
6. Cirrhosis, chronic hepatitis, pancreatitis, nephrotic syndrome. [48 pp.24-8]
7. Premenstrual syndrome, uterine fibroma, endometriosis, cystitis.
8. Disorders of the extremities including tendonitis, joint swelling from infection or trauma, ezcema or psorasis.

X. Contraindications to lymphatic treatment
This includes but is not limited to the following:

The distinction between relative and absolute contraindications to lymphatic technique are unfortunately not well delineated. In fact, the term "absolute contraindication" is not generally used when it comes to lymphatic treatment. Here is an attempt to shed some clarity on the situation. Remember, treat each patient on an individual basis. The following lists are mostly extrapolated from Wallace et al. [1 pp.955-64] and Dowling. [25 p.260]

Relative contraindications to lymphatic treatment:
1. Osseous fractures.
2. Bacterial infections with a temperature greater than 102°F.
3. Abscess or localized infection.
4. Certain stages of carcinoma.
   NOTE: This fact has not been demonstrated. Dowling argues that a case can be made for the delivery of cancerous cells to the body's immune system for clearance and destruction. [25 p.260]

For contraindications to specific lymphatic treatments see Appendix A.

CHAPTER 13 REVIEW QUESTIONS

1. Which of the following structures does not drain into the left (major) duct
    A) Lymph originating from the left eye
    B) Lymph originating from the right leg
    C) Lymph originating from the left upper lobe of the lung
    D) Lymph originating from myocardium

2. Restrictions within Sibson's fascia could produce edema
    A) In the left upper and both lower extremities
    B) In the right upper extremity
    C) In head and neck structures
    D) In both lower extremities.
    E) In the entire body

3. Which of the following is **NOT** true regarding autonomic innervation of the lymphatic system?
    A) The thoracic duct receives most of its sympathetic innervation from T9
    B) The cisterna chyli receives most of its sympathetic innervation from T12
    C) Hypersympathetic tone will initially produce an increase lymphatic return
    D) The role of parasympathetic infuence upon lymph movement is not well understood

4. All of the following are factors that improve lymphatic movement EXCEPT?
    A) Semilunar valves in lymph vessels
    B) Flap valves in terminal lymph capillaries
    C) Increase in interstitial fluid pressure from 0mmHg to 1.3mmHg
    D) Pulmonary respiration
    E) Micropinocytosis

5. All of the following could decrease lymphatic return EXCEPT?
    A) Hypertension
    B) Decreased plasma colloidal osmotic pressure
    C) Severe hypoalbumenemia
    D) Rattlesnake toxin

6. Which of the following correctly outlines the typical sequence for lymphatic treatment.
    A) Rib raising, lymphatic pump, thoraco-abdominal diaphragm release, thoracic inlet release.
    B) Lymphatic pump, thoraco-abdominal diaphragm release, thoracic inlet release, rib raising.
    C) Thoracic inlet release, rib raising, thoraco-abdominal diaphragm release, lymphatic pump
    D) Thoracic inlet release, rib raising, lymphatic pump, thoraco-abdominal diaphragm release.
    E) Lymphatic pump, rib raising, thoraco-abdominal diaphragm release, thoracic inlet release.

7. All of the following are indications for lymphatic treatment EXCEPT?
    A) Upper respiratory tract infection
    B) Abscess
    C) Cirrhosis
    D) Congestive Heart Failure
    E) Nephrotic syndrome

ANSWERS

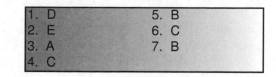

1. D	5. B
2. E	6. C
3. A	7. B
4. C	

CHAPTER 14

COUNTERSTRAIN AND FACILITATED POSITIONAL RELEASE (FPR)

Counterstrain
I. Definition

Counterstrain is a ***passive indirect technique*** in which the tissue being treated is positioned at a point of balance, or ease, away from the restrictive barrier. [1 p. 809] Counterstrain was pioneered by Lawerence H. Jones in 1955. Jones discovered that by placing a patient in a position of ease for 90 seconds he could eliminate "tenderpoints." He initially referred to this new treatment approach as "spontaneous release by positioning". He later called it strain counterstrain, or simply counterstrain.
[1 p.810]

A. What is a tenderpoint?
Tenderpoints are small tense edematous areas of tenderness about the size of a fingertip. [1 p. 811] They are typically located near bony attachments of tendons, ligaments or in the belly of some muscles. Trigger points are also a small, tense, hypersensitive areas of tenderness. *However, trigger points will radiate pain to a specific area when compressed. Tenderpoints do not radiate pain to other locations of the body.*

B. Basic counterstrain treatment steps

1. Locate a significant tenderpoint.
   -Tenderpoints can usually be found at the region of the patient's chief complaint. In addition, tenderpoints may also be located in a corresponding anterior location.
   -Also keep in mind that pain at one location may be induced from a primary strain elsewhere. A common example of this is a patient with a psoas spasm complaining of low back pain. Although tenderness can be elicited at the lumbar spine and sacroiliac regions, a psoas tenderpoint located medial to the ASIS or periumbilical region will be present, and may be the cause of the lumbosacral pain.

2. Palpate the tenderpoints.
   -The pressure used to elicit a tenderpoint is only a few ounces. [1 p.811]
   -To determine if that point is clinically significant, compare the same spot to the other side.
   -If there are multiple areas of tenderness, treat the most tender area first. [1 p.811]

129

3. <u>Place the patient in the position of optimal comfort.</u>
   -Maintaining light contact with the tenderpoint, the physician makes a gross adjustment, **shortening the muscle** being treated.
   -Reapply firm pressure to check for reduction of tenderness.
   -Fine tune the treatment with small areas of motion until at least 70% of the tenderness has been reduced. [1 p.812]

   Maverick Point
   Approximately 5% of tenderpoints will not improve with the expected treatment even with careful fine tuning. These Maverick points are treated by positioning the patient in a position opposite of what would be used typically. [1 p.812]

4. <u>With the patient completely relaxed, maintain the position of comfort for 90 seconds.</u>
   -Ninety seconds is the time required for the proprioceptive firing to decrease in frequency and amplitude. [25 p.88-9]

5. <u>Slow return to neutral.</u>
   -The first few degrees are the most important. [1 p. 813]
   -Make sure the patient is completely relaxed and does not try to help by actively moving.

6. <u>Recheck the tenderpoint.</u>
   -No more than 30% of the tenderness should remain.
   -Tenderness from a viscerosomatic reflex will return within a few hours. [1 p.813]

II. Counterstrain Techniques
A. Cervical Spine

Anterior Cervical Tenderpoints
Location:
   Usually slightly anterior to or on the most lateral aspect of the lateral masses. [1 p.815]

Treatment position:
   Sidebend and rotate the patient's head away from the side of the tenderpoint.

Anterior Cervical Maverick Points
Anterior Seventh Cervical [26 p.47]
Location:
   About 2-3cm. lateral to the medial end of the clavicle. At the lateral attachment of the sternocleidomastoid.

Treatment position:
   Flexion, sidebend toward and rotate away from the side of the tenderpoint.

Posterior Cervical Tenderpoints
Location:
   Usually at the tip of the spinous process or on the lateral sides of the spinous process.

Treatment Position:
   Extend, sidebend (slightly), and rotate away.

Posterior Cervical Maverick Points
Inion (Posterior First Cervical)
Location:
> At the inion (posterior occipital protuberance) or just below

Treatment position:
> Marked flexion.

B. Thoracic Spine

Anterior Thoracic Tenderpoints
Location:
> T1-T6: Located at the midline of the sternum at the attachment of the corresponding ribs.
> T7-T12: Most are located in the rectus abdominus muscle about one inch lateral to the midline on the right or left.

Treatment Position:
> Flex thorax and add a small amount of sidebending and rotation away.

Posterior Thoracic Tenderpoints
Location:
> On either side of the spinous process or on the transverse process.

Treatment Position
> Extend, rotate away and sidebend slightly away.

C. Ribs

Anterior tenderpoints are associated with depressed ribs (also called exhalation ribs, an exhalation dysfunction, or an inhalation restriction). Posterior tenderpoints are associated with elevated ribs (also called inhalation ribs, an inhalation dysfunction, or an exhalation restriction). [56] [p.1011, 25 p.272]

Jones recommends maintaining rib treatment positions for **120 seconds** to allow the patient extra time to relax. [1 p.815]

Anterior Rib Tenderpoints

Location:
> Rib 1: Tenderpoint is located just below the medial end of the clavicle.
> Rib 2: Tenderpoint is 6-8cm lateral to the sternum on rib 2. [26 p.78]
> Ribs 3-6: Tenderpoints are located along the mid-axillary line on the corresponding rib.

Treatment Position:
> Ribs 1 and 2: Flex head, sidebend and rotate towards.
> Ribs 3-6: Sidebend and rotate the thorax toward, encourage slight flexion.

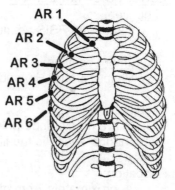

Fig 14.1: Anterior rib tenderpoints

131

Posterior Rib Tenderpoints

Location:
   The angle of the corresponding rib.

Treatment Position:
   Most of these are treated with minimal flexion, sidebend away and rotation away. [26 p.82, 40 p.66]

D. Lumbar Spine

Anterior Lumbar Tenderpoints
Location:
   L1: Medial to the ASIS.
   L2-L4: On the AIIS.
   L5: One cm lateral to the pubic symphysis on the
      superior ramus.

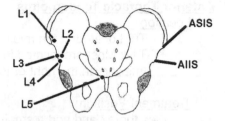

Treatment Position:
   Most are treated with the patient supine, knees and
   hips flexed and markedly rotated away.

Fig 14.2: Anterior lumbar tenderpoints

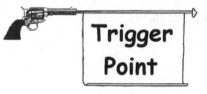

Trigger Point

> The anterior tenderpoint for L5 is located one cm lateral to the pubic symphysis on the superior ramus.

Posterior Lumbar Tenderpoints
Location:
   On either side of the spinous process or on the transverse process. L3 and L4 may be found on the iliac crest. Also, L5 may be found on the PSIS.

Treatment Position:
   Most are treated with the patient prone, extended and sidebent away (rotation may be towards or away).

Posterior Lumbar Maverick Points
Lower Pole Fifth Lumbar
Location:
   Caudad to PSIS as much as one cm.

Treatment position:
   Patient prone. Hip and knee flexed. Leg internally rotated and adducted. [26 p.112]

E. Pelvis
There are many tenderpoints for pelvic muscles and associated structures. Perhaps the most important of these is the iliacus.
Iliacus:
Location:
   Approximately 7 cm medial to the ASIS.

Treatment Position:
   Patient supine with the hip flexed and externally rotated.

Pelvis Maverick Point
   Piriformis
      Location:
         Usually in the piriformis muscle 7 cm medial to and slightly cephalad to the greater trochanter.

      Treatment position:
         Pt prone. Hip and knee flexed. Thigh abducted and externally rotated.

III. Facilitated Positional Release (FPR)

A. Definition

A system of indirect myofascial release treatment developed by Stanley Schiowitz, D.O. The component region of the body is placed into a neutral position, diminishing tissue and joint tension, in all planes, and an activating force (compression or torsion) is added. [1 p.1133] It is easily applied, nontraumatic and only takes 3-4 seconds to induce a release.

FPR Technique can be used to treat:
1. Superficial muscles
2. Deep intervertebral muscles to influence vertebral motion

Typical FPR Procedure
   Superficial Muscle Treatment
1. With the patient in a neutral position, the physician first straightens the AP curvature of the spine (decreasing the kyphosis or lordosis).
2. The physician then applies the facilitating force (compression or torsion, or both).
3. The physician then shortens the muscle to be treated.
4. The position is held for 3 to 4 seconds.
5. The physician releases the position and reevaluates the dysfunction.

   Deep intervertebral muscle treatment (Intervertebral motion treatment)
      Diagnosis C5 ES_RR_R:
1. The patient is supine, with his/her head beyond the end of the table, resting in a pillow in the physician's lap.
2. With the patient in a neutral position, straighten the cervical lordosis by flexing the head slightly.
3. The physician then applies the facilitating force (compression or torsion, or both).
4. The physician will then place C5 in ES_RR_R using the head as a lever.
5. The position is held for 3 to 4 seconds.
6. The physician releases the position and reevaluates the dysfunction.

133

CHAPTER 14 REVIEW QUESTIONS

1. What percentage of tenderpoints are considered to be "maverick"?
   - A. 1%
   - B. 5%
   - C. 7%
   - D. 10%
   - E. 15%

2. When fine tuning position for a counterstrain technique, what is the minimum acceptable reduction of pain?
   - A. 30%
   - B. 60%
   - C. 70%
   - D. 85%
   - E. 95%

3. What region is associated with the greatest number of "maverick" tenderpoints?
   - A. Cervical spine
   - B. Thoracic spine
   - C. Lumbar spine
   - D. Ribs
   - E. Pelvis

4. When utilizing facilitated positional release to a superficial muscle, which is performed first?
   - A. Application of traction
   - B. Application of compression
   - C. Shortening of the muscle
   - D. Straightening of the AP spinal curves
   - E. Fine tuning the position

5. Which of the following is **NOT** correctly matched?
   - A. Counterstrain => Hold 90 seconds
   - B. Facilitated positional release => Hold 30 seconds
   - C. Posterior cervical tenderpoint => Tip of spinous process
   - D. Posterior rib tenderpoint => Angle of rib
   - E. All are correctly matched

6. Which of the following is the correct location for the iliacus tenderpoint?
   - A. On the ASIS
   - B. 1 cm lateral to the ASIS
   - C. 3 cm medial to the ASIS
   - D. 5 cm lateral to the ASIS
   - E. 7 cm medial to the ASIS

ANSWERS

1. B	4. D
2. C	5. B
3. A	6. E

CHAPTER 15

MUSCLE ENERGY

DANIEL G. BERSEN, D.O.

I. Definition

A form of OMT in which the patient actively uses his muscles on request, "from a precisely controlled position in a specific direction, against a distinctly executed counterforce." [1 p.1133]

II. Principles of Muscle Energy Treatment

Muscle energy can be performed as an active direct or active indirect techniques (see Chapter 1, The Basics for further description of these types of treatments).

NOTE: Most forms of muscle energy treatment are direct. Indirect is rarely used.

III. Types of Muscle Energy

1. Postisometric relaxation (direct technique): The physician, after correct diagnosis of the somatic dysfunction, reverses all components in all planes and engages the restrictive barrier.

    The physician then instructs the patient to contract equally against the offered counterforce by the physician. This isometric contraction where the distance between the origin and the insertion of the muscle remains the same as the muscle contracts will stretch the internal connective tissues.
    The Golgi tendon organs senses this change in tension in the muscle tendons and causes a reflex relaxation of the agonist muscle fibers. [1 p.694] Therefore, by reflex relaxation of the agonist muscle, the physician is then able to passively stretch the patient in all planes of motion to the new restrictive barrier.
    For example, if the biceps muscle is in spasm, extend the elbow fully to the restrictive barrier, flex the biceps against resistance for 3-5 seconds, then relax. Extend the elbow to the new restrictive barrier then repeat.

2. Reciprocal inhibition: Another muscle energy technique utilizes the reflex mechanism of reciprocal inhibition when antagonistic muscles are contracted.

    By contracting the antagonistic muscle, signals are transmitted to the spinal cord and through the reciprocal inhibition reflex arc, the agonist muscle is then forced to relax.

    Reciprocal inhibition can be done directly [28 p.311] or indirectly. [28 p.680]

    a. Reciprocal inhibition - direct technique
    If the biceps muscle is in spasm, extend the elbow fully to the restrictive barrier, then have the patient contract his triceps against resistance. This isometric force through reciprocal inhibition allows the biceps muscle to relax and return to a normal resting state.

b. Reciprocal inhibition - indirect technique
If the biceps muscle is in spasm, fully flex the elbow (away from the restrictive barrier), then have the patient contract his triceps against resistance. This isometric force through reciprocal inhibition allows the biceps muscle to relax and return to a normal resting state.

3. Joint Mobilization using muscle force: This type of muscle energy restores normal range of motion of a joint using muscle contraction. [56 p.882] For example, contracting the hip flexors helps pull the innominate anterior in a posterior innominate dysfunction.

4. Oculocephalogyric reflex:: This type of muscle energy uses extraocular muscle contraction to reflexively effect the cervical and truncal musculature. [56 p.883].

5. Respiratory assistance: This type of muscle energy uses the patient's voluntary respiratory motion to restore normal motion. [56 p.883] Most inhalation rib dysfunctions are treated in this fashion.

6. Crossed extensor reflex: This form of muscle energy uses the crossed extensor reflex to achieve muscle relaxation. It is typically used in extremities that are so severly injured or not accessible that direct manipulation is impossible. For example, contraction of the right biceps produces relaxation of the left biceps and contraction of the left triceps. [56 p.883]

V. Typical Muscle Energy Treatment Procedure
1. The physician positions the bone or joint so the muscle group will engage the restrictive barrier (direct treatment) in all planes of motion.
2. The operator instructs the patient to reverse direction in one or all planes of motion.
3. The patient contracts the appropriate muscle(s) or muscle group with the objective of moving the body part through a complete range of motion.
4. The physician maintains an appropriate counterforce so that the contraction is perceived at the **critical** articulation or area for 3-5 seconds.
5. The physician then instructs the patient to relax and the physician also relaxes. Then during the post-isometric relaxation phase, the physician takes up the slack, allowing it to be passively lengthened. Increased range of motion is noted by the physician.
6. Steps 1-5 are repeated for 3-5 times until the best possible increase in motion is obtained.

VI. Localization
Localization of force is more important than intensity of force. Localization depends on the physician's palpatory perception of muscle activation (increased muscle tension) at a specific level. The physician must engage the restrictive barrier in all planes of motion. Such perception enables the operator to make subtle assessments about a dysfunction and to create variations of suggested treatment procedures.

VII. Contraindications
Muscle Energy should not be performed on patients with low vitality who could be further compromised by adding active muscular exertion. Examples of these types of patients are **post-surgical patients** and **intensive care patients**.[1 p.696] Some authors state that only post-isometric relaxation type procedures are contraindicated in the above type patients. These authors report that gentler types of muscle energy such as reciprocal inhibition can be performed on these patients. [56 p.884]

VIII. Muscle Energy Techniques

Cervical Spine

Positional Diagnosis: OA ES$_L$R$_R$

Treatment Position: Supine

1. With the distal pad of one finger, monitor the OA joint, engage the restrictive barrier in all three planes by sidebending right, rotating left and flexing the patient's head until tension is felt under your monitoring finger. This is localization. Direct the patient to use a small amount of force to straighten his head while you exert an equal amount of counterforce.
2. Maintain the forces for 3-5 seconds, repeat 3-5 times, each time re-engaging the new restrictive barrier.
3. Recheck for symmetry of motion.

Positional Diagnosis: AA R$_R$

Treatment Position: Supine

1. Cradle the occiput in your hands and flex the patient's cervical spine 45°, locking out all the facets below the AA joint.
2. Rotate the atlas to the left to the point of initial resistance.
3. Direct the patient to gently rotate his head to the right. Apply an equal counterforce through your fingers and hands.
4. Maintain the forces for 3-5 seconds, repeat 3-5 times, each time re-engaging the new restrictive barrier.
5. Recheck for symmetry of motion.

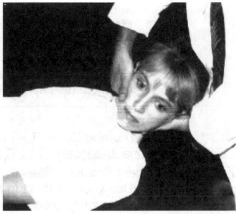

Fig 15.1: Treatment of AA R$_R$

Typical Cervicals (C2-C7)

Positional Diagnosis: C3 ER$_R$S$_R$

1. With the distal pad of one finger on the articular pillar of the dysfunctional segment, engage the restrictive barrier by reversing the somatic dysfunction in all three planes of motion until motion is felt under your monitoring finger. Remember that *rotation and sidebending components are to the same side.*
2. Direct the patient to gently straighten his head while you apply an equal counterforce.
3. Repeat steps 4-5 in the above example.

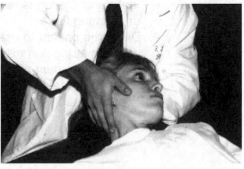

Fig 15.2: Treatment of C3 ER$_R$S$_R$

Thoracic Spine
Upper Thoracic Spine (T1-T4)
Positional Diagnosis: T3 ES$_L$R$_L$
Treatment Position: Seated

1. In the upper thoracic spine the physician will use the head and neck as lever to induce motion at the dysfunctional segment.
2. With one hand monitor the posterior transverse process of T3. Engage the restrictive barrier by flexing, rotating and sidebending right until motion is felt under your monitoring finger.
3. Direct the patient to use a small amount of force to straighten his head while you exert an equal amount of counterforce.
4. Maintain the forces for 3-5 seconds, have the patient relax, the physician relaxes, and re-engage the new restrictive barrier.
5. Repeat step four 3-5 times and then recheck for increased symmetry.

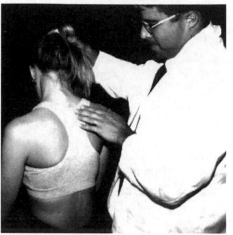

Fig 15.3: Treatment of T3 ES$_L$R$_L$

Lower Thoracic Spine (T5-T12)
Positional Diagnosis: T7 ER$_L$S$_L$
Treatment Position: Seated

1. Use your left hand to monitor the posterior transverse process of T7.
2. Instruct the patient to place his left hand behind his neck, and to grasp his left elbow with his right hand.
3. Reach across the patient's chest with your right arm, sidebending and rotating T7 to the right until motion is felt under your monitoring finger.
4. Direct the patient to use a small amount of force to straighten his body while you exert an equal amount of counterforce.
5. Repeat step four 3-5 times and then recheck for increased symmetry.

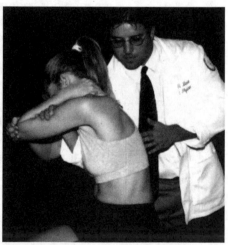

Fig 15.4: Treatment of T7 ER$_L$S$_L$

Ribs

Inhalation Dysfunctions (rib held up)   B1
  Treatment Position: Supine
  Key Rib: Lowest in Group

1. With the patient supine, place one hand on the anterior aspect of the key rib. Flex the patient for pump handle dysfunctions (sidebend the patient for bucket handle dysfunctions) down so that tension is taken off the dysfunctional rib
2. The physician palpates the dysfuncitonal rib.
3. Patient inhales, then exhales deeply. For bucket handle dysfunctions, patient is instructed to reach for his knee on the affected side.
4. The patient is instructed to hold his breath at end-expiratory phase for 3-5 seconds. During this time, the physician adjusts flexion/sidebending to the new restrictive barrier. Physician follows rib shaft into exhalation with his hand during the expiratory phase.
5. On inhalation, the physician resists inhalation motion of the rib.
6. Repeat steps 3-5 a total of 3-5 times. Retest for symmetry of motion.

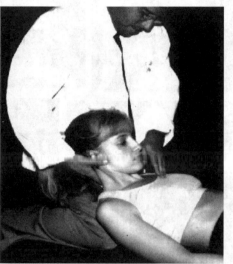
Fig 15.5: Treatment of a Pump-handle dysfunction of Rib 4

Exhalation Dysfunctions (rib held down)   TE
  NOTE: There are many different methods used when treating exhalation dysfunctions. Techniques differ slightly. The important concept of these rib treatments is to keep in mind which muscle is being used to correct the dysfunction. This is summarized in table 15.1 The following muscle energy techniques are as presented in the Foundations of Osteopathic Medicine, first edition.

  Treatment Position: Supine
  Key Rib: Top Rib in Group

1. The patient is instructed to place the forearm on the affected side across his forehead with the palm up.
2. The physician grasps the key rib posteriorly at the rib angle.
3. The patient is instructed to inhale deeply while the physician applies an inferior traction on the rib angle.
4. The patient is instructed to hold his breath at full inhalation while performing one of the following isometric contractions for 3-5 seconds:
   a. Rib 1:
      Patient raises head directly toward ceiling.
   b. Rib 2:
      Patient turns head 30 degrees away from dysfunctional side and lifts head toward ceiling.
   c. Ribs 3-5:
      Patient pushes elbow of affected side toward the opposite ASIS.
   d. Ribs 6-9:
      Push arm anterior.
   e. Ribs 10-12:
      Patient adducts arm.
5. Repeat step 4 a total of 3-5 times and then retest.

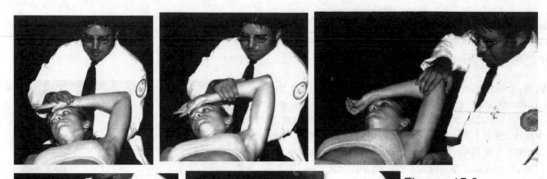

Figures 15.6 a-e
a: (top left) Treatment of exhalation dysfunction of Rib 1 on the left.
b: (top middle) Treatment of exhalation dysfunction of Rib 2 on the left.
c: (top right) Treatment of exhalation dysfunction Ribs 3-5 on the left.
d: (bottom left) Treatment of exhalation dysfunction of Ribs 6-9 on the left.
e: (bottom right) Treatment of exhalation dysfunction of Ribs 10-11 on the left.

Table 15.1 [28 p.565]

Ribs	Muscles
Rib 1	Anterior and Middle Scalenes
Rib 2	Posterior Scalene
Ribs 3-5	Pectoralis Minor
Ribs 6-9	Serratus Anterior
Ribs 10-11	Latissimus Dorsi
Rib 12	Quadratus Lumborum

NOTE: Some osteopathic texts [56] treat ribs 11 and 12 with the quadratus lumborum, whereas others [28] just treat rib 12 with the quadratus lumborum.

Lumbar Spine: Lumbar seated technique
> Positional Diagnosis: $L3ERS_R$
> Same steps as the lower thoracic spine.

Sacrum:
  Unilateral Sacral Flexion
> Positional Diagnosis: Right USF [56 p. 900]
> Treatment Position: Prone
> 1. Place your left hypothenar eminence on the patient's right ILA.
> 2. Ask the patient to inhale and hold his breath, while you push anterior on the ILA. Hold for 3-5 seconds.
> 3. Direct the patient to exhale while you resist any posterior inferior movement of the sacrum.
> 4. Repeat steps two and three 3-5 times and retest.

Unilateral Sacral Extension

Positional Diagnosis: Right USE [56 p.900]

Treatment Position: Prone

1. Place your left hypothenar eminence on the patient's right sacral sulcus.
2. Ask the patient to exhale and hold his breath, while you push anterior and caudad on the superior sulcus. Hold for 3-5 seconds.
3. Direct the patient to inhale while you resist any anterior superior movement of the sacrum.
4. Repeat steps two and three 3-5 times and retest.

Sacral Torsions:

Positional Diagnosis: L on L (Forward Sacral Torsion)

Treatment Position: Left Lateral Sims Position (lying on left side with face down)

Patient day
Physician down ☆

1. Patient lies on his left side (*axis side down*) with his torso rotated so that he is face down.
2. Flex patient's hips until motion is felt at the lumbosacral junction.
3. Drop the patient's legs off the table to induce left sidebending and engage a left sacral oblique axis.
4. Ask the patient to lift his legs toward the ceiling against your equal counterforce for 3-5 seconds. Monitor with other hand the right superior pole for posterior movement.
5. Repeat for 3-5 times and then retest for symmetry.

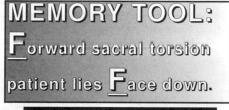

MEMORY TOOL: **F**orward sacral torsion patient lies **F**ace down.

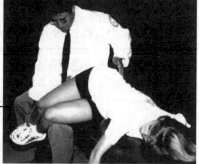

Fig 15.7: Treatment of a L on L, Forward Sacral Torsion

Positional Diagnosis: R on L (Backward Sacral Torsion)

Treatment Position: Left Lateral Recumbent with face up

1. Patient lies on his left side (*axis side down*) with his torso rotated so that he is face up.
2. Grasp patient's left arm and pull through to rotate his torso to the right. Flex patient's hips until motion is felt at the lumbosacral junction.
3. Drop the patient's legs off the table to induce left sidebending and engage a left sacral oblique axis.
4. Ask the patient to lift his legs toward the ceiling against your equal counterforce for 3-5 seconds. Monitor with other hand the right superior pole for anterior movement.
5. Repeat for 3-5 times, each time re-engaging the new restrictive barrier, and retest for symmetry of motion.

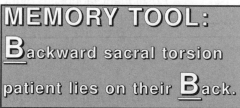

MEMORY TOOL: **B**ackward sacral torsion patient lies on their **B**ack.

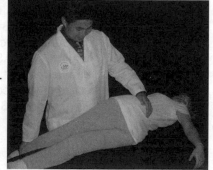

Fig 15.8: Treatment of a R on L, Backward Sacral Torsion.

141

Innominates:
Positional Diagnosis: Right Innominate Anterior

Treatment Position: Supine
1. Flex patient's right hip and knee until resistance is felt.
2. Instruct patient to extend his hip against your counterforce for 3-5 seconds.
3. Wait a few seconds for the tissues to relax, then take up the slack to the new restrictive barrier.
4. Repeat until no restrictive barrier is felt (usually 3-5 times).

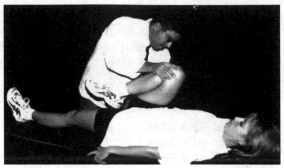

Fig 15.9 Treatment of a Right Innominate Anterior.

Positional Diagnosis: Right Innominate Posterior
Treatment Position: Supine
1. Drop the patient's right leg off the table until resistance is felt. Stabilize the patient's left ASIS with your right hand.
2. Instruct patient to flex his hip against your counterforce for 3-5 seconds.
3. Repeat steps 3 and 4.

Fig 15.10: Treatment of a Right Innominate Posterior.

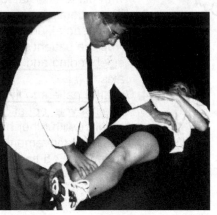

Pubic Shears:
Positional Diagnosis: Right Superior Pubic Shear
Treatment Position: Supine
1. Drop the patient's right leg off the table and abduct until resistance is felt. Stabilize the patient's left ASIS with your right hand.
2. Instruct patient to bring his right knee to his left ASIS (flexion and adduction) against your counterforce for 3-5 seconds.
3. Repeat steps 3 and 4.

Positional Diagnosis: Right Inferior Pubic Shear
Treatment Position: Supine
1. Flex and abduct patient's right hip and knee and until resistance is felt. Stabilize the patient's left ASIS with your right hand.
2. Instruct patient to push his right knee to his left foot (extension and adduction) against your counterforce for 3-5 seconds.
3. Repeat steps 3-4.

Upper Extremities:

Positional Diagnosis: Right forearm has restriction of supination (radial head posterior).
Treatment Position: Seated

1. Place your right hand at the distal end of the patient's right forearm and supinate it to initial resistance as you monitor with the other thumb at the radial head.
2. Direct the patient to pronate the right forearm against equal resistance supplied through your right hand.
3. Maintain the forces long enough to sense the patient's contractile force at the localized segment or area (usually 3-5 seconds).
4. Both the patient and physician relax their forces, and the physician takes up the slack to the new point of initial resistance.
5. Repeat for 3-5 times and then recheck findings.

Positional Diagnosis: Right forearm has restriction of pronation (radial head anterior).
Treatment Position: Seated

1. Support the patient's right elbow with your left hand.
2. Place your right hand at the distal end of the patient's right forearm and pronate it to initial resistance.
3. Direct the patient to supinate the right forearm against an equal counterforce supplied through your right hand.
4. Maintain the force for 3-5 seconds, then both the physician and the patient relaxes. The physician then re-engages the new restrictive barrier. Repeat for 3-5 times and then recheck findings.

Lower Extremities

NOTE: There are many different methods used when correcting fibular head dysfunctions. Techniques differ slightly. The following techniques have been described by Fred Mitchell, D.O. [44]

Positional Diagnosis: Right fibular head anterior [44 p.550]
Treatment Position: Prone

1. With the patient in the prone position and the knee flexed, place your right hand on the lateral side of the patient's foot, cupping the ankle.
2. Plantar-flex and invert the patient's foot to initial resistance.
3. Externally rotate the tibia.
4. Direct the patient to dorsiflex against your isometric counterforce, 3-5 seconds.
5. Relax forces, plantar-flex, invert and externally rotate the tibia to the new barrier. Repeat steps 1-4.

Positional Diagnosis: Right fibular head posterior [44 p.550]
Treatment Position: Prone

1. With the patient in the prone position and the knee flexed, place your right hand on the lateral side of the patient's foot, cupping the ankle.
2. Plantar-flex and invert the patient's foot to initial resistance.
3. Internally rotate the tibia.
4. Direct the patient to dorsiflex against your isometric counterforce, 3-5 seconds.
5. Relax forces, plantar-flex, invert and internally rotate the tibia to the new barrier. Repeat steps 1-4.

CHAPTER 15 REVIEW QUESTIONS

1. Which of the following is a necessary component for any successful muscle energy treatment?
   A. Reciprocal inhibition
   B. Postisometric relaxation
   C. Patient assistance
   D. Direct treatment to the pathologic barrier
   E. Holding the position for 90 seconds

2. Which is true regarding the localization of forces used in all muscle energy technique?
   A. Applied force must address a single plane of motion
   B. The counterforce used by the physician should be greater than the force applied by the patient
   C. The counterforce used by the physician should be less than the force applied by the patient
   D. A few seconds after the patient relaxes, the physician takes up the slack in all planes of motion
   E. None of the above are correct

3. Which joint is treated by the use of rotational force only?
   A. OA
   B. AA
   C. C3
   D. T2
   E. Posterior radial head

4. Which of the following segments is **NOT** treated by inducing the motion of the patient's head?
   A. OA
   B. C2
   C. C7
   D. T6
   E. 2nd rib exhalation dysfunction

5. Which muscle is used to treat an exhalation dysfunction of rib 11 with a muscle energy technique?
   A. Serratus anterior
   B. Serratus posterior
   C. Quadratus lumborum
   D. Ilicostalis
   E. Latissimus dorsi

6. In which patient would muscle energy techniques be contraindicated?
   A. 23 year old paraplegic
   B. 6 year old healthy child
   C. 76 year old healthy man
   D. 38 year old female immediately post MI
   E. 45 year old male with GERD

ANSWERS

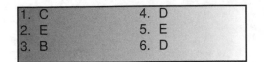

1. C	4. D
2. E	5. E
3. B	6. D

CHAPTER 16

HIGH VELOCITY LOW AMPLITUDE (HVLA)

I. Definition

A **passive, direct technique** which uses high velocity / low amplitude forces to remove motion loss in a somatic dysfunction. After positioning a restricted joint against its restrictive barrier a short (low amplitude) quick (high velocity) thrust is directed to move the joint past the restrictive barrier. HVLA techniques may also be called *thrust techniques, mobilization with impulse treatment.* [1 p.1134]

II. Neurophysiologic mechanism of HVLA

There are 2 theories:

Theory #1 - An HVLA thrust is thought to forcefully stretch a contracted muscle producing a barrage of afferent impulses from the muscle spindles to the central nervous system. The central nervous system reflexively sends inhibitory impulses to the muscle spindle to relax the muscle. [28 p.306]

Theory #2 -An HVLA thrust is though to forcefully stretch the contracted muscle pulling on it's tendon activiating the Golgi tendon receptors and reflexively relaxing the muscle. [28 p.292]

III. General Procedure:

1. After correct diagnosis of a somatic dysfunction, the physician will move the dysfunctional segment in such a way that it is against its restrictive barrier. This is ideally done by reversing all three planes of motion.

   For example, if a segment was FR_LS_L, the physician would extend, rotate and sidebend the spine to the right (ER_RS_R) until motion is felt at the level of the dysfunctional segment.

   NOTE: Due to the facet orientation and biomechanics in certain regions of the spine, it is not always possible to reverse all three planes of motion (i.e. the cervical spine). See specific HVLA techniques for details.

2. The patient then is asked to relax.

   If the patient is not relaxed, the treatment will fail and the corrective thrust may cause soft tissue damage. The exhalation phase of respiration is the relaxation phase, and the final force is often applied during exhalation. [1 p.664]

3. The physician then uses a short, quick thrust to move the dysfunctional segment through the restrictive barrier. Often a pop or click is heard along with an increase in the range of motion. Be sure to remain against the restrictive barrier before applying the thrust, do not back off before the thrust.

4. Re-evaluate range of motion.

145

IV. Indications and Contraindications

A. Indications

1. Treatment of motion loss in somatic dysfunction.

   However, it is not ordinarily indicated for treatment of joint restriction due to pathologic changes such as contractures or advanced degenerative joint disease. [1 p.661-2]

B. Absolute contraindications [1, 2, 14, 28]

1. Osteoporosis
2. Osteomyelitis (including Pott's disease)
3. Fractures in the area of thrust
4. Bone metastasis
5. Severe rheumatoid arthritis - These patients are at particular risk with cervical manipulation. Rheumatoid arthritis may weaken the transverse ligament of the dens, resulting in atlantal-axial subluxation. HVLA manipulation may lead to rupture of this ligament resulting in catastrophic neurologic damage. [28 p.295]
6. Down's Syndrome - Similar to rheumatoid arthritis, laxity may develop in the transverse ligament of the dens, resulting in atlantal-axial subluxation. HVLA manipulation may lead to rupture of this ligament resulting in catastrophic neurologic damage.

C. Relative contraindications [1, 2, 14, 28]

1. Acute whiplash
2. Pregnancy
3. Post-surgical conditions
4. Herniated nucleus propulsus
5. Patients on anticoagulation therapy or hemophiliacs should be treated with great caution to prevent bleeding.
6. Vertebral artery ischemia (positive Wallenberg's test)

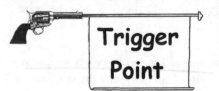

Trigger Point

> **Know the absolute and relative contraindications for HVLA.**

V. Complications [1 p.665]

A. Minor complications:

Most common
   Soreness or symptom exacerbation.

B. Major Complications:

Most common overall
   Vertebral artery injury. These problems usually arise with the use of cervical rotatory forces with the neck in the extended position. [1 p.1020]

Most common in the low back
   Cauda equina syndrome (very rare).

VI. Specific HVLA treatments

A. Cervical

OA FS$_R$R$_L$ (see fig 16.1)

1. The patient supine and the physician at the head of the table.
2. Grasp the patient's head and flex the neck slightly.
3. The MCP joint of the thrusting hand is placed at the base of the occiput.
4. Extend the occiput slightly, make sure that extension is limited to only the OA joint. (NOTE: For an extended OA lesion, flex the head slightly so that flexion is limited to the OA joint).
5. Sidebend the occiput to the left and rotate it to the right to engage the restrictive barrier.
6. Apply a HVLA thrust by translating the occiput to the right. The direction of the thrust should be directed toward the patient's opposite (right) eye.
7. Re-evaluate the range of motion.

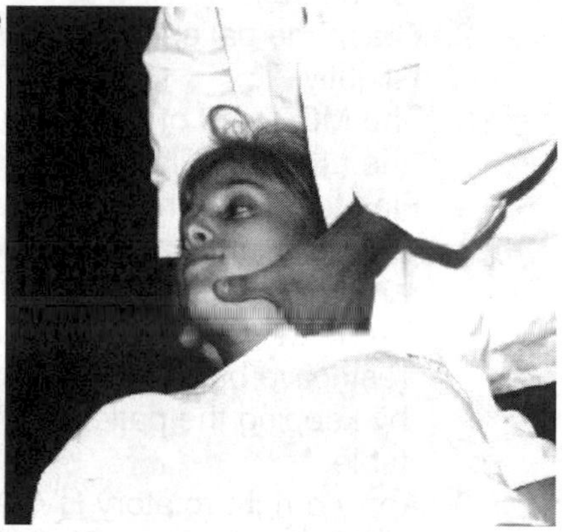

Fig 16.1: Treatment of OA FR$_L$S$_R$

AA rotated right (AAR$_R$) (see fig 16.2) [56 p.858]

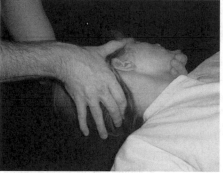

1. The patient supine and the physician at the head of the table.
2. The palm of the physician's left hand grasps the patient's chin.
3. The index finger of the physician's right hand is placed by the soft tissue of the AA joint. The physician's right thumb contacts the patient's right zygomatic process, avoiding the right mandible.
4. The patient is asked to inhale, then exhale fully.
5. At the end of exhalation, the physician applies a left rotational high velocity, low amplitude thrust using the right index finger as a fulcrum
6.. Re-evaluate the range of motion.

Fig 16.2 Treatment of the AA rotated right.

Typical cervical segments (C2 - C7)

These cervical segments can be treated by using either a sidebending or rotatory thrust.

C3 FS$_L$R$_L$ Rotational thrust (see fig 16.3) [56 p.858-859]

1. The patient supine and the physician at the head of the table.
2. Grasp the patient's head and flex the neck slightly.
3. The MCP joint of the thrusting hand is placed at the articular pillar of C3.
4. Flex the head and neck down to C3 and then induce a small amount of extension by applying anterior translation at C3.
5. Rotate the head and neck to the right to the restrictive barrier. Right sidebending is achieved by keeping the patient's right temple close to the table.
6. Apply a right rotatory HVLA thrust using the left MCP as a fulcrum. The direction of the thrust should be directed toward the patient's opposite eye.
8. Re-evaluate the range of motion.

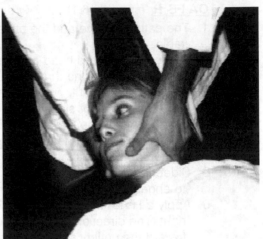

Fig 16.3: Treatment of C3 FR$_L$S$_L$, with a rotational thrust.

C6 ES$_R$R$_R$ Sidebending thrust (see fig 16.4)

1. The patient supine and the physician at the head of the table.
2. The MCP joint of the left hand is placed at the articular pillar of C6.
3. Grasp the patient's head and flex the neck to the C6 - C7 joint. Induce a small amount of extension by applying anterior translation at C6
4. Sidebend the neck to the left until localized at the C6-C7 joint.
5. Rotate the neck to the right to limit motion of (lock) the above facets.
6. Apply a sidebending HVLA thrust by translating C6 to the right. The direction of the thrust should be directed toward the patient's opposite shoulder.
7. Re-evaluate the range of motion.

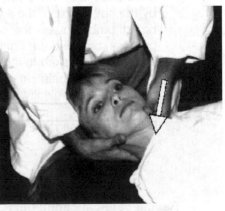

Fig 16.4: Treatment of C6 ES$_R$R$_R$, with a sidebending thrust.

B. Thoracics and Ribs

The thoracic segments and ribs can be treated with HVLA in many positions. The position most commonly taught at osteopathic medical schools has been nicknamed the Kirksville Krunch. This technique is easy to understand and versatile. With very little modification of technique the Kirksville Krunch can treat most thoracic and rib dysfunctions. For other types of thoracic HVLA treatments (prone, seated, etc.), please refer to the Foundations of Osteopathic Medicine, [56] An Osteopathic Approach to Diagnosis and Treatment, [2] or Greenman's Principles of Manual Medicine. [14]

When treating a flexed lesion, the corrective force will be directed at the dysfunctional segment and the thrust is aimed toward the floor. When treating an extended lesion the corrective thrust is directed at the vertebrae **below** the dysfunctional segment and the thrust is aimed 45° cephalad. A neutral lesion is treated the same way as a flexed dysfunction, however sidebend the patient away from you. A purely flexed or extended lesion (no rotation or sidebending) is treated using roughly the same position, except the physician will use a bilateral fulcrum (thenar eminence under one transverse process and a flexed MCP under the other transverse process). Ribs 2-10 can also be treated using the Kirksville Krunch. The difference is that the physician's thenar eminence is under the posterior rib angle of the "key" rib.

T7 FS$_R$R$_R$ (see fig 16.5)

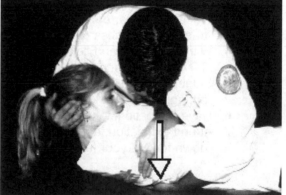

Fig 16.5: Treatment of T7 FR$_R$S$_R$. The arrow in the diagram demonstrates the direction of the thrust.

1. The patient supine and the physician standing on the left side of the patient (stand on the opposite side of the posterior transverse process).
2. The patient will cross his arm over his chest, so that the superior arm is opposite that of the physician. For simplicity this is referred to as "opposite over adjacent".
3. Place the thenar eminence under the posterior transverse process of the dysfunctional segment.
4. With the other hand flex the patient's torso to the T7 -T8 joint space.
5. Sidebend the patient to the left engaging the restrictive barrier.
6. Have the patient take a deep breath in and exhale.
7. At end exhalation, apply a HVLA thrust straight down toward your fulcrum (thenar eminence).

T7 ES$_L$R$_L$ (see fig 16.6)

1. The patient supine and the physician standing on the right side of the patient (stand on the opposite side of the posterior transverse process).
2. Patient crosses arms across chest opposite over adjacent.
3. Place the thenar eminence under the posterior transverse process of the vertebrae **below** the dysfunctional segment.
4. With the other hand, flex the patient's torso to the T7 -T8 joint space.
5. Sidebend the patient to the right engaging the restrictive barrier.
6. Have the patient take a deep breath in and exhale.
7. At end exhalation, apply a HVLA thrust directed 45° cephalad toward your fulcrum (thenar eminence).

149

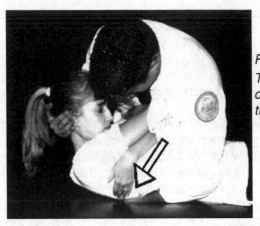

Fig 16.6: Treatment for T7 ES$_L$R$_L$.
The arrow in the diagram
demonstrates the direction of
the thrust.

T7 NS$_L$R$_R$ (see fig 16.7)

1. The patient supine and the physician standing on
   the left side of the patient (stand on the opposite
   side of the posterior transverse process).
2. Patient crosses arms opposite over adjacent.
3. Place the thenar eminence under the posterior
   transverse process of the dysfunctional segment.
4. With the other hand flex the patient's torso to the
   T7 -T8 joint space.
5. Sidebend the patient to the right (away from you)
   engaging the restrictive barrier.
6. Have the patient take a deep breath in and exhale.
7. At end exhalation, apply a HVLA thrust straight
   down toward your fulcrum (thenar eminence).

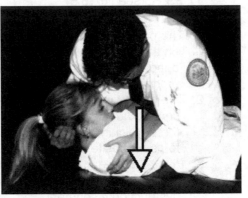

Fig 16.7: Treatment for T7 NS$_L$R$_R$.
Remember to sidebend the patient
away from you to engage the barrier..

Rib 1 Inhalation dysfunction (rib held up)(see fig 16.8)

NOTE: Inhalation dysfunctions of rib one cannot be
    treated using the Kirksville Krunch.

1. The patient prone and the physician at the head of the
   table.
2. Sidebend the head and neck to the side of the
   dysfunctional rib.
3. Rotate the head and neck away.
4. Place the 1st MCP on the tubercle of rib 1.
5. Have the patient take a deep breath in and exhale.
6. At end exhalation, apply a HVLA thrust through the
   thenar eminence. The direction of the thrust should
   be posterioanterior and caudad.

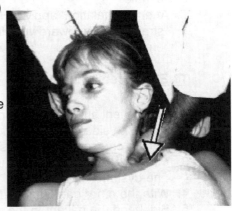

Fig 16.8: Treatment for an
inhalation dysfunction of rib 1.

150

Right Rib 5 Inhalation (rib held up) or Exhalation Dysfunction (rib held down) (inhalation or exhalation rib or exhalation or inhalation restriction). Kirksville Krunch treatment type (Range: ribs 2- 10).

1. The patient supine and the physician standing on the left side of the patient (stand on the opposite side of the dysfunctional rib).
2. Patient crosses arms opposite over adjacent.
3. Place the thenar eminence under the posterior rib angle of the "key" rib (see Chapter 3 for further explanation of "key" rib).
4. With the other hand flex, the patient's torso and slightly sidebend away from the dysfunctional rib.
5. Have the patient take a deep breath in and exhale.
6. At end exhalation, apply a HVLA thrust straight down toward your fulcrum (thenar eminence).

C. Lumbar Spine

T10-L5 may be treated with HVLA using the "lumbar roll". Flexion, extension or neutral lesions can all be treated in the same lateral recumbent position. The physician may treat the patient with the posterior transverse up or the posterior transverse process down. For example, if L3 was FRS_R, the physician can treat the patient in the left lateral recumbent position (posterior transverse process up) or in the right lateral recumbent position (transverse process down). There is only one modification with the patient's position between the two treatments. This modification is italicized in step #6 in the following examples and summarized in table 16.1.

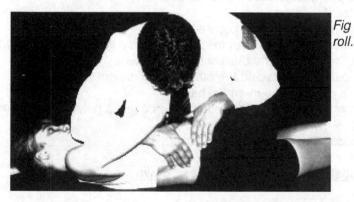

Fig 16.9: Treatment position for a lumbar roll.

Type II (Flexed or Extended) posterior transverse process up
   L3 ER_RS_R
1. Patient in the left lateral recumbent position (posterior transverse process up).
2. Stand in front of the patient.
3. Flex the patient's legs until you palpate motion at L3
4. Straighten the patient's inferior leg.
5. Hook the superior foot in the lower legs popliteal fossa
6. *Pull patient's inferior arm out (toward you) to rotate the torso and down (caudad) to induce left sidebending down to the dysfunctional segment.*
7. Place one arm in the patient's axilla and the other on the patient's iliac crest.
8. Have the patient take a deep breath in and exhale.
9. At end exhalation, apply a HVLA thrust by rotating the patient's pelvis forward and toward the table.
10. Retest the range of motion.

151

Type II (Flexed or Extended) posterior transverse process down
L3 ER$_R$S$_R$

1. Patient in the right lateral recumbent position (posterior transverse process down).
2. Stand in front of the patient.
3. Flex the patient's legs until you palpate motion at L3.
4. Straighten the patient's inferior leg.
5. Hook the superior foot in the lower leg's popliteal fossa.
6. *Pull patient's inferior arm out (toward you) to rotate the torso and up (cephalad) to induce left sidebending down to the dysfunctional segment.*
7. Place one arm in the patient's axilla and the other on the patient's iliac crest.
8. Have the patient take a deep breath in and exhale.
9. At end exhalation, apply a HVLA thrust by rotating the patient's pelvis forward and toward the table.
10. Retest the range of motion.

NOTE: Flexion or extension can also be added to further engage another barrier. With the patient in the lateral recumbent position, anterior motion of the torso will produce flexion, posterior motion will produce extension.

Type I (neutral dysfunctions) posterior transverse process up
L3 NS$_L$R$_R$

1. Patient in the left lateral recumbent position (posterior transverse process up).
2. Stand in front of the patient.
3. Flex the patient's legs until you palpate motion at L3.
4. Straighten the patient's inferior leg.
5. Hook the superior foot in the lower leg's popliteal fossa.
6. *Pull patient's inferior arm out (toward you) to rotate the torso and up (cephalad) to induce right sidebending down to the dysfunctional segment.*
7. Place one arm in the patient's axilla and the other on the patient's iliac crest.
8. Have the patient take a deep breath in and exhale.
9. At end exhalation, apply a HVLA thrust by rotating the patient's pelvis forward and toward the table.
10. Retest the range of motion.

Type I (neutral dysfunctions) posterior transverse process down
L3 NS$_L$R$_R$

1. Patient in the right lateral recumbent position (posterior transverse process down).
2. Stand in front of the patient.
3. Flex the patient's legs until you palpate motion at L3
4. Straighten the patient's inferior leg.
5. Hook the superior foot in the lower leg's popliteal fossa.
6. *Pull patient's inferior arm out (toward you) to rotate the torso and down (caudad) to induce right sidebending down to the dysfunctional segment.*
7. Place one arm in the patient's axilla and the other on the patient's iliac crest.
8. Have the patient take a deep breath in and exhale.
9. At end exhalation, apply a HVLA thrust by rotating the patient's pelvis forward and toward the table.
10. Retest the range of motion.

Table 16.1

Lumbar Roll Treatment

Type II Dysfunction:

If treating the patient with the transverse process up => pull the patient's inferior arm down.

If treating the patient with the transverse process down => pull the patient's inferior arm up.

Type I Dysfunction:

If treating the patient with the transverse process up => pull the patient's inferior arm up.

If treating the patient with the transverse process down => pull the patient's inferior arm down.

CHAPTER 16 REVIEW QUESTIONS

1. Which of the following is **FALSE** regarding HVLA?
   A. The techniques are passive
   B. The techniques are indirect
   C. The techniques involve a short, quick thrust
   D. The thrust is usually performed during exhalation
   E. A pop or click may be heard

2. Which of the following is **NOT** an absolute contraindication for HVLA?
   A. Fracture
   B. Rheumatoid arthritis
   C. Osteoporosis
   D. Tenosynovitis
   E. Pott's disease

3. Which of the following is **NOT** a relative contraindication for HVLA?
   A. Herniated nucleus pulposis
   B. Pregnancy
   C. Vertebral artery insufficiency
   D. Hemophila A
   E. Scoliosis

ANSWERS

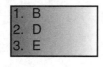

1. B
2. D
3. E

CHAPTER 17

ARTICULATORY TECHNIQUES

I. Definition

Articulatory techniques (also called springing techniques or low velocity / moderate amplitude techniques) are direct techniques that increase range of motion in a restricted joint. The physician engages the restrictive barrier and uses gentle repetitive forces to increase range of motion within that joint. [1 p. 763] Respiratory cooperation and/or muscle energy activation are frequently added to further stretch tight myofascial structures that may limit articular motion.

Post-operative patients and elderly patients find articulatory techniques more acceptable than other vigorous types of direct techniques, since articulating forces are gentle in nature. [1 p.763]

A. Indications:
1. Limited or lost articular motion.
2. Need to increase frequency or amplitude of motion of a body region. For example, the need to increase frequency and amplitude of chest wall motion in a person with respiratory disease.
3. The need to normalize sympathetic activity (rib raising technique). [1 p.450]

B. Contraindications: [1 p.764]
1. Repeated hyper-rotation of the upper cervical spine when positioned in extension may cause damage to the vertebral artery.
2. Acutely inflamed joint especially where the cause of the inflammation may be from an infection or fracture.

C. Typical articulatory procedure
1. Move the affected joint to the limit of all ranges of motion. Once a restrictive barrier is reached slowly and firmly, continue to apply gentle force against it.
2. At this time you may use respiratory cooperation or muscle energy activation to further increase myofascial stretch of tight tissues.
3. Return the articulation to its neutral position.
4. Repeat the process several times.
5. Cease repetition of motion when no further response is achieved.

II. Frequently used articulatory techniques

A. Rib Raising
Purpose:
1. Increase chest wall motion.
2. Normalize sympathetic activity. [1 p.950, 28p.57]
   The thoracic chain ganglia lie directly anterior to the corresponding rib heads. Movement of the chain ganglia by rib raising initially stimulates the sympathetic outflow, but this is followed by long-lasting sympathetic inhibition.
3. Improve lymphatic return.

155

Rib raising is useful for those patients who have a resistant or noncompliant chest wall, such as a patient with viral pneumonia. Since pneumonia (as well as other disease processes [28 p.73]) is associated with hypersympathetic activity, **rib raising will normalize this sympathetic hyperactivity**. Rib raising can be done in the seated or supine position. The supine position is described here.

Procedure: [1 p.950]
1. Patient supine.
2. Physician seated at the side of the patient.
3. Place your hands under the patient's thorax, contacting the rib angles with the pads of your fingers.
4. Apply gentle traction.
5. Raise the patients ribs by pushing your fingertips upwards and lowering your forearms (It is easier to push your fingers upward by using your forearm as a lever).

B. <u>**Spencer Techniques**</u> (Seven Stages of Spencer)

This technique is useful in patients who have developed fibrosis and restriction during a period of inactivity (adhesive capsulitis) following an injury. Such injuries may include a healed rotator cuff tear, or immobilization of the shoulder girdle after a humerus fracture.

The Spencer techniques are performed in 7 stages. In all stages, the patient is in the lateral recumbent position lying with the side of the dysfunctional shoulder up. The physician stands on the side of the table facing the patient, then carefully and slowly moves the upper extremity through the following sequence: [56 p. 848-850]

<u>Stage I:</u>   Stretching tissues and pumping fluids with the arm extended

<u>Stage II</u>:   Glenohumeral extension/flexion with the elbow flexed

<u>Stage III:</u>   Glenohumeral flexion/extension with the elbow extended

<u>Stage IV:</u>   *Broken into 2 parts:*

IVa: Circumduction and slight compression with the elbow flexed/extended.

IVb: Circumduction and traction with the elbow extended.

<u>Stage V:</u>   Adduction and external rotation with the elbow flexed

<u>Stage VI:</u>   Abduction with Internal Rotation with the arm behind the back.

<u>Stage VII:</u>   Stretching tissues and pumping fluids with the arm extended.

<u>NOTE</u>: The purpose of this technique is to improve motion in the glenohumoral joint, therefore, it is important that the physician limits motion at the scapula by placing his hand on the top of the patient's shoulder. Muscle energy techniques can also be utilized at each of the shoulders' restrictive barriers.

CHAPTER 17 REVIEW QUESTIONS

1. Which is true of low velocity / moderate amplitude techniques?
    A. They tend to be rough and are not suitable for elderly patients
    B. They are generally well tolerated post surgically
    C. They require active patient participation
    D. The technique is indirect, and therefore the restrictive barrier is not engaged
    E. If the technique fails to work on the first attempt, other techniques should be tried

2. Which is true about rib raising?
    A. It must be performed in inhalation, as the ribs fall in exhalation
    B. An increase of sympathetic activity is typically incurred after an initial decrease
    C. It is a useful technique in patients with viral pneumonia
    D. The technique is autonomic in nature and has little or no effect on chest wall motion
    E. Rib raising must be done in the supine position

3. Which is **FALSE** regarding Spencer techniques?
    A. They are useful in treating adhesive capsulitis
    B. One of the steps requires extension of the arm to 180°
    C. One step requires abduction and internal rotation
    D. Muscle energy techniques can be employed to enhance the Spencer techniques
    E. All of the above are true

ANSWERS

1. B
2. C
3. B

CHAPTER 18

SPECIAL TESTS

GLENN S. FUOCO, D.O.

I. Cervical spine

A. Spurling Test (Compression Test)

Narrowing of the neural foramina can cause referred pain into the ipsilateral arm upon compression of the cervical spine, due to nerve root compression. With the patient seated, the physician extends and sidebends the C-spine to the side being tested, and pushes downward on the top of the patient's head. The test is positive if pain radiates into the ipsilateral arm. The pain's distribution can help localize the affected nerve root. [5 p.50-51, 6 p.127, 24 p.411]

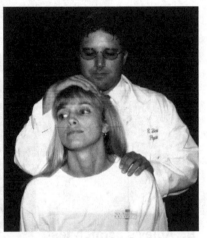

B. Wallenberg's Test

To test for vertebral artery insufficiency, in a supine position the physician flexes the patient's neck, holding it for ten seconds, then extends the neck holding it for ten seconds. The same is done for head and neck rotation to the right and left, head and neck rotation right and left with the neck in the extended position, and in positions that the physician would attempt to mobilize the C-spine. A positive test results when the patient complains of dizziness, visual changes, lightheadedness, or eye nystagmus occurs. [5 p.53-54]

It is important to detect vertebral artery insufficiency, as a result similar tests to Wallenberg's test have been described in the medical literature. These tests are essentially variations of Wallenberg's test. One particular test that has been described in the osteopathic literature is **Underberg's test**. this test is perfomed with the neck backward bent and the head fully rotated to either side. If the patient develops vascular or neurologic symptoms, HVLA is contraindicated. [28 p.586]

II. Shoulder

A. Thoracic Outlet Syndrome Tests

1. Adson's Test

The neurovascular bundle can be compromised by tight scalene muscles. While monitoring the patient's pulse, the arm is extended at the elbow, the shoulder is extended, externally rotated, and slightly abducted. The patient is then asked to take a deep breath and turn his/her head toward the ipsilateral arm. The test is positive with a severely decreased or absent radial pulse. [1 p.588, 6 p.127, 5 p.122, 28 p.528]

2. Wright's test [5 p.120] (a.k.a. arm hyperextension test) [28 p.529]

This neurovascular bundle can be compromised as it passes under the pectoralis minor muscle at the coracoid process. This test entails hyperabducting the arm above the head with some extension. The test is positive with a severely decreased or absent radial pulse.

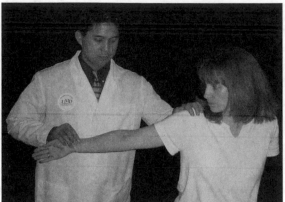

Adson's test

3. Costoclavicular syndrome test [5 p.122] (a.k.a. Military Posture Test) [28 p.528]

The neurovascular bundle can be compromised between the clavicle and the first rib. The examiner palpates the radial pulse while depressing and extending the shoulder. The test is positive with a severely decreased or absent radial pulse.

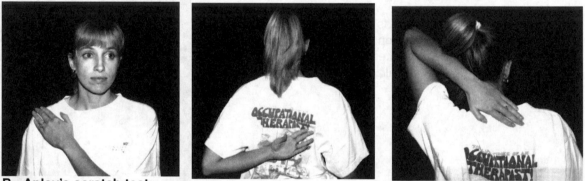

B. Apley's scratch test

This test is used to evaluate the range of motion of the shoulder. To test abduction and external rotation, ask the patient to reach behind the head and touch the opposite shoulder. To evaluate internal rotation and adduction, ask the patient to reach in front of the head and touch the opposite shoulder. Next, to further evaluate internal rotation and adduction, instruct the patient to reach behind the back and touch the inferior angle of the opposite scapula. Observe the patient's movement for any asymmetry or any limitations of movement.

Another way to evaluate range of motion of both shoulders at once is to ask the patient to abduct the arms to 90°, then supinate the forearms and continue abduction until the hands touch overhead. This will compare bilateral abduction. Next, to test abduction and external rotation, ask the patient to interlock the hands behind the head and push the elbows posterior. Finally, instruct the patient to place the hands behind the back as high as possible as if to touch the ipsilateral inferior angle of the scapula. [1 p.559, 6 p.21]

C. Drop Arm Test

This test detects tears in the rotator cuff. The patient is instructed to abduct the shoulder to 90°, and then to slowly lower the arm. A positive test results if the patient cannot lower the arm smoothly, or if the arm drops to the side from 90°. [1 p.558, 5 p.118]

D. Speed's Test

    This test assesses the biceps tendon in the bicipital groove. The patient fully extends the elbow, flexes the shoulder and supinates the forearm. The physician resists the flexion of the shoulder. A positive test occurs with tenderness in the bicipital groove. [5 p.117]

E. Yergason's Test

    This test determines the stability of the biceps tendon in the bicipital groove. The patient flexes the elbow to 90° while the physician grasps the elbow with one hand and the wrist with the other hand. While pulling downward on the patient's elbow, the physician externally rotates the forearm as the patient resists this motion. A positive test results when pain is elicited as the biceps tendon pops out of the bicipital groove. [1 p.558, 6 p. 32, 5 p.117]

III. Wrist

A. Allen's Test

    This test assesses the adequacy of blood supply to the hand by the radial and ulnar arteries. The patient is instructed to open and close the hand being tested several times and then to make a tight fist. The physician occludes the radial and ulnar arteries at the wrist. The patient is then asked to open the hand; the palm should be pale. The physician releases one of the arteries and assesses the flushing of the hand. If it flushes slowly, or not at all, then the released artery is not adequately supplying the hand. This procedure is repeated for the other artery. [1 p.559, 6 p.102-3]

B. Finkelstein Test

    To test for tenosynovitis in the abductor pollicis longus and extensor pollicis brevis tendons at the wrist (De Quervain's disease), the patient makes a fist with the thumb tucked inside the fingers. The physician stabilizes the patient's forearm and deviates the wrist ulnarly. A positive test results when the patient feels pain over the tendons at the wrist. [5, p.189; 6 p.76-77]

C. Phalen's Test

    This test aides in the diagnosis of carpal tunnel syndrome. The physician maximally flexes the patient's wrist and holds this position for one minute. If a "tingling" sensation is felt in the thumb, index finger, middle and lateral portion of the ring fingers, the test is positive and is indicative of carpal tunnel syndrome. [1 p.559, 6 p.83, 5 p.194]

D. Reverse Phalen's Test (Prayer's test)

    Also used in the diagnosis of carpal tunnel syndrome, this test has the patient extend the wrist while gripping the physician's hand. If after one minute, the same symptoms are seen as in Phalen's test, the reverse Phalen's test is positive. [5 p.194]

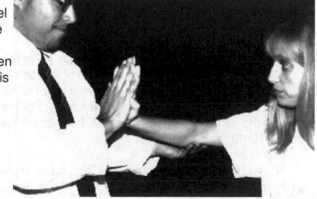

E. Tinel's Test

This test is used in the diagnosis of carpal tunnel syndrome. The physician taps over the volar aspect of the patient's transverse carpal ligament. A positive test will cause tingling or paresthesia into the thumb, index, middle and lateral half of the ring finger. [1 p.559, 5. p.194, 6 p.82]

> NOTE: Tinel's test may also be used in the diagnosis of other neuropathies, such as ulnar nerve entrapment at the elbow; peroneal compression at the fibular head and posterior tibial nerve entrapment at the ankle. [6 p.57, 5 p.484]

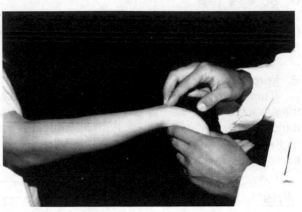

Tinel's test at the wrist

IV. Lumbar spine

A. Hip-drop Test

This test assesses the sidebending ability of the lumbar spine and thoracolumbar junction. With the patient standing, the physician locates the most superior and lateral aspect of the iliac crests. The patient is instructed to bend one knee without lifting the heel from the floor. Normally, the lumber spine should sidebend toward the side contralateral to the bending knee, producing a smooth convexity in the lumbar spine on the ipsilateral side. The ipsilateral iliac crest should drop more than 20-25°. A positive test is indicated by anything less than a smooth convexity in the lumbar spine, or a drop of the iliac crest of less than 20-25°, and alerts the physician to a somatic dysfunction of the lumbar or the thoracolumbar spine. [1 p.497-8]

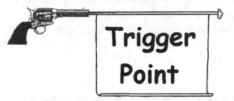

Trigger Point

The purpose of the hip-drop test is to evaluate sidebending (lateral flexion) of the lumbar spine

B. Straight Leg Raising Test (Lasegue's Test)

This test is used in the evaluation of sciatic nerve compression. The patient lies supine. The physician grasps the leg being tested under the heel with the hand, and to keep the knee extended, places the other hand on the anterior aspect of the knee. The physician then lifts the leg upward, flexing the hip. The leg is lifted until the patient feels discomfort. Normally, the leg can be raised to about 70-80° of hip flexion.

If the patient experiences pain, the cause most likely will be due to hamstring tightness or due to problems with the sciatic nerve. Once the patient feels pain upon lifting the leg, the physician lowers the leg just beyond where the pain was felt, and then dorsiflexes the foot (Braggard's Test). This stretches the sciatic nerve. If no pain is elicited, the pain from the leg-raising is probably from tight hamstrings and the test is considered negative. If pain is felt all the way down the leg, this indicates a sciatic origin, and the straight leg raising test is considered positive. [5 p.267, 6 p.256]

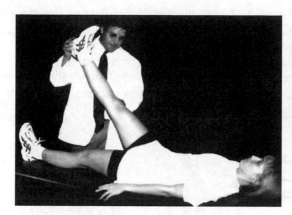

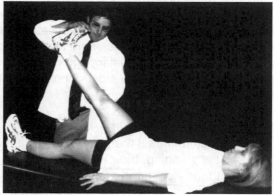

Straight leg raising test   Braggard's test

V. Sacrum and Innominates

A. Seated Flexion Test

This test assesses **sacroiliac motion**. It evaluates somatic dysfunction in the pelvis, most commonly in the sacrum. [1 p.100] The patient is seated with both feet flat on the floor. The physician locates the patient's PSIS's and places his thumbs on the inferior notch. The patient is instructed to bend forward and the physician assesses the level of the PSIS's as this motion is completed. A positive test occurs when, at the termination of forward bending, the PSIS's are not level. Somatic dysfunction is present on the side of the superior PSIS. [1 p.498]

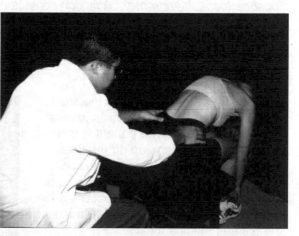

B. Standing Flexion Test

This test assesses **iliosacral motion**. It evaluates the possibility of somatic dysfunction in the leg or pelvis, most commonly the innominate. [1 p.496] With the patient standing, the physician locates the patient's PSIS's and places his thumbs on the inferior notch. The patient is instructed to bend forward and the physician assesses the level of the PSIS's as this motion is completed. A positive test occurs when, at the termination of forward bending, the PSIS's are not level. Somatic dysfunction is present on the side of the superior PSIS. [1 p.496]

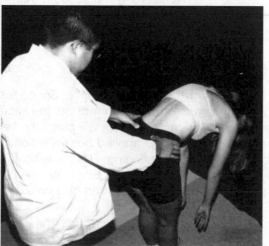

C. ASIS Compression Test

This test helps determine the side of a SI dysfunction. It is particularly helpful when the standing or seated flexion tests are equivocal. With the patient in the supine position, the physician comes in contact with the ASIS's and applies a posterior compression to each ASIS while stabilizing the other. There is usually an ease of posterior compression (some authors [28] describe this as a sense of "resiliency"). If there is a resistance to compression (that side did not have "resiliency") then the test is considered positive on that side. A positive test indicates dysfunction of the sacrum, innominate or pubic bones. [1 p.616]

D. Pelvic side shift test [1 p.498]

This test determines if the sacrum is in the midline. With the patient standing, the physician stabilizes the shoulders with the right hand and pushes the pelvis to the right with the left hand. The hands are then switched and the pelvis is translated to the left. The test is positive on the side of freer translation. This indicates that the pelvis is shifted to that side.

It is often seen in a flexion contracture of the iliopsoas (psoas syndrome). A flexion contacture of the right iliopsoas will cause a positive pelvic shift test to the left and vice versa. [1 p.597, 28 p. 486]

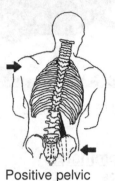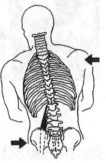

Positive pelvic shift test to the left.

Positive pelvic shift test to the right.

E Trendelenberg's Test

This test assesses gluteus medius muscle strength. The physician stands behind the patient. The patient is instructed to pick one of the legs up off the floor. Normally, the gluteus medius muscle should pull up the unsupported pelvis to keep it level. A positive test occurs when the pelvis falls, which indicates weakness in the gluteus medius muscle. [5 p.323, 6 p.164]

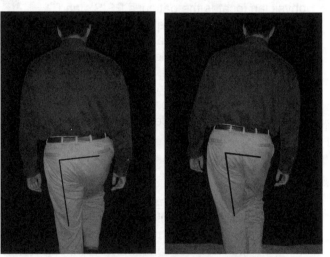

Negative Trendelenberg (left)
Positive Trendelenberg (right) indicates left gluteus medius weakness

F. Lumbosacral spring test (a.k.a. Spring test) [56 p.1251]

This test assesses whether or not the sacral base is tilted posterior. With the patient in the prone position, the physician will place the heel of the hand over the lumbosacral junction. Gentle and rapid springing is applied downward onto the lumbosacral junction. The test is positive when there is little or no springing. This is indicative of the sacral base moving posterior. This test is postive in a unilateral sacral extension, sacral margin posterior, sacral base posterior and when the sacrum rotates backward on an oblique axis.

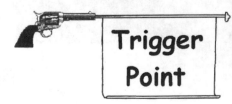

Trigger Point

The lumbosacral spring test will be positive in all the dysfunctions in which the sacral base moves posterior.

G. Backward bending test [1 p.616] (a.k.a. The Sphinx Test)

This test determines if the sacral base has moved posterior or anterior. The test is positive if a part of the sacral base moves posterior (a unilateral sacral extension, sacral margin posterior and when the sacrum rotates backward on an oblique axis).

With the patient prone, the physician places his thumbs on the superior sulci. If asymmetry is present, either one side of the sacrum has moved posterior, or the other side has moved anterior. To determine between the two, have the patient prop up on their elbows (sphinx position). Normally, this movement (lumbar extension) causes the sacral base to move anterior. If one side of the sacral base is anterior, it will move more anterior with lumbar extension and consequently the physician's thumbs will become more symmetrical. However, if part of the sacral base is posterior, it will resist anterior movement with lumbar extension and consequently the physician's thumbs will become more asymmetric.

- *If the physician's thumbs become more symmetric with lumbar extension, part of the sacral base moved anterior.*
- *If the physician's thumbs become more asymmetric with lumbar extension, part of the sacral base has moved posterior.*

VI. Hips

A. Ober's Test

This test detects a tight tensor fascia lata and iliotibial band. The patient lies on the side opposite the iliotibial band being tested. The physician stands behind the patient and flexes the knee on the side being tested to 90°, abducts the hip as far as possible, and slightly extends the hip while stabilizing the pelvis to keep the patient from rolling. Slight hip extension is necessary to ensure that the iliotibial band passes directly over the greater trochanter. The physician slowly allows the thigh to fall to the table. The test is positive if the thigh remains in the abducted position, indicating a tight iliotibial band. [5 p.354, 6 p.167]

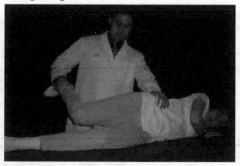
Negative Ober's test

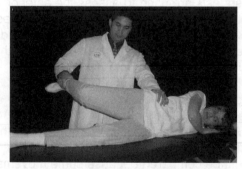
Positive Ober's Test

B. Patrick's Test (FABERE Test)

This test is used to assess pathology of the sacroiliac and hip joint, especially osteoarthritis of the hip. The term FABERE indicates the positioning of the hip being tested. Flexion, Abduction, External Rotation, then Extension. The patient's hip is flexed, abducted, and externally rotated into a figure-4 position. Any pain in or around the hip joint indicates general pathology of that hip joint. At this point, the physician places one hand on the contralateral ASIS and the other hand on the knee of the testing leg. Pressure is placed downward on both points, the most important motion being the further extension of the hip. Pain will be accentuated by any arthritic changes in the hip or sacroiliac joint. [1 p.627, 5 p. 343, 6 p.262]

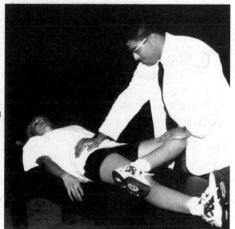

C. <u>Thomas Test</u>

This test assesses the possibility of a flexion contracture of the hip, usually of iliopsoas origin. The patient lies supine and the physician checks for exaggerated lumbar lordosis, common in hip flexion contractures. The physician flexes one hip so that knee and anterior thigh touches the patient's abdomen. If a flexion contracture is not present, the patient's opposite leg will remain flat on the table. If present, a contracture of the iliopsoas will cause the opposite leg to lift off of the table. [5 p.152, 6 p.155]

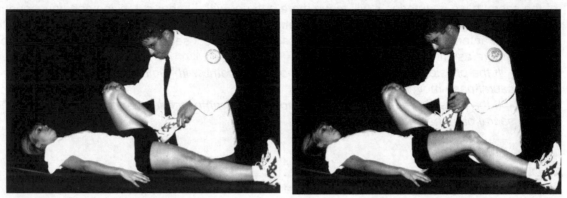

Negative Thomas Test   Positive Thomas Test

VII. <u>Knee</u>

A. <u>Anterior and Posterior Draw Tests</u>

These tests are used to assess the anterior and posterior cruciate ligaments. The patient lies supine with the hip flexed to 45° and knee flexed to 90°. The physician sits on the patient's foot of the knee being tested, wraps both hands around behind the tibia, and places one thumb on the medial joint line and one on the lateral joint line. The tibia is then pulled anteriorly (anterior draw) to test the ACL. If the tibia slides out from under the femur, the test is positive for an ACL tear. Both sides must be compared because some movement may be possible in some patients. The physician then pushes posteriorly on the tibia to check the PCL (posterior drawer). After comparing both knees, the test is positive if the tibia excessively moves backward under the femur. [6 p.186, 5 p.400-2]

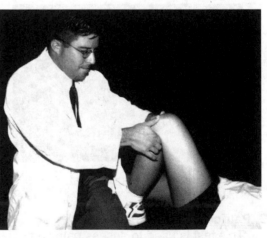

B. <u>Bounce Home Test</u>

This test evaluates problems with full knee extension, usually due to meniscal tears or joint effusions. The patient is supine and the physician grasps the heel. The knee is flexed completely. Then, the knee is allowed to drop into extension. Normally, the knee should "bounce home" into full extension to a sharp end-point, without restriction. The test is positive if extension is incomplete or there is a "rubbery" feel to end-point extension. [1 p.630, 5 p.413, 6 p.194]

C. Apley's Compression and Distraction Tests

These tests evaluate the meniscus and ligamentous structures of the knee. The patient lies prone and the knee is flexed to 90°. The compression part of the test is performed with the physician pressing straight down on the heel, and internally and externally rotating the tibia in this position. Pain indicates a meniscal tear. Then, the physician pulls upward (the "distraction" part) on the foot, and internally and externally rotates the tibia. Pain this time indicates ligamentous injury, usually the medial and/or lateral collateral ligaments. [6] p.193, 5 p.413

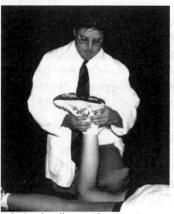
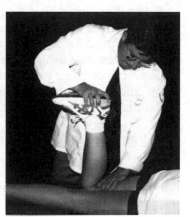

Apley's distraction test   Apley's compression test

D. Lachman's Test

This test also assesses the stability of the ACL and is somewhat more accurate than the Draw tests. The patient lies supine. The physician grasps the proximal tibia with one hand and the distal femur with the other hand. The knee is flexed to about 30°. The tibia is then pulled forward by the grasping hands. Both sides are compared, and the test is positive if the tibia excessively moves out from under the femur. [1] p.631, 5 p.397

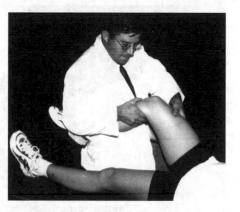

E. McMurray's Test

This test detects tears in the posterior aspect of the menisci. To test the medial meniscus, the patient's knee is fully flexed. The physician's fingers palpate the medial knee joint line. The tibia is then externally rotated and a valgus stress is placed on the knee. Maintaining this position, the knee is then slowly extended. If a palpable or audible "click" is noticed, the test is positive for a posterior tear of the medial meniscus. To test the lateral meniscus, the same procedure is used with internal rotation of the tibia and a varus stress on the knee. [1] p.632, 5 p.413, 6 p.191

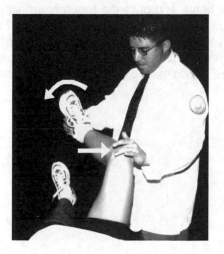
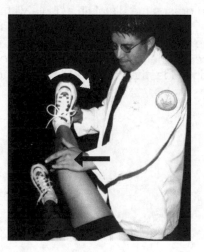

F. Patellar Grind Test

This test assesses the posterior articular surfaces of the patella and the possibility of chondromalacia patellae, commonly seen with patello-femoral syndrome. The patient lies supine with knees fully extended and relaxed. The physician pushes the patella distally, then instructs the patient to contract the quadriceps muscles. Any roughness of the articular surfaces will grind, and be palpable and painful when the quadriceps contract and move the patella. The test is positive if the patient feels pain with contraction of the patella. [6 p.194, 5 p.418]

G. Valgus and Varus Stress Tests

These tests are used to assess the stability of the collateral ligaments. With the patient lying supine or sitting on the table, the knee is flexed just enough to unlock it from full extension. The physician stabilizes the ankle with one hand while the other pushes against the knee, first medially then laterally. Pushing the knee medial (with a **L**ateral force) is the va**L**gus stress test. If there is gapping on the opposite side, then the medial collateral ligament is torn. To test the lateral collateral ligament, the physician pushes the knee laterally (varus stress test). If there is any gapping of the lateral joint line, the test is positive.

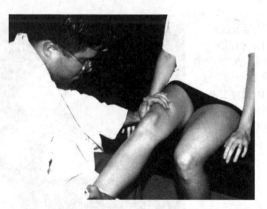

Valgus Stress Testing

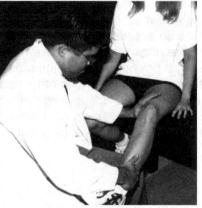

Varus Stress Testing

VIII. Ankle

A. Anterior Draw Test of the Ankle

This test is used to assess the medial and lateral ligaments of the ankle, mainly the anterior talofibular ligament, but also the superficial and deep deltoid ligaments. The patient lies supine. The physician grasps the distal tibia/fibula with one hand, and pulls the foot forward with the other hand grasping the posterior aspect of the calcaneus. The foot should be held in 20° of dorsiflexion the entire time. If, after comparing both sides, excessive movement of the talus under the tibia/fibula occurs, then a bilateral injury has occurred to the mentioned ligaments. If there is deviation to one side, then only the ligaments to the opposite side of the foot are damaged. [5 p.480]

CHAPTER 18 REVIEW QUESTIONS

1. Stenosis of the intervertebral foramen, resulting in a radiculopathy, which radiates into the upper extremity can be most effectively assessed using which test?
     A. Spurling's test.
     B. Wallenberg's test.
     C. Adson's test.
     D. Roos test.
     E. Speed's test

2. Which one of the following tests will be positive in vertebral artery insufficiency?
     A. Spurling's test.
     B. Wallenberg's test.
     O. Adson's test.
     D. Roos test.
     E. Speed's test.

3. Af patient comes to your office with left sided shoulder pain. You suspect an overuse injury. In order to evaluate shoulder range of motion you would perform which one of the following tests?
     A. Apley's compression test.
     B. Apley's distraction test.
     C. Apley's scratch test.
     D. Adson's test.
     E. Roos test

4. A positive Adson's test will indicate which of the following?
     A. Decreased muscle strength the gluteus medius.
     B. A flexion contracture of the iliopsoas.
     C. Instability of the biceps tendon in the bicipital groove.
     D. Thoracic outlet syndrome.
     E. A rotator cuff tear.

5.. A positive Yergason's test will indicate which of the following?
     A. Decreased muscle strength the gluteus medius.
     B. A flexion contracture of the iliopsoas.
     C. Instability of the biceps tendon in the bicipital groove.
     D. Thoracic outlet syndrome.
     E. A rotator cuff tear

6. Which one of the following is true concerning de Quervain's disease?
     A. It results in a flexion contracture of the palmar fascia.
     B. It results from damage to the radial nerve.
     C. It is also known as iliotibial band syndrome.
     D. It results from an inflammation of the abductor pollicis longus and/or extensor pollicis brevis tendons.
     E. It often results from repetitive and strenuous supination of the forearm.

7. A positive phalen's test in a patient complaining of paresthesia in the upper extremity may lead the practitioner to the diagnosis of:
    A. Thoracic outlet syndrome.
    B. Carpal tunnel syndrome.
    C. A rotator cuff tear.
    D. De Quervain's disease.
    E. Tennis elbow.

8. The hip drop test will be positive in which one of the following conditions?
    A. A group somatic dysfunction in the lumbar spine.
    B. Sciatic nerve root compression.
    C. Neuropathy involving the superior gluteal nerve.
    D. Congenital hip dislocation.
    E. A sacral torsion.

9. The trendelenberg test will assess which one of the following muscle groups.
    A. The hip extensors.
    B. The hip flexors.
    C. The hip abductors.
    D. The hip adductors.
    E. The hip external rotators.

10. A 45 year old male presents to your office with left sided low back pain. He states the pain is worsened by standing up straight after prolonged sitting. The pain radiates to his groin. On examination, you notice that L1 is FR_LS_L, and the he has a tenderpoint medial to his left ASIS. You believe the problem lies within the left hip flexor. Which one of the following tests may aid in confirming your diagnosis?
    A. The hip drop test.
    B. The Thomas test.
    C. Ober's test.
    D. Hoover's test.
    E. The Trendelenberg test.

11. A 32 year old female injured her knee one hour ago playing basketball. As the ER physician, you notice a small joint effusion. She has a positive McMurray's test, and a positive Apley's compression test. Apley's distraction, anterior drawer, and valgus and varus tests are negative. Based on the above information, which one of the following choices is the most likely diagnosis?
    A. Chondromalacia patella.
    B. A medial collateral tear.
    C. A lateral collateral tear.
    D. An anterior cruciate tear.
    E. A medial meniscal tear.

12. Excessive anterior movement of the tibia on the femur is indicative of which one of the following conditions?
    A. An ACL injury.
    B. A PCL injury.
    C. A meniscal injury.
    D. A medial collateral injury.
    E. A lateral collateral injury.

13. Which one of the following statements is true concerning Apley's compression test?
    A. Pain elicited with Apley's compression indicates pathology on the posterior surface of the patella.
    B. Apley's compression will be positive in meniscal injuries.
    C. Apley's compression will be positive in ligamentous injuries.
    D. Apley's compression will be positive in both ligamentous and meniscal injuries.
    E. Apley's compression will be positive in rotator cuff tears.

ANSWERS

1. A	8. A
2. B	9. C
3. C	10. B
4. D	11. E
5. C	12. A
6. D	13. B
7. B	

APPENDIX A

COMMON TECHNIQUES FOR VISCERAL AND SYSTEMIC DYSFUNCTIONS

Chapman's Reflexes [35 p.200]
Objective - Decrease sympathetic tone, improve lymphatic return and increase myofascial motion associated with visceral dysfunction.
Indications - Visceral dysfunction

Sphenopalatine Ganglion Treatment [35 p.223]
Objective - Enhances parasympathetic activity which decreases goblet cells thus encourages thin watery secretions.
Indications - Thick secretions associated with an upper respiratory tract infection (URI).

Rib Raising [35 p.195-98]
Objective -
  Decrease sympathetic activity
  Improve negative intrathoracic pressure for maximum inhalation
  Improve lymphatic return
Indications -
  Hypersympathetic tone associated with visceral dysfunction
  Decreased respiration
  Fever
  Lymphatic congestion
Contraindications -
  Recent spinal surgery
  Rib fracture
  Spinal fracture

Paraspinal Inhibition
Procedure - Paraspinal pressure (similar to rib raising) at L1 and/or L2.
Objective - Mainly used with rib raising to decrease sympathetic tone associated with an ileus.
Indications - Ileus
Contraindications -
  Recent spinal surgery
  Rib fracture
  Spinal fracture

Celiac Ganglion Release [35 p.199-200]
    Objective - Reduce sympathetic tone at T5 - T9.
    Indications - Upper GI dysfunction
    Contraindications -
        Aortic aneurysm
        Nearby surgical wound

Superior Mesenteric Ganglion Release [35 p.199-200]
    Objective - Reduce sympathetic tone at T10 - T11.
    Indications -
        GI dysfunction from jejunum to mid-transverse colon
        GU dysfunction
    Contraindications -
        Aortic aneurysm
        Nearby surgical wound

Inferior Mesenteric Ganglion Release [35 p.199-200]
    Objective - Reduce sympathetic tone at T12 - L2.
    Indications -
        Lower GI dysfunction
        GU dysfunction
        Pelvic dysfunction
    Contraindications -
        Aortic aneurysm
        Nearby surgical wound

Sacral Inhibition [56 p.829, 35 p.224]
    Procedure - With patient in prone position apply deep direct pressure at the sacrum for 2 minutes.
    Objective - Inhibit sacral motion, increasing parasympathetic activity to the left colon and pelvic organs.
    Indications -
        Dysmenorrhea
        Diarrhea
    Contraindications - Nearby infections or incisions

Sacral rocking [56 p.828]
    Procedure - With the patient in the prone position, apply gentle pressure at the sacrum with rocking motion. The rocking motion augments flexion and extension phases associated with respiration or with the cranial rhythmic impulse (CRI).
    Objective - Relaxes the muscles of the lumbosacral junction
    Indications - Tight lumbosacral paraspinals
    Contraindications - Nearby infections or incisions

NOTE: Some authors [35] make no distinction between sacral inhibition and sacral rocking while others [56] do.

Thoracic Inlet Release [1 p.948]
    Objective - Improve lymphatic return in left and right lymphatic ducts.
    Indications - Lymphatic congestion
    Contraindications -
        Upper rib fracture
        Clavicle fracture
        Lymphatic system malignancy (controversial) (see chapter 13 Lymphatics)

Redoming the Diaphragm [35 p.215]

<u>Objective</u> - Increase thoracoabdominal diaphragm excursion improving respiration and improve lymph return.

<u>Indications</u> -

Decreased diaphragmatic excursion

Lymphatic congestion

<u>Contraindications</u> -

Local rib fracture

Nearby incision

Lymphatic system malignancy (controversial) (see chapter 13 <u>Lymphatics</u>)

Pelvic Diaphragm Release

<u>Objective</u> - Improve pelvic diaphragm excursion and improve lymph return.

<u>Indications</u> -

Decreased diaphragmatic excursion

Lymphatic congestion

<u>Contraindications</u> -

Local rib fracture

Nearby incision

Lymphatic system malignancy (controversial) (see chapter 13 <u>Lymphatics</u>)

Thoracic Pump [1. 955]

<u>Objective</u> - Augment thoracic range of motion and affect intrathoracic pressure gradients, improving lymphatic return.

<u>Indications</u> -

Lymphatic congestion

Chest congestion

Fever

Infection

<u>Contraindications</u> -

Osteoporosis (relative contraindication)

Rib or spinal fracture

Malignancy of lymphatic system (controversial) (see chapter 13 <u>Lymphatics</u>)

Pectoral Traction [1 p.955, 35 p.219]

<u>Objective</u> - Augments thoracic range of motion via pectoralis minor stretch, improving lymphatic return.

<u>Indications</u> -

Lymphatic congestion

Works well in patients that cannot tolerate thoracic pump. [1 p.955]

<u>Contraindictions</u> -

Nearby surgical wound

Abdominal pump [56 p.1069]

<u>Objective</u> -

Augments thoraco-abdominal pressure gradients improving lymphatic return.

Massages thoracic duct at cisterna chyli.

<u>Indications</u> -

Upper and lower GI dysfunctions

CHF

COPD, asthma, URI

Hiatial hernia

Decreased motion of L-spine and thoracic cage

<u>Contraindications</u> -
>> Rib or spinal fracture
>> Traumatic disruption of liver or spleen
>> Nearby surgical incision
>> A full stomach
>> Lymphatic system malignancy (controversial) (see chapter 13 <u>Lymphatics</u>)

Liver and Spleen Pumps [1 p.957, 35 p.219-20]

<u>Objective</u> - Augments pressure gradient to improve lymphatic movement thus, enhancing immune function and remove toxins
<u>Indications</u>
>> Right sided CHF
>> Liver and splenic congestion
>> Infection
>> Parenchymal disease of the liver and/or spleen
<u>Contraindications</u> -
>> Spinal or rib fracture
>> Acute hepatitis or friable liver
>> Traumatic disruption of liver or spleen
>> Lymphatic system malignancy (controversial) (see chapter 13 <u>Lymphatics</u>)

Pedal (Dalrymple) Pump [1 p.956-7, 35p. 218-19]

<u>Objective</u> - Augments thoraco-abdominal pressure gradients improving lymphatic return.
<u>Indications</u> -
>> Same as abdominal pump.
>> Better suited in patients that cannot tolerate thoracic pump [35 p.229]
<u>Contrindications</u> -
>> DVT
>> Lower extremity fractures
>> Recent abdominal surgery

APPENDIX B

NEUROLOGIC EXAM

I. Neurological evaluation:

A basic neurologic examination consists of muscle strength testing, sensation testing and deep tendon reflex testing. A detailed neurologic exam consisting of upper motor neuron signs is not in the scope of this text.

A. Muscle strength recording

Table B.1 shows the standard method for recording motor strength

Table B.1 [1 p.552]

Grade	Diagnosis	Definition
5	Normal	Full range of motion (FROM) against gravity and resistance
4	Good	FROM against gravity with some resistance
3	Fair	FROM against gravity with no resistance
2	Poor	FROM with gravity eliminated
1	Trace	Evidence of slight contractility
0	Zero	No evidence of contractility

B. Deep tendon reflex evaluation

Although differences may be subtle, table B.2 shows the standard way to record the amplitude of a reflex. [1 p.552]

Table B.2

Grade	Definition	Injury
4/4	Brisk with sustained clonus	Upper Motor Neuron
3/4	Brisk with unsustained clonus	Normal/UMN
2/4	Normal	Normal
1/4	Decreased but present	Normal/LMN
0/4	Absent	Lower Motor Neuron

II. Peripheral nerve distribution in the upper extremity

Table B.3 [5, 50]

Nerve Root	Sensation	Motor	Reflex
C1	vertex of skull		none
C2	temple and occipital area		none
C3	supraclavicular fossa		none
C4	superior aspect of shoulder		none
C5	lateral aspect of elbow	elbow flexors	biceps reflex
C6	lateral forearm and thumb	wrist extensors	brachioradialis reflex
C7	middle finger	elbow extensors	triceps reflex
C8	little finger and middle forearm	deep finger and wrist flexors	none
T1	medial elbow and medial arm	finger abduction	none

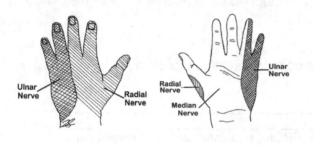

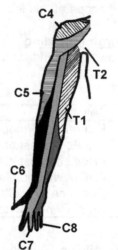

Fig B.1: Dermatomes of the upper extremity.

Figs B.2 and B.3: Posterior (above left) and anterior (above right) view of the cutaneous distribution for the radial, ulnar, and median nerves.

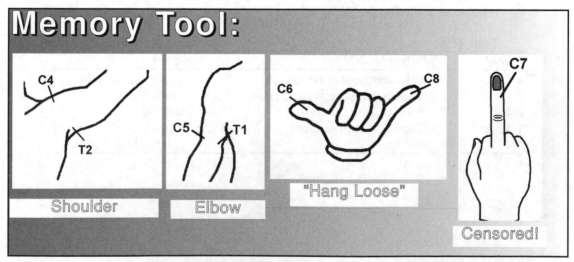

The above table and memory tool depicts dermatome locations as outlined in the International Standards for Neurological Classification of Spinal Cord Injury. [50]

III: Muscles of the shoulder

Table B.4

Muscle	Origin	Insertion	Innervation	Action
Deltoid	Lateral clavical, acromion, spine of scapula	Deltoid tuberosity of the humerus	Axillary nerve (**C5**, C6)	Abducts, adducts, flexes, extends shoulder
Supraspinatus	Supraspinous fossa of scapula	Gr. Tubercle of the humerus	Suprascapular nerve (C4,**C5**,C6)	Abducts arm
Infraspinatus	Infraspinous fossa of scapula	Gr. Tubercle of the humerus	Suprascapular nerve (C4,**C5**,C6)	Externally rotates arm
Subscapularis	Subscapula fossa	Lesser tubercle of the humerus	Upper and lower subscapular nerve (C5,**C6**,C7)	Internally rotates arm
Teres Major	Dorsal surface of inferior angle of scapula	Intertubercular groove of humerus	Lower sub scapular nerve (**C6**,C7)	Adducts and internally rotates arm
Teres Minor	Lateral border of scapula	Gr. Tubercle of the humerus	Axillary nerve (**C5**,C6)	Externally rotates arm
Lat. Dorsi	SP of T7 - T12, thoracolumbar fascia, iliac crest, ribs 9-12	Floor of bicipital groove of humerus	Thoracodorsal nerve (**C6,C7**,C8)	Adducts, extends shoulder Internally rotates arm

IV. Muscles of the Arm

Table B.5

Muscle	Origin	Insertion	Innervation	Action
Coracobrachialis	Coracoid process of scapula	Middle third of medial surface of humerus	Musculocutaneous nerve (C5,**C6**,C7)	Flexes and adducts arm
Biceps brachii	*Long head:* Glenoid labrum, *Short head:* coracoid process	Radial tuberosity of radius	Musculocutaneous nerve (C5,**C6**)	Flexes elbow and supinates forearm
Brachialis	Lower anterior humerus	Coronoid proc. and ulnar tuberosity	Musculocutaneous nerve (C5,**C6**)	Flexes elbow

Table abbreviations
IO -= interosseous membrane
IP = Interphalangeal joint
CMC = carpometacarpal joint
PIP = proximal interphalangeal joint

DIP = distal interphalangeal joint
VB = vertebral body
SP = spinous process
IT = ischial tuberosity

V. <u>Muscles of the Arm</u> (con't)
Table B.5 (con't)

Muscle	Origin	Insertion	Innervation	Action
Triceps	Long Head: lateral edge of scapula Lateral head: humerus (superior to radial groove) Medial head: humerus (inferior to radial groove)	Olecranon process	Radial nerve (C6,**C7,C8**)	Extends elbow
Anconeus	Lateral epicondyle Proximal, median humerus	Olecranon process and ulna	Radial nerve (C7,C8,T1)	Extends elbow

VI. <u>Muscles of the Anterior Forearm</u>
Table B.6

Muscle	Origin	Insertion	Innervation	Action
Pronator teres	Medial epicondyle and coronoid process of ulna	Middle of lateral side of radius	Median nerve (C6,**C7**)	Pronates forearm
Flexor carpi radialis	Medial epicondyle	Base of 2nd and 3rd metacarpals	Median nerve (C6,**C7**)	Flexes and abducts hand
Palmaris longus	Medial epicondyle	Flexor retinaculum palmar aponeurosis	Median nerve (C7,C8)	Flexes hand
Flexor carpi ulnaris	Medial epicondyle and olecranon	5th metacarpal, pisiform, hamate	Ulnar nerve (C7,**C8**)	Flexes and adducts hand
Flexor digitorum superficialis	Medial epicondyle, coronoid process and radius	Middle phalanges (PIP's)	Median nerve (C7,**C8**,T1)	Flexes PIP's also flexes hand
Flexor digitorum profundus	Ulna and interosseous membrane	Distal phalanges (DIP's)	Median nerve (1 & 2 fingers)[C8,T1] Ulnar nerve (3 & 4 fingers)[C8,T1]	Flexes DIP's
Flexor pollicis longus	Radius, ulna and interosseous membrane	Distal phalanx of thumb	Median nerve (**C8**,T1)	Flexes thumb
Pronator quadratus	Anterior surface of distal ulna	Anterior surface of distal radius	Median nerve (**C8**,T1)	Pronates forearm

MEMORY TOOL:
The **D**eep finger flexors (Flexor digitorum profundus)
attach to the **DIP's**

VII. Muscles of the Posterior Forearm

Table B.7

Muscle	Origin	Insertion	Innervation	Action
Brachioradialis	Supracondylar ridge of humerus	Base of radial styloid process	Radial nerve (C5,**C6**,C7)	Flexes forearm
Extensor carpi radialis longus	Supracondylar ridge of humerus	Base of 2nd metacarpal	Radial nerve (C6,C7)	Extends and abducts hand
Extensor carpi radialis brevis	Lateral epicondyle	Base of 3rd metacarpal	Radial nerve (**C7**,C8)	Extends and abducts hand
Extensor digitorum	Lateral epicondyle	Extensor expansion of PIP's and DIP's	Radial nerve (**C7**,C8)	Extends MCP's and wrist
Extensor digiti minimi	Lateral epicondyle	Extensor expansion of PIP and DIP of 5th digit	Radial nerve (**C7**,C8)	Extends 5th digit at PIP and DIP
Extensor carpi ulnaris	Lateral epicondyle and posterior ulna	Base of 5th metacarpal	Radial nerve (**C7**,C8)	Extends and adducts hand and wrist
Supinator	Lateral epicondyle, radial collateral and annular ligaments	Lateral proximal 3rd of radius	Radial nerve (C5,**C6**)	Supinates forearm
Abductor pollicis longus	Posterior radius, ulna and IO membrane	Base of 1st metacarpal	Radial nerve (C7,**C8**)	Abducts thumb and extends thumb at CMC
Extensor pollicis longus	Posterior ulna and IO membrane	Base of distal phalanyx of thumb	Radial nerve (C7,**C8**)	Extends IP and MCP of thumb
Extensor pollicis brevis	Posterior radius and IO membrane	Base of proximal phalanx of thumb	Radial nerve (C7,**C8**)	Extends CMC of thumb
Extensor indicis	Posterior ulna and IO membrane	Extensor expansion of PIP and DIP of 1st finger	Radial nerve (C7,**C8**)	Extends index finger

181

VIII. Muscles of the Hand
Table B.8

Muscle	Origin	Insertion	Innervation	Action
Abductor polllcis brevis	Flexor retinaculum scaphoid and trapezium	Lateral side of proximal phalanx	Median nerve (**C8**,T1)	Abducts thumb
Flexor pollicis brevis	Flexor retinaculum trapezium	Lateral side of proximal phalanx	Median nerve (**C8**,T1)	Flexes thumb
Opponens pollicis	Flexor retinaculum and trapezium	Lateral side of 1st metacarpal	Median nerve (**C8**,T1)	Opposes thumb and other digits
Adductor pollicis	Capitate and 2nd , 3rd metacarpals	Medial side of proximal phalanx	Ulnar nerve (C8,**T1**)	Adducts thumb
Abductor digiti minimi	Pisiform	Medial proximal phalanx of 5th digit	Ulnar nerve (C8,**T1**)	Abduct little finger
Flexor digitorum mimimi brevis	Flexor retinaculum and hook of hamate	Medial proximal phalanx of 5th digit	Ulnar nerve (C8,**T1**)	Flexes PIP of little finger
Opponens digiti minimi	Flexor retinaculum and hook of hamate	Medial side of 5th metacarpal	Ulnar nerve (C8,**T1**)	Opposes little finger with thumb
Lumbricals	Flexor digitorum profundus tendon	Extensor expansions of fingers	Median nerve (1 & 2)(C8,**T1**) Ulnar nerve (3 & 4)(C8,**T1**)	Flexes MCP's and extends IP's
Dorsal interossi (4)	Metacarpals	Extensor expansions and proximal phalanges	Ulnar nerve (C8,**T1**)	Abducts digits
Palmar interossi (3)	Metacarpals	Extensor expansions and proximal phalanges	Ulnar nerve (C8,**T1**)	Adducts digits

IX. Peripheral nerve distribution in the lower extremity
Table B.9 [50]

Nerve Root	Sensation	Motor	Reflex
L1	anterior thigh just below inguinal ligament	hip flexors	none
L2	middle and anterior thigh	hip flexors & adductors	none
L3	anterior thigh just above knee	knee extensors	none
L4	**medial malleolus**	**ankle dorsiflexors**	**patella reflex**
L5	**dorsal aspect of foot and big toe**	**toe extensors**	none
S1	**lateral malleolus**	**ankle plantar flexors**	**achilles reflex**

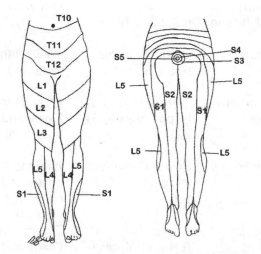

Fig B.4: Dermatomes of the lower extremity

X. Muscles of the Anterior Thigh
Table B.10

Muscle	Origin	Insertion	Innervation	Action
Iliopsoas	VB's of T12 - L5 and Iliac fossa	Lesser trochanter of femur	Femoral nerve (**L1, L2**, L3)	Flexes hip
Sartorius	ASIS	Upper medial side of tibia	Femoral nerve (L2 and L3)	Flexes abducts, and externally rotates thigh
Rectus femoris	AIIS and groove of acetabulum	Base of patella	Femoral nerve (L2, **L3, L4**)	Flexes hip and extends knee
Vastus medialis	Medial lip of femur	Base of patella	Femoral nerve (L2, **L3, L4**)	Extends knee
Vastus lateralis	Gr. trochanter and body of femur	Base of patella	Femoral nerve (L2, **L3, L4**)	Extends knee
Vastus inter-medius	Body of femur	Base of patella	Femoral nerve (L2, **L3, L4**)	Extends knee

XI. Muscles of the Medial and Posterior Thigh

Table B.11

Muscle	Origin	Insertion	Innervation	Action
Adductor longus	Body of pubis	Middle 1/3 of linea aspera of femur	Obturator nerve (L2, **L3**, L4)	Adducts, flexes and internally rotates thigh
Adductor brevis	Body of inferior pubic ramus	Pectineal line, upper part of linea aspera	Obturator nerve (L2, **L3**, L4)	Adducts, flexes and internally rotates thigh
Adductor magnus	IT, inferior pubic ramus	Linea aspera, adductor tubercle, supracondylar line	Obturator and sciatic nerve (L2, **L3, L4**)	Adducts, flexes and extends thigh
Gracilis	Body and inferior pubic ramus	Superior part of medial tibia	Obturator nerve (**L2**, L3)	Adducts thigh, flexes leg
Semitendinosis	Ischial tuberosity (IT)	Superior part of medial tibia	Sciatic nerve (tibial portion)(**L5, S1**, S2)	Extends thigh, flexes and internally rotates leg
Semimembranosis	Ischial tuberosity (IT)	Medial condyle of tibia	Sciatic nerve (tibial portion)(**L5, S1**, S2)	Extends thigh, flexes and internally rotates leg
Biceps femoris	*Long head:* IT *Short head:* posterior femur	Head of fibula	Sciatic (LH = tibial, SH = peroneal)(L5, **S1**, S2)	Extends thigh, flexes and externally rotates leg
Gluteus maximus	Ilium, sacrum, coccyx, sacrotuberus ligament	Gluteal tuberosity and iliotibial tract	Inferior gluteal nerve (L5, **S1, S2**)	Extends hip
Gluteus medius	Ilium	Greater trochanter	Superior gluteal nerve (**L5**, S1)	Abducts hip
Tensor fascia lata	Iliac crest and ASIS	Iliotibial tract	Superior gluteal nerve (L4, L5)	Flexes, abducts hip
Piriformis	Anterior sacrum and sacrotuberus ligament	Greater trochanter	Sacral nerve (**S1**, S2)	Externally rotates leg

XII. Muscles of the Anterior and Lateral Leg
Table B.12

Muscle	Origin	Insertion	Innervation	Action
Tibialis anterior	Lateral tibial condyle, IO membrane	1st cuneiform, 1st metatarsal	Deep peroneal nerve (**L4**, L5)	Dorsiflexes and inverts foot
Extensor hallucis longus	IO membrane, anterior fibula	Distal phalanx of big toe	Deep peroneal nerve (L5, S1)	Extends big toe, dorsiflexes foot
Extensor digitorum longus	Tibial condyle, IO membrane, fibula	Middle and distal phalanges	Deep peroneal nerve (L5, S1)	Extends digits 2-5, dorsiflexes foot
Peroneus longus	Lateral side and fibula head	base of 1st metatarsal, medial cuneiform	Superficial peroneal nerve (**L5, S1**, S2)	Everts and plantarflexes foot
Peroneus brevis	Lower lateral fibula	Base of 5th metatarsal	Superficial peroneal nerve (**L5, S1**, S2)	Everts and plantarflexes foot
Peroneus tertius	Distal 1/3 of fibula and IO membrane	Base of 5th metatarsal	Deep peroneal nerve (L5, S1)	Dorsiflexes and everts foot

XIII. Muscles of the Posterior Thigh
Table B.13

Muscle	Origin	Insertion	Innervation	Action
Gastrocnemius	Lateral and medial femoral condyles	Posterior aspect of calcaneus	Tibial nerve (**S1**, S2)	Flexes knee, plantar-flexes foot
Soleus	Tibia and upper fibular head	Posterior aspect of calcaneus	Tibial nerve (**S1**, S2)	Plantar-flexes foot
Plantaris	Lower lateral supracondylar line	Posterior aspect of calcaneus	Tibial nerve (S1, **S2**)	Weakly assists gastrocnemius
Popliteus	Lateral condyle of femur	Upper posterior side of tibia	Tibial nerve (**L4, L5**, S1)	Unlocks knee and flexes knee
Flexor hallucis longus	Lower 2/3 of fibula, IO membrane	Distal phalanx of big toe	Tibial nerve (**S2**, S3)	Flexes great toe, plantar-flexes foot
Flexor digitorum longus	Middle posterior tibia	Base of distal phalanges	Tibial nerve (**S2**, S3)	Flexes toes 2-5, plantar-flexes foot
Tibialis posterior	IO membrane, proximal tibia and fibula	Navicular, cuneiforms, cuboid, metatarsals 2-4	Tibial nerve (L4, L5)	Plantar-flexes and inverts foot.

XIV. Muscles of the Foot
Table B.14

Muscle	Origin	Insertion	Innervation	Action
Extensor digitorum brevis	Dorsal surface of calcaneus	Tendons of extensor digitorum longus	Deep peroneal nerve (L5,S1)	Extends toes
Extensor hallucis brevis	Dorsal surface of calcaneus	Proximal phalanyx of big toe	Deep peroneal nerve (L5,S1)	Extends big toe
Abductor hallucis	Medial tubercle of calcaneus	Proximal phalanyx of big toe	Medial plantar nerve (S2,**S3**)	Abducts and flexes big toe
Flexor digitorum brevis	Medial tubercle of calcaneus	Middle phalanyx of toes 2-5	Medial plantar nerve(S2,**S3**)	Flexes middle phalanx of toes 2-5
Abductor digiti minimi	Medial and lateral tubercles of calcaneus	5th proximal phalanyx	Lateral planter nerve(S2,**S3**)	Abducts little toe
Quadratus plantae	Medial and lateral surface of calcaneus	Tendon of flexor digitorum longus	Lateral planter nerve (S2,**S3**)	Assists flexor digitorum in flexing toes
Lumbricals	Tendons of flexor digitorum longus	Proximal phalanges of 2-5 and extensor expansion	Medial and lateral planter nerves (S2,**S3**)	Flexes proximal phalanges & extend distal phalanges of toes 2-5
Flexor hallucis brevis	Cuboid and lateral cuneiform	Proximal phalanx of big toe	Medial plantar nerve (S1,**S2**)	Flexes big toe
Adductor hallucis	Distal and proximal metatarsals	Proximal phalanx of big toe	Lateral plantar nerve (S2,**S3**)	Adducts big toe
Flexor digiti minimi brevis	Base of 5th metatarsal	Proximal phalanx of little toe	Lateral plantar nerve (S2,**S3**)	Flexes little toe
Plantar interossei	Medial sides of metatarsals 3-5	Medial base of proximal phalanges of 3-5	Lateral plantar nerve (S2,**S3**)	Adducts toes and flexes MTP's
Dorsal interossei	Adjacent sides of metatarsals	Base of proximal phalanx 2-4	Lateral plantar nerve (S2,**S3**)	Abducts toes and flexes MTP's

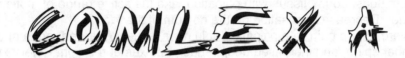

COMLEX A
EXAMINATION

COMLEX A Examination

1. A patient presents with a neurological deficit resulting in an absent triceps tendon reflex and weakness in the extensors of the hand, wrist and elbow. Which nerve is most likely involved?

   A) Musculocutaneous
   B) Median
   C) Radial
   D) Ulnar
   E) Axillary

2. A 45-year-old male with a history of diabetes comes to the emergency department with acute onset of low back pain. The pain started suddenly when he was sliding into home plate during a softball game earlier today. The pain is severe and radiates into his right lower extremity. He describes an electric type pain shooting into his right foot. What are some findings you would expect to see when examining him?

   A) Edematous, boggy tissue with palpation, and full active range of motion of the lumbar spine. Decreased sensation on the dorsum of the foot.
   B) Severe, sharp pain with palpation of lumbar tissues, guarded range of motion of the lumbar spine, and increased deep tendon reflexes of the right lower extremity.
   C) Warm tissue texture changes, hypertonic muscles, and decreased range of motion of the lumbar spine.
   D) Little to no edema or erythema, cool dry skin to palpation, ropy and fibrotic muscles, and decreased range of motion of the lumbar spine.
   E) Dull pain with palpation. Positive straight leg raising test.

3. A 56-year-old male is complaining of low back pain. On examination you notice transverse process of L5 is posterior on the right. Extending L5 worsens the asymmetry while flexion restores rotational symmetry. Which one of the following is the best statement regarding this patient's somatic dysfunction?

   A) Due to the non-neutral L5 somatic dysfunction, a group dysfunction of the high lumbar region will be present.
   B) This patient has a right-sided psoas syndrome.
   C) L5 will resist left rotation in the extended position.
   D) When employing a muscle energy (post-isometric relaxation) technique the patient would be asked to rotate his torso to the left against isometric contraction.
   E) Extending L5 will greatly limit its sidebending to the right

4. A 35-year-old male is in the intensive care unit after a recent motorcycle accident. He fractured C6, C7 and his left tibia. As a result, he has a spinal cord injury. He underwent surgical spine stabilization, but is awaiting surgical stabilization for his tibia fracture. Which one of the following osteopathic treatments is contraindicated in this individual?

   A) Thoraco-abdominal diaphragm release
   B) Thoracic rib raising and paraspinal inhibition
   C) Pedal lymphatic pump
   D) Myofascial release
   E) Counterstrain

5. In a patient with low back pain, the dysfunctional T12 segment is found to have restriction in a transverse plane and around a transverse axis. Which of the following dysfunctions best describes the position of T12?

    A) T12 is flexed
    B) T12 is sidebent right
    C) T12 is rotated left
    D) T12 is neutral sidebent right, rotated left
    E) T12 is extended rotated right, sidebent right

6. In a patient with neck pain, the atlas is rotated to the left. Given this information what else would you expect to find on this patient?

    A) The OA joint will resist translation to the left.
    B) C2 will resist anterior glide on the right
    C) C2 will resist right sidebending
    D) The lower cervical segments will be rotated to the right to compensate for the somatic dysfunction of this upper segment
    E) With the patient's neck flexed to 45 degrees, he will be able to turn his head further left than right.

7. A 20-year-old male presents with low back pain following a fall onto a concrete floor. The patient gives a history of episodic aching of the lumbar region prior to the fall. Examination of the patient in the prone position reveals a deep sacral sulcus on the left, a posterior/inferior ILA on the right when compared to the opposite side, and a lumbosacral junction that springs freely upon compression. The most likely diagnosis is?

    A) A forward sacral torsion on a right oblique axis
    B) A forward sacral torsion on a left oblique axis
    C) A backward sacral torsion on a left oblique axis
    D) A left unilateral sacral flexion
    E) Bilateral sacral extension

8. A 4-year-old child with asthma is brought to the ED by his father. The child developed an upper respiratory tract infection 48 hours ago. Over the past hour his breathing has become increasingly labored and he has started to develop respiratory distress. His father has administered one albuterol treatment via a nebulizer one hour ago; there was slight improvement in the patient's symptoms. On examination, respiratory rate = 50. Inspection of the chest wall reveals sub-costal retractions and evidence of accessory muscle use. Which of the following can be done initially to improve the patient's symptoms?

    A) Oxygen, oral albuterol, intravenous corticosteroids, and thoracic manipulation to stimulate sympathetics.
    B) Oxygen, inhaled albuterol, intravenous corticosteroids and seated thoracic pump technique.
    C) Oxygen, inhaled albuterol, zafirlukast, and manipulation to the cervical spine to normalize vagal tone.
    D) Oxygen, oral corticosteroids, and HVLA to rib 3.
    E) Oral albuterol, cromolyn sodium, and CV4 technique.

9. The first cervical segment has the greatest degree of freedom in which plane(s)?

   A) Transverse
   B) Coronal
   C) Sagittal
   D) Oblique
   E) Transverse and Coronal

10. Which of the following is common in lumbar stenosis with neurogenic claudication, but is not typical in peripheral vascular disease with vascular claudication?

   A) Pain relief with sitting
   B) Increased pain when treating a typical posterior lumbar tenderpoint
   C) Absence of lower extremity weakness
   D) Increased lower extremity pain with walking
   E) Posterior calf pain

11. Which of the following is considered to be the most common congenital anomaly in the lumbar spine?

   A) Sacralization
   B) Lumbarization
   C) Facet hypertrophy
   D) Facet tropism
   E) Spina bifida occulta

12. A mildly obese patient comes to your office complaining of buttock pain. She fell on her buttocks about one week ago and she still has some residual pain. Inspection of her lumbar spine and gluteal region reveals a decreased lumbar lordosis. Standing flexion test and seated flexion test show no evidence of asymmetry. Sacral sulci are equal in depth. The lumbosacral junction does not spring. Based on the information given what is the most likely diagnosis?

   A) Bilateral sacral extension
   B) Forward sacral torsion on a left oblique axis
   C) Anterior sacral base
   D) Unilateral extended sacrum on the right
   E) Unilateral extended sacrum on the left

13. In a patient with acute onset of low back pain, structural examination reveals a positive seated flexion test on the right. The left sacral base is anterior when compared to the right. The spring test is positive. Given the above information what is the most likely sacral diagnosis?

   A) Left sacral rotation on a right oblique axis
   B) Right sacral rotation on a right oblique axis
   C) Right sacral rotation on a left oblique axis
   D) Right unilateral sacral flexion
   E) Extended sacral base

14. A patient has a sacral torsion that resulted in a right anterior sacral base and a negative lumbosacral spring test. Based on the information given, what is the expected somatic dysfunction at L5?

   A) L5 $NS_L R_R$
   B) L5 $NS_R R_L$
   C) L5 $ER_R S_L$
   D) L5 $FR_L S_L$
   E) L5 $FR_R S_L$

15. A 46-year-old male presents to your office complaining of chronic lumbo-sacral pain. There is a negative standing flexion test and a positive seated flexion test. Structural examination reveals a deep sacral sulcus on the left, posterior/inferior ILA on the right, and the lumbosacral junction springs freely upon compression. The most likely diagnosis is:

   A) Right sacral rotation on a right oblique axis
   B) Left sacral rotation on a left oblique axis
   C) Right sacral shear
   D) Right sacral rotation on a left oblique axis
   E) Left sacral rotation on a right oblique axis

16. A 45-year-old female with new onset left upper extremity weakness, miosis, anhydrosis and ptosis was seen by her primary care physician two weeks ago. Diagnostic work-up revealed a Pancoast tumor in the left upper lobe. The tumor appears to be invading the inferior trunk of the brachial plexus. This is the likely etiology of her upper extremity weakness. Based on the tumor's location in the brachial plexus, what physical exam findings would you expect this patient to have?

   A) Winging of the scapula
   B) Weakness with finger abduction
   C) Weakness with arm abduction
   D) Weakness with elbow flexion
   E) Numbness of the lateral aspect of the forearm

17. Nerve entrapment at Guyon's canal is likely to produce:
   A) Wrist adduction weakness
   B) Wrist flexion weakness
   C) Finger abduction weakness
   D) Thumb abductor weakness
   E) Weakness with flexion of the 4th and 5th DIP's

18. A 67-year-old female fell on some ice while walking into her house. She slipped backward landing on her buttock as well as the palm of her hand. She fell in such a way that her right forearm was supinated and her shoulder, elbow and wrist were extended. Based on the above mechanism of injury, which dysfunction is most likely to be seen in this patient?

   A) Left on Left sacral torsion
   B) Right on Right sacral torsion
   C) Right anterior radial head somatic dysfunction
   D) Right posterior radial head somatic dysfunction
   E) Right adducted ulna

19. Which of the following statements is true regarding the biomechanics of the lower extremity?

    A) Anterior glide of the talus provides talocrural stability
    B) The head of the femur will glide posterior with external rotation of the hip
    C) Patella femoral syndrome has been associated with an increase of the femoral neck angle.
    D) Restriction within the subtalar joint will limit internal and external rotation of the leg while the foot is fixed
    E) Somatic dysfunctions of the ankle most commonly occur when the foot Is dorsiflexed

20. Which of the following statements is true of a left cranial torsion of the sphenobasilar synchondrosis?

    A) The sphenoid rotates about an AP axis so that the left greater wing is inferior
    B) The sphenoid and occiput will rotate in the opposite directions about an AP axis
    C) The sphenoid will rotate left about a vertical axis
    D) The occiput will rotate left about a vertical axis
    E) The sphenoid will rotate anterior about a transverse axis

21. A 16-year-old female is experiencing low, midline, wave-like cramping pelvic pain that occurs with menses. The pain has been present for 3 months and has been getting progressively worse. Pain frequently radiates to her lumbar spine and is associated with frequent nausea. In addition to appropriate oral medications, which osteopathic manipulative technique will most effectively decrease the patient's symptoms by altering sympathetic tone?

    A) Rib raising and paraspinal inhibition to the thoraco-lumbar junction
    B) Celiac ganglion release
    C) Pelvic diaphragm release
    D) Muscle energy to T10
    E) Sacral inhibition

22. A 65-year-old female comes to your office with frequent burning substernal and epigastric pain. The pain is associated with fatty meal intake and is relieved with over the counter anti-acids. The pain has been present for one year but has gotten worse over the past several weeks. Based on the above diagnosis, palpatory changes are likely to arise at which of the following vertebral levels?

    A) C5
    B) T3
    C) T6
    D) T10
    E) T12

23. A 45-year-old diabetic male has chronic renal insufficiency. Structural examination is likely to reveal:

    A) Ropy paraspinals at C3
    B) Severe sharp tenderpoints at T5 and T6
    C) Fibrotic paraspinals T8 and T9
    D) Ropy paraspinals at T10 - L1
    E) Fibrotic tissue texture changes at the sacrum

24. An 88-year-old male with chronic peptic ulcer disease may have changes related to viscerosomatic reflexes in which of the following areas?

    A) T1 - T4
    B) T5 - T7
    C) T9 - T11
    D) T11 - L2
    E) L3 - L5

25. A 29-year-old female in her 36th week of pregnancy is having some leg edema. The most effective initial treatment is?

    A) Pedal pump
    B) Thoracic inlet release
    C) Rib raising to the thoraco-lumbar junction
    D) Place the patient in the Trendelenberg position
    E) Muscle energy to L1 - L3

26. A 36-year-old female complains of abdominal pain that is associated with anorexia, fatigue, and weakness. Physical exam reveals an area of hyperpigmentation in the palmar creases, and sparse axillary hair. Lab results reveal low sodium, and elevated potassium, and calcium levels. At what spinal level would you expect to find tissue texture changes due to a viscerosomatic response from the above condition?

    A) T2
    B) T4
    C) T8
    D) T10
    E) L2

27. Which of the following techniques best evaluates inferior motion of the clavicles at the sternum?
    A) Patient prone, index fingers on the anterior aspect of the clavicular heads near sternum, patient shrugs shoulders
    B) Patient supine, index fingers on the superior aspect of the clavicular heads near sternum, patient depresses the shoulders
    C) Patient supine, index fingers on the superior aspect of the clavicular heads near sternum, patient shrugs shoulders
    D) Patient supine, index fingers on the anterior aspect of the clavicular heads near sternum, patient protracts the shoulders
    E) Patient supine, index fingers on the anterior aspect of the clavicular heads near sternum, patient retracts the shoulders

28. A 63-year-old female fell off a chair and landed on her buttocks. She complains of severe, unrelenting low back pain. There is point tenderness to percussion of the spinous process of L3. A lumbar spine X-ray confirms your diagnosis. The most likely etiology of the pain is:

    A) Tumor
    B) Herniated nucleus pulposus
    C) Cauda equina syndrome
    D) Spinal stenosis
    E) Compression fracture

29. A 34-year-old female complains of dysuria and odd smelling urine. Physical examination reveals suprapubic tenderness. At what spinal levels would you expect to find the tissue texture changes related to a viscerosomatic reflex that would confirm the diagnosis?

    A) T2-T4
    B) T5-T7
    C) T8-T10
    D) T11-L1
    E) L2-L5

30. A patient who recently had a parathyroid adenoma removed should have what spinal level examined for a viscerosomatic reflex?

    A) T1-T3
    B) T5-T6
    C) T7-T9
    D) T10-T12
    E) T12-L2

31. While evaluating a mid thoracic somatic dysfunction, your left thumb is more anterior than your right. Your thumbs become symmetric when the patient is in flexion, however you cannot examine the patient in extension because the pain is too great. The most likely diagnosis is

    A) FR_LS_L
    B) ER_LS_L
    C) NR_RS_L
    D) FR_RS_R
    E) ER_RS_R

32. A patient is diagnosed with a right anterior innominate rotation. About which sacral axis does this rotation occur?

    A) Inferior transverse
    B) Oblique
    C) Middle transverse
    D) Sagittal
    E) Superior transverse

33. A female patient complains of progressively worsening low back pain. The pain is located at the lumbosacral junction. Two days ago, she vaginally delivered a 9lbs. 2oz baby boy. On examination the seated flexion test is negative. The most likely diagnosis is:

    A) Left on left sacral torsion
    B) Bilateral sacral flexion
    C) Right innominate anterior
    D) Bilateral sacral extension
    E) Right inferior pubic shear

34. A patient presents with right forearm and wrist pain after a fall. There are no neurologic deficits. X-ray of the cervical spine and right arm are normal. Physical exam reveals an increased carrying angle on the right, the hand and wrist are adducted and the olecranon process prefers medial glide. The most likely diagnosis is:

    A) Posterior radial head dysfunction
    B) Adduction dysfunction of the ulna
    C) Abduction dysfunction of the ulna
    D) Anterior radial head dysfunction
    E) Medial epicondylitis

35. A patient complains of right leg pain for two days. The patient noticed the pain while running; the pain is located on the leg just below the knee joint on the lateral side. The right fibular head resists anterior springing; the left foot dorsiflexes more than the right. The most likely diagnosis is:

    A) Anterior talar dysfunction on the left
    B) Dorsiflexion dysfunction of the talus on the right
    C) Anterior fibular head dysfunction on the left
    D) Posterior fibular head dysfunction on the right
    E) Posterior fibular head dysfunction on the left

36. A patient with dysmenorrhea would like osteopathic treatment for relief of her pain. Which of the following statements concerning the autonomic nervous system effects on the uterus are true?

    A. Parasympathetic stimulation results in constriction of the uterine fundus.
    B. Parasympathetic stimulation results in relaxation of the cervix.
    C. Parasympathetic stimulation results in relaxation of the uterine fundus.
    D. Sympathetic stimulation results in relaxation of the uterine fundus.
    E. Sympathetic stimulation results in constriction of the cervix.

37. A male complains of right foot pain for several weeks. He remembers having the pain before. The pain is located between the third and fourth metatarsal heads. The pain is described as 8/10 in intensity, and burning in nature. What is the most likely diagnosis?

    A) Hammer toes
    B) Claw toes
    C) Morton's neuroma
    D) Bunion
    E) Corns

Case 38-40

A 33-year-old patient with new onset left-sided low back pain comes into your office. Pain stems from the low back and radiates to the left knee. Structural examination reveals the following:
>   A tenderpoint located at the right transverse process of L5
>   L5 neutral, rotated right and sidebent left
>   Positive seated and standing flexion test on the right
>   Deep right sacral sulcus, Left inferior lateral angle is posterior and inferior
>   Springing at the lumbosacral junction is present
>   PSIS on the right is caudad compared to the left PSIS with the patient in the prone position
>   Apparent shorter leg on the right

38. What is the most likely innominate diagnosis?

    A) Right innominate anterior
    B) Right innominate posterior
    C) Right superior innominate subluxation
    D) Right inferior innominate subluxation
    E) There is not enough information in the question to differentiate from the above

39. What is the accepted muscle energy treatment patient position for the above sacral diagnosis?

    A) Right lateral Sims position
    B) Right lateral recumbent with the torso turned left
    C) Left lateral Sims position
    D) Left lateral recumbent with the torso turned right
    E) Patient prone with right lower extremity slightly abducted

40. The correct typical counterstrain position to treat the above tenderpoint is:

    A) Lumbar flexion
    B) Lumbar extension
    C) Left leg adduction
    D) Left leg abduction
    E) Left lumbar sidebending

Case 41-44

A 67-year-old obese diabetic male comes to the emergency room with severe shortness of breath. He appears slightly anxious. He denies any chest pain. Dyspnea worsens when he lies flat on his back. Dyspnea improves when he is placed in a semi-Fowlers position. He admits to a recent 20lbs weight gain, he has developed swelling of the legs, and has nocturia. He has a history of two myocardial infarctions. On examination, he is 5 foot 8 inches tall and weighs 290 pounds. BP 150/80, HR 105, RR 32 and shallow, Temp. 98.6o. On auscultation, there is an S3 gallop rhythm, rales are present in the lower lung fields, abdominal examination reveals a soft and enlarged liver and grade 4 pretibial edema. EKG demonstrates normal sinus rhythm with no changes when compared to his previous hospital admission's EKG 2 months ago.

41. Which of the following is the most appropriate for initial management of this patient's symptoms in the emergency room?

A) Intravenous furosemide
B) Oxygen, intravenous fluids and cardiac monitoring
C) Oxygen and digitalis
D) Intravenous tissue plasminogen activator
E) Placement of a Swan-Ganz Catheter

42. Treatment of which area would most likely decrease hypersympathetic tone to this patient's heart?

A) Occipito-atlantal joint
B) C4
C) T2
D) T6
E) T7

43. In this patient, treatment of which area would have the greatest effect on renal function?

A) Occipito-atlantal
B) T5
C) T8
D) T11
E) The sacrum

44. Which of the following lymphatic techniques listed would be the most appropriate initial treatment in this patient?

A) Liver pump
B) Abdominal pump
C) Classic thoracic pump
D) Thoracic inlet release
E) Pedal pump

Case 45-48

A 44-year-old female with severe rheumatoid arthritis comes to your office with neck pain. She has a history of chronic neck pain, however recently her pain has increased. She denies any trauma and does not recall any specific event that would cause her neck pain to increase. On examination, she has severely diminished range of motion. Palpation of her cervical paraspinals reveals areas of fibrotic tissue with some tenderness noted in the sub-occipital region. The third cervical segment is sidebent left. Neurologic examination is normal.

45. Which of the following describes an appropriate osteopathic technique for C3?

   A) C3 is sidebent to the left and rotated to the right against the restrictive barrier, the patient then rotates to the left against the physician's counter force for 3-5 seconds, then the physician passively rotates the cervical spine farther to the left.
   B) C3 is sidebent and rotated to the right against the anatomic barrier, the patient then rotates to the left against the physician's counter force for 3-5 seconds, then the physician passively rotates the cervical spine farther to the right.
   C) C3 is sidebent and rotated to the right against the restrictive barrier, the patient then rotates to the left against the physician's counter force for 3-5 seconds, then the physician passively rotates the cervical spine farther to the right.
   D) The patient's neck is sidebent to the left and rotated to the left, a high velocity, low amplitude right rotational thrust is applied to the third cervical segment.
   E) The patient's neck is sidebent and rotated to the right, a high velocity, low amplitude right sidebending thrust is applied to the third cervical segment.

46. What is the theorized neurophysiologic mechanism by which the correct answer in the above question achieves its effect?

   A) The Golgi tendon organs senses a change in tension from the isometric muscle contraction, this causes a reflex relaxation of the agonist muscle fibers. Therefore, by reflex relaxation of the agonist muscle, the physician is then able to passively stretch the patient to the new restrictive barrier.
   B) Contracting the agonist muscle causes local prostaglandin release; this produces a localized muscle relaxation and analgesia.
   C) Contracting the antagonistic muscle, signals are transmitted to the spinal cord and through the reciprocal inhibition reflex arc; the agonist muscle is then forced to relax.
   D) An HVLA thrust is thought to forcefully stretch a contracted muscle producing a barrage of afferent impulses from the muscle spindles to the central nervous system. The central nervous system reflexively sends inhibitory impulses to the muscle spindle to relax the muscle.
   E) An HVLA thrust is thought to forcefully stretch the contracted muscle pulling on its tendon, activating the Golgi tendon receptors and reflexively relaxing the muscle.

47. In addition to osteopathic treatment, patient education, and a short course of physical therapy, you decide to prescribe a non-steroidal anti-inflammatory medication. A significant concern regarding long-term use of this medication is:

   A) Osteoporosis
   B) Upper gastrointestinal bleed
   C) Diverticulitis
   D) Irreversible hepatocellular toxicity
   E) Renal failure

Question #48 refers to the case on the previous page

48. Complications from the adverse effect in the previous question can be avoided by?

A) Yearly bone densiometry
B) Concomitant use of misoprostol
C) Yearly colonscopy
D) Frequent monitoring of liver enzymes
E) Frequent monitoring of blood urea nitrogen and serum creatinine

Case 49-51

A 54-year-old nurse complains of paresthesias in her left hand. She describes intermittent numbness that worsens while sleeping. Ibuprofen improves her symptoms. She has difficulty handling small objects and buttoning shirts. On examination, she has decreased sensation on the palmar aspect of her second and third digit when compared to the fifth digit. There is mild atrophy of the left thenar eminence. Tenderpoints are present in the left anterior scalene. The first rib on the left has limited exhalation movement. The lower cervical segments are restricted in left sidebending.

49. The primary reason for treating the cervical somatic dysfunction in the above patient is?

A) To remove possible sites of additional neurologic compression and improve brachial plexus function
B) To improve lymphatic drainage from the upper extremity thus decreasing distal nerve compression
C) To improve vascular drainage from the upper extremity thus decreasing distal nerve compression
D) To decrease sympathetic tone in the upper extremity
E) Due to the distal site of injury in this patient, treatment of the axial spine will not further decrease this patient's symptoms.

50. Treatment to which structure will result in the greatest reduction of excessive autonomic tone in the upper extremity?

A) The occiput
B) C3
C) C7
D) T3
E) T9

51. Which of the following studies is considered the gold standard for diagnosis of the above condition?

A) Magnetic resonance imaging
B) Arteriography
C) Plain x-ray
D) Nerve conduction studies/Electromyography
E) Bone scan

Case 52-56

A 30-year-old athletic male presents to your office complaining of low back pain. He states that the pain started soon after playing baseball. The pain is localized to his low back. He denies any radiation of pain, paresthesias or weakness in the lower extremities. There is no previous history of low back pain. Physical exam reveals no focal neurologic deficits. X-rays of the lumbar spine are normal. There is marked spasm of the paraspinal musculature on the right. There appears to be a group dysfunction from L1-L5 that is markedly rotated right and sidebent left. There is a positive seated flexion test on the right, and the right sulcus is deeper.

52. Which of the following is the most likely diagnosis?

    A) Lumbar spinal stenosis
    B) Cauda equina syndrome
    C) Acute lumbar strain
    D) Herniated nucleus pulposus
    E) Spondylolisthesis

53. If the patient had reported decreased sensation on the medial aspect of the ankle, absent patellar reflex and marked weakness of ankle dorsiflexion and knee extension, what would the most likely diagnosis be?

    A) Spondylolisthesis
    B) Lumbar spinal stenosis
    C) Herniated nucleus pulposus
    D) Acute lumbar strain
    E) None of the above are likely diagnoses

54. If the above patient had a sacral torsion present, based on the above findings what is the most likely diagnosis?

    A) Left torsion on Right oblique axis
    B) Right torsion on Left oblique axis
    C) Left torsion on Left oblique axis
    D) Right torsion on Right oblique axis
    E) Cannot determine based on the limited information

55. The patient is found to have a tenderpoint 1cm lateral to the pubic symphysis on the right superior pubic ramus. This tenderpoint correlates to somatic dysfunction of which vertebra?

    A) L1
    B) L2
    C) L3
    D) L4
    E) L5

56. Which of the following is the correct treatment position for the above tenderpoint?

    A) Patient prone, right knee and hip extended, rotated to contralateral side
    B) Patient prone, knees and extended, rotated to ipsilateral side
    C) Patient left lateral recumbent position, right knee flexed, hips extended
    D) Patient supine, left knee and hip flexed, sidebent and rotated to ipsilateral side
    E) Patient supine, both knees flexed and hips flexed to about 90 degrees

Case 57-61

A 34-year-old female enters your office complaining of hip pain following a fall off of a stepladder 4 days earlier. X-rays taken in the emergency department revealed no fracture, and the patient has been very uncomfortable since the fall. The pain is localized on the left, and does not radiate down the thigh. The left ASIS is cephalad, the left PSIS is caudad and the pubes are level. While performing a standing flexion test, you note that the left PSIS demonstrated greater excursion than the right.

57. Which additional palpatory finding is most likely to be present in this patient?

    A) Resistance to posterior compression of the right ASIS
    B) Backward sacral torsion on a left axis
    C) Longer leg on the right
    D) L5 neutral sidebent left, rotated right.
    E) Exquisite pain upon palpation of the pubic symphysis

58. What is the innominate somatic dysfunction?

    A) Left innominate anterior
    B) Left innominate posterior
    C) Right innominate anterior
    D) Right innominate posterior
    E) Not enough information to determine

59. Which of the following soft tissue dysfunctions is the most likely cause of this innominate dysfunction?

    A) Tight quadriceps
    B) Tight hip adductors
    C) Tight hip abductors
    D) Tight hamstrings
    E) Tight piriformis

60. Which of the following is the best statement regarding typical muscle energy treatment for this innominate dysfunction?

    A) Hip flexors are isometrically contracted to provide the necessary force to correct this dysfunction.
    B) The patient is best treated in a seated position.
    C) The patient is treated with her hip flexed and slightly abducted
    D) Hamstrings are activated by the patient to correct the dysfunction
    E) Muscle energy treatment is relatively contraindicated in the above patient

61. If a right-sided psoas syndrome is suspected in this patient, which lumbar dysfunction is likely to be present?

    A) L1 Neutral sidebent left and rotated right
    B) L2 Extended, sidebent left and rotated left
    C) L1 Flexed, sidebent right and rotated right
    D) L2 Flexed, sidebent left and rotated left
    E) L4 Neutral sidebent right rotated left.

Case 62-65

You are examining a 29-year-old male presenting to the emergency room complaining of right-sided flank pain. The pain is intermittent, excruciating and radiates to the right testicle.

<u>Physical exam reveals</u>:
   Vitals:
      Temp: 98.60F, Heart Rate: 105 Respiratory Rate: 20 Blood pressure 140/90 Pain: 10/10

<u>Abdomen</u>: There is no rebound tenderness or signs of peritoneal irritation. There is costovertebral angle tenderness on the right.

<u>Laboratory data</u>:
   Urinalysis: RBC's: too numerous to count, small leukocytes, nitrite negative. The CBC is normal.

<u>Radiological data</u>:
   KUB demonstrates a 6 mm well circumscribed radio-opaque mass approximately 10 cm superior to the middle of the right pubic ramus. IVP confirms the presence and location of the stone with severe hydronephrosis.

62. Which of the following is true regarding osteopathic treatment for the above patient?

   A) All osteopathic treatment is absolutely contraindicated in the above patient, until the patient's pain is controlled.
   B) Due to the patient's excruciating pain, osteopathic treatment should be limited to gentle techniques such as rib raising and paraspinal inhibition only.
   C) High velocity thrust to the thoraco-lumbar junction will decrease ureterospasm via a CNS inhibitory reflex.
   D) Pain would decrease with the treatment of a posterior tenderpoint.
   E) Post-isometric relaxation muscle energy is indicated.

63. Which of the following soft tissue dysfunctions has been specifically associated with ureterolithiasis?

   A) Psoas spasm
   B) Abdominal rectus spasm
   C) Piriformis tenderpoint
   D) Paraspinal spasm
   E) Quadratus lumborum spasm

64. What is the primary reason for treating the thoraco-lumbar junction in the above patient?

   A) To decrease this patients pain
   B) To increase function of the contralateral kidney
   C) To decrease ureterospasm and increase glomerular filtration rate
   D) To decrease bladder spasm
   E) To decrease this patient's blood pressure

65. What is the most likely composition of the mass in the KUB?

   A) Struvite
   B) Uric acid
   C) Calcium oxalate
   D) Cystine
   E) Bile pigment

Case 66-70

A 63-year-old-male with COPD is complaining of right shoulder and arm pain. The patient has noticed that the pain gets worse during exacerbation of his COPD, especially, when he has difficulty breathing. Physical examination reveals bilateral rhonchi with decreased breath sounds. Weakness and paresthesias of the right arm and a diminished right radial pulse occur when the right arm is abducted, extended and the patient turns his head to the right side. There is hypertrophy of respiratory accessory muscles and no lymphadenopathy noted. EKG showed a right axis deviation, low voltage complexes, and poor R wave progression. Chest, cervical spine and right shoulder X-rays are negative.

66. The most likely diagnosis is:

    A) Myocardial infarction
    B) Cervical disk herniation
    C) Cervical radiculopathy
    D) Pancoast's tumor
    E) Thoracic outlet syndrome

67. The most likely etiology of the pain is:

    A) Cervical rib
    B) Ischemic myocardium
    C) Hypertrophied scalene muscles
    D) Herniated nucleus pulposus
    E) Shoulder dislocation

68. The most appropriate treatment for the pain would be:

    A) Muscle energy treatment of the first rib
    B) HVLA treatment of the cervical rib
    C) Reduction of the shoulder
    D) Counterstrain treatment of the scalene muscles
    E) Morphine and nitrates

69. At what spinal level would you expect to find tissue texture changes related to this patient's COPD?

    A) C0-C2
    B) T2-T6
    C) T7-T10
    D) T11-L2
    E) L3-L5

70. The increased sympathetic tone would cause which of the following in a COPD patient?

    A) Thinning of secretions
    B) Bronchoconstriction
    C) Thickening of secretions
    D) Decreased tissue congestion
    E) Vasodilatation of the pulmonary vasculature

Case 71-73

The mother of a 3 year-old female complains that her child limps when she walks. Originally, she thought that her daughter had foot pain because she had worn new shoes. After a thorough inspection of the feet, the mother found that the pain was located in her left hip. Her daughter has also had a runny nose for seven days without a fever. Physical examination reveals a playful child with a limp that favors the right side. Hips have full range of motion bilaterally but the child guards all motion of the left hip. There are no neurologic deficits noted. Laboratory tests and X- rays of the hip are normal.

71. What is the most likely diagnosis?

    A) Septic arthritis
    B) Legg-Calve Perthes disease
    C) Slipped capital femoral epiphysis
    D) Developmental dislocation of the hip
    E) Transient synovitis of the hip

72. Which treatment will help decrease the symptoms associated with the above condition?

    A) Antibiotics
    B) Corticosteroids
    C) Non-steroidal anti-inflammatory drugs
    D) Surgical fixation
    E) Hip manipulation

73. The most likely etiology for the above condition is:

    A) Idiopathic
    B) Bacterial
    C) Developmental
    D) Viral
    E) Obesity

Case 74-76

A 53-year-old male complains of chronic pyrosis and regurgitation after meals for several years. The patient has been taking antacids and over-the-counter famotidine, but they are no longer relieving his symptoms. The patient admits to drinking five to six beers and four cups of coffee a day, and smoking half a pack of cigarettes a day.

74. These symptoms are typical of:

A) Dyspepsia
B) GERD
C) Peptic ulcer disease
D) Zollinger-Ellison syndrome
E) Mallory Weiss syndrome

75. Chronic pyrosis and regurgitation would most likely cause paraspinal tissue texture changes from a viscerosomatic reflex at which spinal level?

A) C3-C6
B) T1-T4
C) T3-T8
D) T10-T11
E) L1-L3

76. Treatment of the anterior Chapman reflex point for this patient's hyperacidity would be directed just lateral to the sternum at the interspace of:

A) Ribs 4 and 5 on the left side
B) Ribs 5 and 6 on the right side
C) Ribs 5 and 6 on the left side
D) Ribs 6 and 7 on the right side
E) Ribs 6 and 7 on the left side

Case 77-78

A 24-year-old female presents for a routine physical examination. While assessing her posture from the side you observe that an imaginary plum line dropped from the ceiling to the floor would fall posterior to the apex of the coronal suture, through the external meatus, through most of the bodies of the cervical vertebrae, through the shoulder joint, through the bodies of the lumbar vertebrae, just posterior to the axis of the hip, slightly anterior to the axis of the knee joint and slightly anterior to the lateral malleolus.

77. Which of the following best describes this patient's posture

    A) Military posture
    B) Swayback posture
    C) Ideal posture
    D) Flat back posture
    E) Anterior postural deviation

78. A week later, the patient returns with low back pain. Her head is now located forward of the plum line. She has a slight increase in her cervical lordosis. Her thoracic spine is slightly kyphotic in the upper segments with a flattening of the lumbar spine. Her lumbar vertebrae are straightened and have moved posterior relative to the plum line. Which of the following best describes this patient's new posture?

    A) Military posture
    B) Swayback posture
    C) Posterior postural deviation
    D) Flat back posture
    E) Anterior postural deviation

Case 79-82

A patient complains of neck pain. After a thorough exam you find that there are several muscles in spasm. The most painful muscle originates from the transverse processes of the cervical vertebra and inserts onto rib 1.

79. Which muscle is it?

    A) Platysma
    B) Longus colli
    C) Posterior scalene
    D) Sternocleidomastoid
    E) Anterior scalene

80. A tenderpoint is located 2cm lateral to the medial end of the left clavicle at the attachment of the inserting neck muscle. What is the counterstrain treatment position for this anterior cervical tenderpoint?

    A) Head and neck rotated left, sidebent right
    B) Head and neck rotated right, sidebent right
    C) Head and neck rotated left, sidebent left
    D) Head and neck rotated right, sidebent left
    E) Head and neck rotated right, and flexed

81. Spasm of the muscle in question 79 could result in which one of the following conditions?

    A) 1st rib dysfunction
    B) Left cervical rotation
    C) Second rib elevation
    D) Thoracic outlet syndrome
    E) Torticollis

82. Further examination of the patient reveals that ribs 2 - 6 lag behind with inhalation. What muscle would be used to treat this dysfunction if you used a muscle energy treatment?

    A) Anterior scalene
    B) Middle scalene
    C) Posterior scalene
    D) Pectoralis minor
    E) Serratus anterior

Case 83-84

A patient with low back pain has a right on left sacral torsion.

83. Which of the following is associated with a right on left sacral torsion?

    A) A non-neutral dysfunction of L5 that is rotated left and sidebent left; and a positive seated flexion test on the right
    B) A non-neutral dysfunction of L5 that is rotated right and sidebent right; and a positive seated flexion test on the left
    C) A neutral dysfunction of L5 that is rotated right and sidebent left; and a positive seated flexion test on the right
    D) A neutral dysfunction of L5 that is rotated left and sidebent right; and a positive seated flexion test on the left
    E) A flexed dysfunction of L5 that is rotated right and sidebent right; and a positive seated flexion test on the right

84. Which sacral region in the above dysfunction will spring freely?

    A) Left superior sulcus
    B) Right superior sulcus
    C) Left inferior lateral angle
    D) Right inferior lateral angle
    E) Sacral base

Matching 85-90

Directions: For each numbered item (characteristic) select the one lettered heading (treatment type) most closely associated with it. Each lettered heading may be selected once, more than once, or not at all.

A. Dalrymple pump
B. Galbreath technique
C. Thoracic pump
D. Splenic pump
E. Liver pump

85. Contraindicated in acute hepatitis
86. Increases fluid flow from middle ear structures via the eustachian tube
87. Contraindicated in deep venous thrombosis
88. Indicated for pneumonia
89. Contraindicated in infectious mononucleosis
90. Helps decongest the medial pterygoid plexus

COMLEX A
ANSWERS

COMLEX A Answers

1. Answer C: The radial nerve innervates the extensors of the upper extremity [elbow (triceps), wrist and hand]. An absent triceps (C7) reflex and wrist drop will indicate radial nerve pathology.

The musculocutaneous nerve innervates the biceps, brachialis, and coracobrachialis. A patient with a musculocutaneous nerve injury presents with a loss of the biceps reflex (C5, C6). **Answer A**

The median nerve innervates forearm pronators, wrist and finger flexors and thenar muscles. **Answer B**

The ulnar nerve innervates flexor carpi ulnaris, hypothenar muscles and the adductor pollicis. **Answer D**

The axillary nerve innervates the teres minor and deltoid muscles. Injury to the axillary nerve results in atrophy of the deltoid and weakness with shoulder abduction and flexion. **Answer E**

2. Answer C: The above patient has an acute somatic dysfunction of the lumbar spine. He also herniated one of his lumbar discs. Acute somatic dysfunctions are associated with severe sharp pain (especially with palpation). Acute tissue texture changes are usually described as edematous, erythematous, and boggy. There is increased moisture on the overlying skin and associated hypertonic muscles. The muscle contraction and guarding will cause a limited range of motion of the involved areas.

Answer A did not contain the limited range of motion in the lumbar spine that is consistent with this type of injury. **Answer A**

An acute herniated disc results in decreased reflexes of the effected lower extremity. **Answer B**

This patient likely has a positive straight leg raising test and decreased sensation somewhere on the foot, secondary to a herniated disc. Answers D and E included these findings however, they were coupled incorrectly with descriptors of a chronic somatic dysfunction. Chronic tissue texture changes include cool dry skin; flaccid, doughy, or mushy muscles; and firm, ropy, thickened, fibrotic interstitial tissues. Decreased range of motion is secondary to fibrotic tissues or possibly contractures. **Answers D and E**

3. Answer C: The patient in the above question has L5 flexed, rotated right, and sidebent right. If the spine is extended symmetry is worsened, and L5 will resist left rotation.

A non-neutral L5 dysfunction does not always cause a high lumbar group dysfunction or a right-sided psoas syndrome. **Answers A and B**

Post-isometric relaxation muscle energy technique is an example of a direct technique in which the patient is positioned toward the barrier and is asked to turn away from the barrier. In this case the patient would be positioned with his torso rotated to the left and he would be asked to rotate his torso to the right. **Answer D**

Extending L5 will limit its sidebending to the left, not right. **Answer E**

4. Answer C: The above patient has a lower extremity that is awaiting surgical stabilization. The rhythmic motion of the pedal pump will exert forces at the still unstable fracture site.

There are several different techniques to release the thoraco-abdominal diaphragm. Some are very gentle and can be performed on individuals with several concurrent medical or surgical conditions. **Answer A**

Thoracic rib raising and paraspinal inhibition will not harm the recent surgical site in the cervical spine or the lower extremity fracture. **Answer B**

Although myofascial release and counterstrain would be contraindicated in some areas for the above individual, the modalities are not specifically contraindicated and thus not the best answers. **Answers D and E**

5. Answer E: Vertebral motion around a transverse axis is flexion or extension. So therefore T12 must be either flexed or extended. Vertebral motion in a transverse plane is rotation. So therefore T12 must also be rotated. Understanding Fryette's principles one must conclude if a vertebrae is flexed or extended and rotated it must be sidebent toward the same side.

T12 has restricted motion around a transverse axis, therefore it is flexed or extended, not neutral. **Answer D**

Answers A, B and C only comment on one plane of motion.

6. Answer E: Rotation of the atlas (on the axis) is the AA joint. Flexing the patient's head will lock out rotation of C2 - C7 and will isolate rotation to the AA joint. Since the AA joint is rotated to the left, the patient should be able to turn his head further left than right.

The AA joint will not necessarily affect motion of the occiput on the atlas (OA joint) or C2 on C3. **Answers A, B and C**

Motion at the AA joint will not necessarily cause compensation or somatic dysfunction of the lower cervical units. **Answer D**

7. Answer A: In a patient with a deep left sulcus and a negative lumbosacral spring test the left portion of the sacrum has moved anterior. Since the above patient has a posterior/inferior ILA on the right this indicates that this portion of the sacrum has moved posteriorly. A forward sacral torsion on a right oblique axis (i.e. a right rotation on a right oblique axis) is the only answer that would be consistent with the above findings.

In a forward sacral torsion on a left oblique axis (left on left) the right sulcus would be deeper and the left ILA would be posterior/inferior. **Answer B**

In a backward sacral torsion or a bilateral sacral extension, the lumbosacral spring test would be positive (i.e. the lumbosacral junction would not spring). **Answers C and E**

In a unilateral sacral flexion on the left, the left ILA would be posterior and significantly inferior. **Answer D**

213

8. Answer B: Acute management of asthma includes supplemental oxygen, inhaled bronchodilators (albuterol) and intravenous corticosteroids. Osteopathic techniques that have been used successfully for asthma include the seated thoracic pump technique, CV4 technique, and cervical spine manipulation to normalize the vagus. [35 p.49]

Although the patient did not respond to one treatment of inhaled albuterol, additional doses can be administered every 20 minutes. Oral albuterol is not rocommended if inhaled medications can be administered. [34] **Answer A**

Zafirlukast is an oral leukotriene receptor agonist. It is useful for patients with mild to moderate symptoms, however it's onset of action is delayed for approximately 2 weeks. **Answer C**

Oral corticosteroids may be effective, however the preferred route of administration is IV. The asthmatic patient will usually present with a rib 3 or 4 dysfunction, however, as with most viscero-somatic reflexes, it responds poorly to HVLA. **Answer D**

Cromolyn sodium is a medication that is useful in patients with mild asthma, especially allergic asthma. [34] However, onset of action is delayed several weeks. **Answer E**

9. Answer A: Motion in the transverse plane is rotation. Segmental motion is conventionally defined as the specified segment on the one below. Since rotation is the main motion of the first cervical segment (the AA joint-the atlas on the axis) it has the greatest degree of freedom in the transverse plane.

Motion in the coronal plane is sidebending. **Answer B**

Motion in the sagittal plane is flexion/extension. **Answer C**

The oblique plane is not a true description of a plane. **Answer D**

Vertebral motion in the transverse and coronal planes refer to rotation and sidebending respectively. There is a slight amount of flexion allowed at the atlas, but no sidebending. The AA joint essentially allows rotation only. **Answer E**

10. Answer B: Spinal extension decreases the size of the intervertebral foramina and it decreases the AP diameter of the spinal column. Spinal extension is necessary when treating a typical posterior lumbar tenderpoint. Extension increases pain associated with spinal stenosis, but will not affect the patient with vascular claudication since the patient is at rest.

Sitting flexes the spinal column, thus decreases pain associated with neurogenic claudication. Sitting (resting) will also decrease the symptoms associated with vascular claudication. **Answer A**

Lower extremity weakness is seen in patients with neurogenic claudication, but not in patients with vascular claudication. **Answer C**

Symptoms of lumbar spinal stenosis (pain, numbness and sometimes weakness in the lower extremities) typically increased with extension of the spinal column (standing, walking). Symptoms of peripheral vascular disease, (leg pain and cramping) increases with activity and decreases with rest. Walking produces symptoms in both vascular and neurogenic claudication. **Answer D**

Posterior calf pain is common in both neurogenic and vascular claudication. **Answer E**

11. Answer D: Facet tropism is a misalignment of the facet joint. According to Osteopathic Principles in Practice [28 p.449] it is the most common anomaly of the lumbar spine.

Sacralization occurs in approximately 3.5% of the population. **Answer A**

Lumbarization occurs in <1% of the population. **Answer B**

Facet hypertrophy is not a congenital anomaly. It is a condition often seen with degenerative changes. **Answer C**

Spina bifida occulta occurs in about 10% of the population. **Answer E**

12. Answer A: The above patient has a bilateral sacral extension (a.k.a. sacral base posterior or a posterior sacral base). The examiner will notice that the sacral sulci are equal in depth and there is no springing at the lumbosacral junction (i.e. the lumbosacral spring test is positive). The seated flexion test will be FALSELY negative - Why? Since both SI joints are restricted, asymmetry will not be appreciated.

In a forward sacral torsion (left-on-left or right-on-right) the seated flexion test would be positive, the sulci would appear asymmetric, and the lumbosacral spring test would be negative. **Answer B**

In an anterior sacral base (a.k.a. bilateral sacral flexion or sacral base anterior), the findings will be the same, except that the lumbosacral junction would spring (lumbosacral spring test is negative). **Answer C**

In a unilateral extended sacrum on the right the seated flexion test will be positive on the right, the right sulcus will appear shallow (posterior) and the lumbosacral spring test will be positive. **Answer D**

In a unilateral extended sacrum on the left, the seated flexion test will be positive on the left, the left sulcus will appear shallow (posterior) and the lumbosacral spring test will be positive. **Answer E**

13. Answer C: In a sacral torsion (or sacral rotation on an oblique axis) the seated flexion test is positive on the opposite side of the axis. In this case the right positive seated flexion test indicates a left oblique axis. A positive spring test (a.k.a. lumbosacral spring test) indicates that part of the sacral base has moved posterior. Since the left sacral base is anterior (i.e. the left sulcus is deep), then this must indicate that the right sacral base has moved posterior. Out of all the answers listed the only possible one that would correlate with the above findings is right sacral rotation on a left oblique axis.

In left sacral rotation on a right oblique axis, and right sacral rotation on a right oblique axis there would be a positive seated flexion test on the left. **Answers A and B**

In a right unilateral sacral flexion the right sulcus would be deeper, and the lumbosacral junction would spring freely. **Answer D**

In an extended sacral base the seated flexion test would be falsely negative, and the sulci would appear symmetric. **Answer E**

14. **Answer A**: If a sacral torsion is present, a right sacral base anterior (a deep right sulcus) and a negative lumbosacral spring test indicate a left on left torsion. Using the rules of L5 on the sacrum and Fryette's principles one can figure out the dysfunction of L5.

Rules of L5:
1) When L5 is rotated, the sacrum rotates in the opposite direction.
   - Sacrum rotated left, L5 must be rotated right.
2) When L5 is sidebent, a sacral oblique axis is engaged on the same side as the sidebending.
   - Sacrum has a left oblique axis, L5 must be sidebent left.

Fryette's principle I:
   If L5 is rotated right and sidebent left, L5 must be in the neutral plane (L5 NS$_L$R$_R$).

15. **Answer A:** Right sacral rotation on a right oblique axis. A right sacral rotation on a right oblique axis will result in a deep sacral sulcus on the left, a posterior/inferior ILA on the right, and the lumbosacral junction springs freely upon compression.

A left rotation on a left oblique will result in a deep sacral sulcus on the right and a posterior/inferior ILA on the left. **Answer B**

A right sacral shear can either be a right unilateral sacral flexion or a right unilateral sacral extension. A right unilateral sacral extension will result in a positive lumbosacral spring test. A right unilateral sacral flexion will result in a deep sacral sulcus on the right (not left). **Answer C**

A backward sacral torsion (right-on-left or a left-on-right) will result in a positive lumbosacral spring test (i.e. the lumbosacral junction will not spring freely). **Answers D and E**

16. **Answer B:** The inferior trunk is formed by the C8 and T1 nerve roots. As a result, this will produce weakness with the intrinsic muscles of the hand (interossi) and deep finger flexors. It will also likely produce numbness in the little finger (C8) and medial elbow (T1).

The winging of the scapula is due to injury to the long thoracic nerve, which is formed by the C5 - C7 nerve roots. **Answer A**

The deltoid and supraspinatus is primarily responsible for arm abduction. The supraspinatus (suprascapular nerve) receives innervation from the superior trunk. The deltoid (axillary nerve) receives innervation from posterior cord, specifically from C5 and C6 nerve roots. The axillary nerve does not receive contributions from the inferior portion of the brachial plexus. **Answer C**

Numbness at the lateral aspect of the forearm and elbow flexion (musculocutaneous nerve) would not be affected since it stems from the superior trunk of the brachial plexus. **Answers D and E**

17. **Answer C**: Guyon's (pisohamate) canal is located at the wrist. The medial border is the pisiform bone, lateral border is the hamate, roof is the flexor retinaculum and floor is the pisohamate ligament. [53] [p.315] The ulnar nerve runs through the Guyon's canal. Nerve entrapment would produce weakness in the hypothenar muscles, adductor pollicis, interossi, and 3rd and 4th lumbricals. The interossi are responsible for abduction and adduction of the fingers.

Wrist adductors and wrist flexors originate in the forearm and would not be affected with entrapment at the wrist. **Answer A and B**

The median nerve innervates the abductor pollicis brevis. The radial nerve innervates the abductor pollicis longus. **Answer D**

Weakness with flexion of the 4th and 5th DIP's (ulnar portion of flexor digitorum profundus) would be due to injury to the ulnar nerve proximal to the wrist (most likely at the cubital tunnel). **Answer E**

18. Answer C: The patient has an anterior radial head somatic dysfunction. Radial head somatic dysfunction can often be caused by a fall on an outstretched arm and can result in wrist and elbow pain. Specifically, an anterior radial head somatic dysfunction is usually caused by a fall on an outstretched supinated arm. Supination of the wrist and forearm physiologically causes the radial head to glide anteriorly.

A left on left torsion as well as a right on right torsion can be due to trauma, however "falling on the buttocks" is too nonspecific to indicate either dysfunction. **Answers A and B**

A posterior radial head somatic dysfunction can be due to a fall forward on an outstretched pronated arm. Pronation of the wrist and forearm physiologically causes the radial head to glide posteriorly. At the impact of the fall, the arm is positioned with the shoulder flexed, elbow and wrist extended and the forearm pronated. **Answer D**

Abducted ulna is not associated with trauma from falling backward on an outstretched arm. **Answer E**

19. Answer D: The subtalar joint acts mostly as a shock absorber and allows internal and external rotation of the leg while the foot is fixed. Restriction within this joint will limit this motion.

The talocrural joint (a.k.a. tibiotalar joint) is composed of the articulation of the trochlea of the talus and the ankle mortise. Posterior glide of the talus (dorsiflexion) provides stability to this joint. This joint is relatively unstable in plantar flexion (anterior glide of the talus), and allows the greatest degree of inversion/eversion in this position. **Answer A**

The head of the femur will glide anterior with external rotation of the hip, and posterior with internal rotation of the hip. **Answer B**

It is believed that an increase in the Q angle is associated with patello-femoral syndrome (a.k.a. lateral patella femoral tracking syndrome). Changes in this angle can result in genu valgum or genu varum. Changes in the femoral neck angle are associated with coxa valga and coxa vara. **Answer C**

Somatic dysfunctions of the ankle most commonly occur when the foot is supinated because of the relative instability of the ankle in this position. **Answer E**

20. Answer B: In a cranial torsion of the SBS (which is the same as a cranial torsion- just a different way of saying it) the sphenoid and occiput rotate in opposite directions about an AP axis. Specifically in a left cranial torsion, the sphenoid will rotate so that the left greater wing is superior.

In a left cranial torsion, the sphenoid will rotate so that the left greater wing of the sphenoid is superior, not inferior. **Answer A**

The sphenoid and occiput rotate about vertical axes in lateral strains. **Answers C and D**

The sphenoid will rotate about a transverse axis with flexion and extension phases of the CRI. **Answer E**

21. Answer A: The above patient has signs and symptoms of dysmenorrhea. Pain is produced by uterine vasoconstriction, anoxia, and sustained contractions mediated by prostaglandins. 38 The uterus receives sympathetic innervation from T10 - L2 segments. Rib raising and paraspinal inhibition will decrease sympathetic tone, therefore these techniques will most effectively enhance blood flow and relax the uterus, thus decreasing pain.

The purpose of the celiac ganglion release is to calm sympathetics from T5 - T9. [35 p.227] This technique will not affect autonomic tone to the uterus. **Answer B**

The pelvic diaphragm release will not effectively normalize sympathetic tone in the uterus. **Answer C**

Although manipulative techniques at vertebral levels could alter autonomic function, muscle energy at T10 will not greatly affect sympathetic tone in the uterus because treatment of one segment is less likely to be as effective as compared to treatment of a few levels. **Answer D**

Parasympathetic flow to the uterus originates in the pelvic splanchnic nerves (S2-S4). Treatment directed at the sacrum will influence parasympathetic tone, not sympathetic tone. **Answer E**

22. Answer C: This patient is likely to have a gastric ulcer or GERD. Unlike duodenal ulcers, gastric ulcers symptoms typically worsen after eating. Abnormal stimuli from the gastric mucosa will enter the spinal cord at the T5 - T9 level and facilitate these segments. This may result in abnormal efferents to somatic structures leading to palpatory changes at these levels.

Since C5 is not closely associated with autonomic innervation to the upper GI tract. **Answer A**

Efferents from T3 affects sympathetic tone in the heart, lung and head. **Answer B**

In the GI system T10 - T11 is associated with sympathetic tone in portions of the duodenum and the pancreas, jejunum, ileum and proximal 2/3 of transverse colon. **Answer D**

In the GI system T12 - L2 is associated with sympathetic tone in the distal 1/3 of the transverse colon and rectum. **Answer E**

23. Answer D: Renal insufficiency has been associated with tissue texture changes at the thoraco-lumbar junction. [35 p.129] Key terms that describe chronic tissue texture changes are ropy and fibrotic.

The parasympathetics, which supply the kidney and upper ureter, originate from the vagus nerve and are influenced by the occiput, C1 and C2, not C3. Although it is not known how the parasympathetics affect the kidney, they do maintain normal peristaltic waves in the ureters. [35 p.126] **Answer A**

T5 and T6 are not segmentally related to the kidney. **Answer B**

Sympathetic fibers arising from T8 - T9 do not supply the kidney. **Answer C**

Parasympathetics from the pelvic splanchnic supply the lower ureter and bladder. **Answer E**

24. Answer B: Sympathetic control for the upper GI tract is via T5 - T9 visceral efferents. Abnormal stimuli from visceral afferents enter the spinal cord, sensitize interneurons and produce an exaggerated motor response (a process called facilitation) at these segments.

Head and neck = T1 - T4. **Answer A**

T9 - L2 = left colon and pelvic structures. **Answers C and D**

L3 - L5 = Nothing!!! **Answer E**

25. Answer B: Prior to lymphatic pumping techniques, the thoracic inlet should be released to remove any impedance into the thoracic duct and ultimately the central circulation.

The thoracic inlet should be released first before a lymphatic pump is attempted. **Answer A**

Edema in the lower extremities is due to the mechanical effect of the uterus and abdominal contents pushing against the inferior vena cava. Rib raising to the thoraco-abdominal junction will normalize sympathetics, but in the above case sympatheticonia (increased sympathetic tone) is not the cause of the edema. **Answer C**

Placing the patient in the Trendelenberg position will increase the pressure against the diaphragm and may make the patient short of breath. Therefore, it is not appropriate. **Answer D**

Muscle energy will do little to improve this patient's lower extremity edema. **Answer E**

26. Answer D: This patient has Addison's disease, which is a disease of the adrenal gland and would cause a viscerosomatic response at T10. [35 p.192]

T2 and T4 receive sympathetic innervation from the head and neck, heart esophagus and lungs, not the adrenal medulla. **Answers A and B**

T8 would receive sympathetic innervation for the upper GI tract. **Answer C**

L2 would receive innervation from the lower GI tract, uterus and cervix, penis, clitoris and legs. **Answer E**

27. Answer C: The clavicle moves in three different planes. First, it moves superior and inferior with shrugging and depressing the shoulder. Second, it moves anterior and posterior with retraction and protraction of the shoulder. Third, it rotates anteriorly and posteriorly with internal and external rotation of the arm when it is abducted at 90°. [28 p.163] Shrugging the shoulder causes the lateral end of the clavicle to move superior, this causes the medial end to move inferior, via a "see-saw" motion. This motion is easily observed with the patient in the supine position.

The clavicle cannot be properly evaluated in the prone position. **Answer A**

Patient supine, index fingers on the superior aspect of the clavicular head near sternum, patient depresses the shoulders. This will move the clavicle superior at the sternum, if no somatic dysfunction is present. **Answer B**

Patient supine, index fingers on the anterior aspect of the clavicular head near sternum, patient protracts the shoulders. This will move the clavicle posterior at the sternum, if no somatic dysfunction is present. **Answer D**

Patient supine, index fingers on the anterior aspect of the clavicular head near sternum, patient retracts the shoulders. This will move the clavicle anterior at the sternum, if no somatic dysfunction is present. **Answer E**

28. **Answer E**: This is the classic presentation of a compression fracture. The key findings are spinous process point tenderness to percussion with confirmation on X-ray. X-rays primarily identify bony and some soft tissue problems.

A tumor would usually be painless, not result from trauma, and it is unlikely to be visible on X-ray unless it obscures a structure or displaces it. **Answer A**

Herniated nucleus pulposus and cauda equina syndrome would not be visible on X-ray, and do not fit the case history. **Answers B and C**

Spinal stenosis would be visible on X-ray, but pain is not usually localized to the spinous process, or elicited with percussion of the spinous process. **Answer D**

29. **Answer D**: This patient most likely has a urinary tract infection, and would have tissue texture changes from a viscerosomatic reflex at T11-L1.

T2-T4 receives sympathetic innervation from the head and neck. **Answer A**

T5-T7 receives sympathetic innervation from the upper GI tract. **Answer B**

T8-T10 receives sympathetic innervation from the upper and middle GI tract. **Answer C**

The spinal cord stops at L2; therefore the lowest possible segment to receive sympathetic innervation is L2. **Answer E**

30. **Answer A**: The parathyroid glands are structures in the neck, and could have caused viscerosomatic reflex changes at the spinal level T1-T4.

T5-T6 spinal levels are associated with the viscerosomatic reflex from the heart, lungs and esophagus. **Answer B**

T7-T9 spinal levels are associated with the viscerosomatic reflex from the upper GI tract. **Answer C**

T10-T12 spinal levels are associated with the viscerosomatic reflex from the middle GI tract and the gonads. **Answer D**

T12-L2 spinal levels are associated with the lower GI tract. **Answer E**

31. **Answer D**: Flexed, rotated right, sidebent right is the correct diagnosis. On the board exams it may be abbreviated as FR_RS_R. The static evaluation in the neutral position shows that the left thumb is more anterior, which means the segment is rotated right. Since the asymmetry at the segment resolved with flexion, the freedoms of motion are flexion, right rotation and left sidebending.

In a FR$_L$S$_L$ (flexed rotated left, sidebent left) somatic dysfunction your left thumb would be posterior, not anterior. **Answer A**

In an ER$_L$S$_L$ (extended rotated left, sidebent left) somatic dysfunction your left thumb would be posterior, not anterior, and symmetry would be restored in extension. **Answer B**

In a NR$_R$S$_L$ (neutral, rotated right, sidebent left) somatic dysfunction symmetry would not be restored in flexion. **Answer C**

In an ER$_R$S$_R$ (extended, rotated right sidebent right) somatic dysfunction symmetry would be restored in extension. **Answer E**

32. Answer A: The innominates rotate about an inferior transverse sacral axis with ambulation, and in posterior and anterior innominate somatic dysfunctions.

Sacral rotation occurs about 2 oblique axes with ambulation and with sacral torsions. **Answer B**

Postural motion occurs about a middle transverse sacral axis. **Answer C**

Sacral margin somatic dysfunctions rotate about a vertical axis. **Answer D**

Respiration and craniosacral motion occur about the superior transverse sacral axis. **Answer E**

33. Answer B: A bilateral sacral flexion occurs during the delivery phase of childbirth when the sacrum nutates (sacral base moves anteriorly) to allow more space for the fetus to pass through the pelvic outlet into the birth canal. If the sacrum fails to counternutate (sacral base moves posteriorly), a bilaterally sacral flexion dysfunction remains. Due to birth mechanics, bilateral sacral flexion is a common dysfunction in the post-partum patient. [56 p.781] Since the sacrum is bilaterally flexed it would cause a falsely negative seated flexion test.

A left on left sacral torsion would have a positive seated flexion test on the right. **Answer A**

Right innominate anterior and a right inferior pubic shear are not specifically associated with childbirth. **Answers C and E**

A bilateral sacral extension would have a falsely negative seated flexion test. However, it has not been specifically associated with childbirth. **Answer D**

34. Answer C: This is the presentation of an abduction dysfunction of the ulna.

A posterior radial head dysfunction would cause the forearm to prefer pronation, and the radial head would resist anterior glide. This dysfunction is caused by falling on a pronated forearm. The carrying angle is not affected in radial head dysfunctions. **Answer A**

An adducted dysfunction of the ulna would have a decreased carrying angle, the hand and wrist would be abducted and the olecranon process would prefer lateral glide. **Answer B**

An anterior radial head dysfunction would cause the forearm to prefer supination and the radial head would resist posterior glide. Falling backward on a supinated forearm can cause this dysfunction. **Answer D**

Medial epicondylitis (also known as golfer's elbow) is a strain of the flexor muscles of the forearm near the medial epicondyle. It is associated with pain at the medial epicondyle; it is not associated with a change in the carrying angle. **Answer E**

35. Answer D: In a posterior fibular head dysfunction the foot will prefer supination and the proximal fibular head will resist springing anteriorly. Since there is pain in the right leg, pain can be used as the indicator of laterality or sidedness of the dysfunction in the extremities.

An anterior talar dysfunction is associated with resistance to posterior glide, a foot that prefers plantar flexion and has restriction to dorsiflexion. **Answer A**

An posterior talar dysfunction is associated with resistance to anterior glide, a foot that prefers dorsiflexion and has restriction to plantar flexion. **Answer B**

In an anterior fibular head dysfunction the foot prefers pronation. The proximal fibular head will resist springing posteriorly. In addition, the patient's history does not indicate a problem with the left foot. **Answer C**

In a posterior fibular head dysfunction the foot will prefer supination. The proximal fibular head will resist springing anteriorly. The patient had pain in the right leg, indicating it was a right-sided dysfunction, not left. **Answer E**

36. Answer C: Parasympathetic stimulation of the uterus causes relaxation of the fundus and constriction of the cervix. **Answers A and B**

Sympathetic stimulation of the uterus causes constriction of the fundus and relaxation of the cervix. **Answers D, and E**

37. Answer C: Morton's neuroma is a fibroneuromatous reaction between the heads of the third and fourth metatarsals. [25 p. 336] Pain is present at the forefoot at the site of the neuroma it is often accompanied with dysesthesia or burning plantar pain. [32 p.455]

A hammer toe is a condition in which the proximal interphalangeal (PIP) joint is hyperflexed. Typically there is an obvious deformity and the patient may have pain at the PIP when wearing shoes. [32 p.447] **Answer A**

Claw toe is a fixed flexion deformity of the proximal interphalangeal joints associated with hyperextension of the metatarsophalangeal articulations. All toes, especially the lesser toes, tend to be effected. [32 p.408] **Answer B**

A bunion, also called hallux valgus, is a lateral deviation of the proximal phalanx of the first toe associated with soft tissue changes, pain, swelling, and inflammation at the aspect of the head of the first metatarsal, which is angled medially. **Answer D**

Soft corns are hyperkeratotic lesions found between the toes, usually the fourth and fifth toes; they are extremely painful. Hard corns are associated with hammer or claw toes. [25 p. 337] **Answer E**

Case 38-40

38. Answer B: In a right posterior innominate the standing flexion test is positive on the right, the right ASIS is cephalad, the right PSIS is caudad and there is a relative short leg on the right.

In an anterior rotated innominate the PSIS on the right would be cephalad compared to the left PSIS. **Answer A**

In a right superior innominate subluxation (a.k.a. innominate upslip, superior innominate shear [56, 33]) the right leg would be shorter and the right PSIS would be cephalad. **Answer C**

In a right inferior innominate subluxation (a.k.a. innominate downslip, inferior innominate shear [56, 33]) the right PSIS would be caudad and the right leg would appear longer. **Answer D**

There is enough information provided to choose one of the above diagnoses. **Answer E**

39. Answer C: The patient in the above question has a left on left sacral torsion. The accepted muscle energy treatment position of the patient is the left lateral Sims position. [56 p.899, 33 p.203] In this position the patient is lying in the left lateral recumbent position and the torso is turned to the left so the patient is lying face down.

The right lateral Sims position would be used to treat a right on right sacral torsion. [56 p.899, 33p.203] **Answer A**

The right lateral recumbent position with the torso turned left would be used to treat a left on right sacral torsion. [56 p.899] **Answer B**

The left lateral recumbent position with the torso turned right would be used to treat a right on left sacral torsion. [56 p.899] **Answer D**

This position could be used to treat a sacral shear. [1 p.735] **Answer E**

40. Answer B: According to Yates [26 p.106] the typical treatment position for a tenderpoint at the transverse process of L5 is lumbar extension, sidebending away with rotation either toward or away. Jones just specifies lumbar extension. [40 p.71]

Case 41-44

41. Answer A: Treatment of acute congestive heart failure includes oxygen and IV furosemide. Nitroglycerine, which also can be used, is a venodilator that can potentiate the effect of furosemide. Other agents include morphine (reduces anxiety and dilates pulmonary and systemic veins [34 p.120]) and nitroprusside (a useful adjunct in the treatment of CHF due to acute valvular regurgitation or hypertension).

Although oxygen and cardiac monitoring would be wise choices, additional intravenous fluids will worsen his congestive heart failure, the goal of initial treatment would be to remove excess fluid. **Answer B**

Digitalis is useful in the long-term management of heart failure. It is not typically used in the treatment of acute congestive heart failure. **Answer C**

Thrombolytic therapy (tissue plasminogen activator) is not used in congestive heart failure. **Answer D**

Placing a Swan-Ganz Catheter may be helpful in cases in which a prompt response to therapy does not occur. [34] **Answer E**

42. **Answer C:** The sympathetic innervation to the heart generally stems from T1 - T5. Treatment to this area may decrease sympathetic tone in this patient.

The OA (atlanto-occipital) joint has a direct influence on the function of the vagus nerve (parasympathetic innervation to the heart). Therefore treatment of the OA (atlanto-occipital) joint may alter parasympathetic tone to the heart. **Answer A**

Manipulation of the cervical spinal segments near the cervical chain ganglia may influence sympathetic tone to head and neck structures, not the heart. **Answer B**

Although some texts list T6 as a level for sympathetic influence to the heart, not all texts agree. However, they all do agree on T2, therefore T6 is not the best answer. **Answer D**

T7 is not considered to have sympathetic influence to the heart. **Answer E**

43. **Answer D:** The kidneys receive sympathetic innervation from segments T10 - T11. Therefore, treatment of these segments would be most likely to decrease excessive sympathetic tone to the kidneys. This will improve the glomerular filtration rate and increase urinary output.

Although the occipito-atlantal joint will influence the vagus nerve, it is not known how the parasympathetic nervous system affects the kidney. **Answer A**

The kidney does not receive sympathetic innervation from T5 or T8. **Answers B and C**

Although treatment of the sacrum will influence the pelvic splanchnic nerve, the kidney does not receive innervation from the pelvic splanchnic nerve. **Answer E**

44. **Answer D:** As a general rule, it is best to release any diaphragms, especially the thoracic inlet, prior to starting any pumping techniques. Once the diaphragms are free of restriction and sympathetic tone is normalized, lymphatic pumps will help return lymph through open channels.

Case 45-48
45. **Answer C:** This is an example of direct muscle energy using post-isometric relaxation technique.

Sidebending and rotation in the third cervical segment are always toward the same side (type II mechanics). When positioning a patient for a muscle energy technique, C3 should be sidebent and rotated toward the same side. **Answer A**

C3 is sidebent and rotated to the right against the restrictive (not anatomic) barrier, the patient then rotates to the left against the physician's counter force for 3-5 seconds, then the physician passively rotates the cervical spine farther to the right. **Answer B**

Since the patient has severe rheumatoid arthritis HVLA is relatively contraindicated and therefore it is not the most appropriate technique. In addition, the patient is not correctly positioned for an HVLA technique in answers D and E. **Answers D and E**

46. **Answer A:** This correctly describes the neurophysiologic mechanism of the post-isometric relaxation type of muscle energy.

Prostaglandins are not released with active muscle contraction and do not result in local muscle relaxation. Prostaglandins typically cause pain and inflammation; some anti-inflammatory medications block the release of prostaglandins. **Answer B**

This correctly describes the neurophysiologic mechanism of the reciprocal inhibition type of muscle energy, not the post-isometric relaxation type of muscle energy. **Answer C**

There are two theories by which HVLA is thought to achieve its effects. They are described by choices D and E. **Answers D and E**

47. **Answer B:** NSAID-associated gastropathy is one of the most prevalent serious drug toxicities in the United States. Approximately 1 - 2% of patients using NSAIDS for three months and approximately 2 - 5% of patients using NSAIDS for one year have gastrointestinal ulcers, bleeding or perforation. [42 p. 424]

NSAID use has not been linked to osteoporosis or diverticulitis. Although long term use of corticosteroids will lead to osteoporosis. **Answers A and C**

NSAIDS have been linked with reversible hepatocellular toxicity. Liver enzymes usually revert to normal after the drug is discontinued. As a result, it is recommended that liver enzymes are checked periodically in patients on long term NSAIDS. [42 p. 425] **Answer D**

NSAIDS may increase serum creatinine concentrations in some patients. However, renal failure is uncommon in patients without underlying renal impairment. **Answer E**

48. **Answer B:** In a double blind, randomized, placebo-controlled study 51 misoprostol decreased serious gastrointestinal complications by 40%.

Since NSAID use has not been linked to osteoporosis or diverticulitis, yearly bone densitometry or yearly colonoscopy will not prevent NSAID induced complications. **Answers A and C**

NSAIDS have been associated with reversible (not irreversible) hepatocellular toxicity and renal failure is uncommon; therefore these are not the best answers. However, it is recommended that a complete blood count, liver function tests, renal function as well as stool guiac testing be done every 4 months in patients on long term NSAIDS. [42 p.169] **Answers D and E**

Case 49-51

49. **Answer A:** The above patient has carpal tunnel syndrome. Osteopathic treatment for carpal tunnel syndrome includes: [1 p.560]

1. Treating rib and upper thoracic somatic dysfunctions to decrease sympathetic tone in the upper extremity.
2. Treating cervical somatic dysfunctions and myofascial restrictions to enhance brachial plexus function and remove potential sites of additional compression.
3. Treating the carpal tunnel with direct release techniques to increase the space in the carpal tunnel.

50. Answer D: The above patient has carpal tunnel syndrome (CTS). This condition is due to a compression of the median nerve, usually at the transverse carpal ligament. However, cervical or rib dysfunction as well as anterior scalene hypertonicity may further complicate CTS. Ipsilateral upper thoracic and rib dysfunction will result in increased upper extremity sympathetic tone producing arm and hand symptoms. Decreasing sympathetic tone is an integral part of OMT treatment for CTS. The upper thoracic segments (specifically T2 - T8) supply sympathetics to the upper extremity.

Sympathetic innervation arises from the thoracic and lumbar regions. Treatment of the occiput, C3, and C7 will not alter the sympathetic tone in the upper extremity. **Answers A, B and C**

T9 is a segment that generally receives sympathetic fibers from structures below the diaphragm. **Answer E**

51. Answer D: Nerve conduction studies/electromyography is considered to be the gold standard for the diagnosis of carpal tunnel syndrome. Nerve conduction studies will identify if there has been any damage to the myelin or axon of the median nerve. Electromyography will identify if this damage is severe enough to cause denervation of the distal muscles innervated by the median nerve.

Other studies listed have essentially no role in the diagnosis of carpal tunnel syndrome. **Answers A, B, C and E**

Case 52-56

52. Answer C: An acute lumbar strain is low back pain without focal neurological deficits. The pain may be sharp or dull, and usually localized to the low back, although it may radiate in a non-dermatomal type of fashion.

Spinal stenosis is a chronic joint disease characterized by slowly developing joint pain, usually resulting from intervertebral narrowing, foraminal encroachment and/or spinal canal compression. Often this occurs in elderly patients and the neurologic examination will reveal some deficits. **Answer A**

Cauda equina syndrome is compression of the distal spinal cord. This will result in paresthesias and weakness as well as incontinence. **Answer B**

A herniated nucleus pulposus (herniated disc) will often result in neurologic deficits therefore making this a less likely diagnosis. **Answer D**

Spondylolisthesis is a forward slippage of the lumbar vertebrae. Radiographic findings in this patient are normal making this an unlikely diagnosis. **Answer E**

53. Answer C: Herniated nucleus pulposus. A herniated disc at L4 will result in the decreased sensation, the decreased deep tendon reflexes and lower extremity weakness described.

Radiographic findings on the patient were normal making spondylolisthesis unlikely. **Answer A**

Spinal stenosis is usually due to intervertebral narrowing and degenerative joint disease. Although neurological deficits are common, spinal stenosis is usually seen in the elderly population. **Answer B**

Neurologic exam is negative in acute lumbar strains. **Answer D**

54. Answer C: In sacral torsions, specific L5 findings are present. L5 will influence the sacrum in the following ways: if L5 is rotated, the sacrum will rotate in the opposite way on an oblique axis. If L5 is sidebent, the sacral oblique axis is engaged on the same side. Since the patient's L5 was NS_LR_R, the sacrum is rotated left on a left oblique axis. If the reader is not aware of these "rules of sacral torsions", then the palpatory finding and seated flexion test are still consistent with a left on left sacral torsion.

55. Answer E: Anterior lumbar tenderpoints are located around the pelvis. L5 is located approximately 1 cm lateral to the pubic symphysis on the superior rami.

L2, L3 and L4 tenderpoints are located near the AIIS. **Answers B, C and D**

L1 tenderpoint is located medial to the ASIS. **Answer A**

56. Answer E: An anterior L5 somatic dysfunction is treated with the patient in the supine position. The knees and hips flexed. Jones reports flexion of both hips to about 135 degrees. [40] Yates reports flexion of both thighs to 60 - 90 degrees with sidebending and rotation away. [26 p.132]

Case 57-61

57. Answer C: The patient is has a left innominate posterior. A shorter leg on the ipsilateral side (in this case, the left leg) will be present in this dysfunction. Consequently, the contralateral leg (in this case, the right leg) will appear longer.

Resistance to posterior compression is describing the ASIS compression test. This test will confirm the findings of the seated or standing flexion test. [56 p.776] Since there is a somatic dysfunction on the left side, posterior compression on the right is likely to demonstrate adequate resiliency (i.e. it will have normal springing motion). **Answer A**

A backward torsion on a left axis (right on left) is a specific sacral somatic dysfunction and not necessarily associated with an innominate dysfunction. **Answer B**

L5 neutral, sidebent left, rotated right is also not necessarily associated with a left innominate posterior. **Answer D**

Exquisite pain upon palpation of the pubic symphysis could be present with a pubic rami fracture or pubic symphysis somatic dysfunction. It is not necessarily present in a left innominate posterior. **Answer E**

58. Answer B: A positive standing flexion test on the left indicates a left innominate problem. The left ASIS is cephalad and the left PSIS is caudad, these findings are indicative of a posterior innominate on the left.

In a left innominate anterior, the left ASIS would be caudad and the left PSIS cephalad. **Answer A**

In a right innominate anterior or a right innominate posterior, the standing flexion test will be positive on the right. **Answers C and D**

59. Answer D: The most common cause of a left innominate posterior is tight hamstrings. The hamstrings attach to the ischial tuberosity and contraction can cause the innominate to rotate posteriorly.

The most common cause of a left innominate anterior is tight quadriceps. The quadriceps have attachments to the AIIS and contraction can cause the innominate to rotate anteriorly. **Answer A**

Hip adductors are attached to the pubic bones and femur. Tight hip adductors can cause an inferior pubic shear. **Answer B**

Tight hip abductors and piriformis tightness has not been specifically linked with innominate dysfunction. **Answers C and E**

60. Answer A: Hip flexors are used to correct the dysfunction. The treatment position to correct a left innominate posterior is as follows: With the patient supine, drop the left leg off the table to engage the restrictive barrier. Instruct the patient to flex their hip against your counterforce for 3-5 seconds.

In the typical muscle energy treatment, for this dysfunction the patient should be supine, not seated. **Answer B**

Hamstrings are hip extensors and would be used to correct an anterior innominate dysfunction. **Answer D**

Since the patient is not critically ill, muscle energy is not contraindicated in this patient. **Answer E**

61. Answer C: In psoas syndrome a high lumbar dysfunction is likely to be present. Specifically the lumbar dysfunction will be flexed, sidebent and rotated to the side of the tight psoas. In this case, L1 would be flexed, rotated right and sidebent right. [56 p. 748]

Case 62-65

62. Answer B: Initial management of ureterolithiasis includes rib raising and paraspinal inhibition to decrease hypersympathetic tone. [35 p.138] Other OMT should be delayed until at least partial pain management has been achieved. [35 p.139]

Not all osteopathic treatment is contraindicated in the above patient provided standard medical protocols are followed. **Answer A**

High velocity thrust and post-isometric relaxation muscle energy is contraindicated in the above patient, due to the nature of the illness and level of patient's pain. **Answers C and E**

Treatment of a posterior tenderpoint is likely to worsen this patient's pain, because it typically requires the patient to be in extension. In addition, treating the cause of the pain (ureteral stone) would decrease the patient's pain, not just counterstrain. **Answer D**

63. **Answer A**: Due to the close proximity of the ureter to the psoas muscle, ureterospasm has been associated with iliopsoas dysfunction and psoas syndrome.

Abdominal rectus spasm and a piriformis tenderpoint are not likely due to the fact that these muscles are not local to the site of irritation. **Answers B and D**

Paraspinal muscle spasm may be seen in patients with ureteral stones, especially patient's with costovertebral angle tenderness, however paraspinal muscle spasm can occur in many different dysfunctions and has not been specifically associated with ureterospasm. **Answer C**

The quadratus lumborum lies posterior to the iliopsoas and would less likely be affected with a ureteral stone. **Answer E**

64. **Answer C**: Ureterolithiasis is associated with ureterospasm. In addition, patient's with unilateral renal disease associated with ureteral stones have a decreased glomerular filtration rate. [35 p.138] This is probably because hypersympathetic tone to the kidneys will decrease GFR. [35 p.125] Treating the thoracic spine will decrease sympathetic tone to the kidneys (T10 - T11) and treating the lumbar region will decrease sympathetic tone to the ureters associated with ureterospasm.

Although controlling the patient's pain is important, pain management is usually controlled with medication; osteopathic treatment should be limited to the reduction of sympathetic tone. Paraspinal inhibition and rib raising have been suggested techniques. [35 p.138] **Answer A**

Treatment to the thoraco-lumbar junction cannot increase function of the normally functioning contralateral kidney. **Answer B**

Since the obstruction is proximal to the bladder, spasm is not the primary concern in the above patient; therefore it is not the primary reason for treating the thoraco-lumbar junction. **Answer D**

Although the patient does have some high blood pressure, it is a result of the patient's diagnosis. Treating the thoraco-lumbar junction to decrease the blood pressure is treating a symptom, not the cause. **Answer E**

65. **Answer C**: Approximately 80% of all renal stones are calcium oxalate and can be visualized on KUB x-ray, 5% are uric acid and 1% is cystine, the remainders are magnesium, ammonium phosphate or calcium phosphate. Also, uric acid and cystine stones are not easily visualized on a KUB.

Case 66-70

66. **Answer E**: The patient has thoracic outlet syndrome. The patient has a classic presentation of this syndrome. This is characterized by weakness and paresthesias with a decreased radial pulse when the arm is abducted, extended when the patient takes a deep breath and turns his head towards the effected shoulder (Adson's test) [25 p. 436-437]

Myocardial infarction is unlikely since acute changes, such as ST elevation or depression are not present in the EKG. The EKG changes in the question are associated with cor pulmonale. [43 p.1087] COPD is the most common cause of cor pulmonale. **Answer A**

Cervical disc herniation and radiculopathy would result in weakness and paresthesias in the upper extremity, however it will not result in a decreased peripheral pulse. In addition, C-spine x-rays are negative; therefore radiculopathy from cervical stenosis is unlikely. **Answers B and C**

Pancoast's tumor is located at the pulmonary apex. The tumor may cause shoulder and arm pain with paresthesia, however, the chest x-ray would show a density in the right upper lobe. **Answer D**

67. **Answer C**: Based on the history, the most likely etiology is hypertrophied scalene muscles. One of the areas that causes neurovascular compression of the upper extremity is between the anterior and middle scalene. Chronic COPD can result in hypertrophy or increased tension of the scalene muscles. [25] p. 436

Although cervical ribs can cause thoracic outlet syndrome, it would have been reported on the cervical spine x-ray. [25 p. 436] **Answer A**

Ischemic myocardium is associated with a myocardial infarction, not with thoracic outlet syndrome. **Answer B**

Herniated nucleus pulposus is not an etiology of thoracic outlet syndrome, but is the cause of cervical radiculopathy. **Answer D**

Shoulder dislocation is not an etiology of thoracic outlet syndrome and was ruled out by the shoulder X-ray report. **Answer E**

68. **Answer D**: Counterstrain of the hypertrophied scalene would cause reduced compression on the neurovascular bundle, and is the appropriate treatment.

Although the patient may have a rib 1 dysfunction, the primary etiology of this patient's symptoms is due to scalene hypertrophy. Therefore treatment of rib 1 is not the best answer. **Answer A**

Since this patient does not have a cervical rib this would not be the best answer. In addition, a 63-year-old COPD patient may have osteopenia, which would be a contraindication for HVLA. **Answer B**

Reduction of the shoulder is the treatment for a shoulder dislocation. **Answer C**

Morphine and nitrates are the treatment for a myocardial infarct. **Answer E**

69. **Answer B**: T2-T7 is the spinal level for the sympathetic reflex of the lungs.

Answers A and E have no sympathetic innervation. C0 is another term for the occiput.

T7-T10 is the sympathetic innervation for the upper to middle GI tract. **Answer C**

T11-L2 is the sympathetic innervation for the middle to lower GI tract. **Answer D**

70. **Answer C**: Increased sympathetic tone in a COPD patient will cause a thickening of pulmonary secretions via increased goblet cell production. [35 p.37-38]

Thinning of secretions is due to an increase in parasympathetic tone or a decrease in sympathetic tone. **Answer A**

Increased sympathetic tone will also result in bronchiole dilation, not bronchoconstriction. [35 p.37-38] **Answer B**

Pulmonary vasoconstriction from increased hypersympathetic tone could result in increased tissue congestion and possibly the development of pneumonia. **Answer D**

Increased sympathetic tone will also result in vasoconstriction, not vasodilatation of the pulmonary vasculature. [35 p.37-38] **Answer E**

Case 71-73

71. Answer E: Transient synovitis of the hip (also known as toxic synovitis) is a nonspecific, common, unilateral (5% bilateral) inflammatory arthritis involving the hip joint, which occurs in children under 10 years of age (typically 3-6 years of age). It is the most common cause of limp with hip pain in children. The male to female ratio is 3-5:1. There may be a history of a preceding upper respiratory tract infection. Pain may be present in the hip, antero-medial aspect of the thigh and the knee. Occasionally, a low-grade fever of 100-101F may be present. X-ray of the hip is normal.

Septic arthritis is a serious pyogenic infection of the joint space. It occurs most often in children less than 3 years old. The joint is swollen, and effusion, erythema, tenderness, pain and warmth are evident. The child may have a history of a recent bacterial infection. Septic arthritis is usually accompanied by a fever. The knee is the most commonly affected joint followed by the hip, elbow, and ankle. **Answer A**

Legg-Calve-Perthes disease is a juvenile idiopathic avascular necrosis of the femoral head. The onset is insidious taking weeks to months, which does not fit the case history. **Answer B**

Slipped capital femoral epiphysis represents a displacement of the femoral head from the femoral neck due to a stress fracture through the femoral capital epiphyseal growth plate. It is classically seen in obese adolescent males. This would have been diagnosed by the X-ray of the hip. **Answer C**

Developmental dislocation of the hip encompasses the severity spectrum from mild acetabular dysplasia to frank dislocation. Hip X-ray would have demonstrated a shallow acetabulum with a completely or partially subluxed femoral head. **Answer D**

72. Answer C: Most children can be treated symptomatically with bed rest at home and non-steroidal anti-inflammatory medication to decrease pain and inflammation. [32 p.668]

Antibiotics would be indicated for septic arthritis. **Answer A**

Corticosteroids are not indicated for any of these conditions. **Answer B**

Surgical fixation is indicated for slipped capital femoral epiphysis. [32 p.653] **Answer D**

Hip manipulation has not been shown to improve the symptoms or shorten the duration of transient synovitis of the hip. **Answer E**

73. Answer A: The etiology of transient synovitis of the hip is idiopathic, but mild trauma at an age when the socket or acetabulum is not fully developed is a proposed theory. [32 p.667]

Bacterial would be the etiology of septic arthritis. **Answer B**

Transient synovitis of the hip is not a developmental disorder. **Answer C**

Although one theory proposes a viral etiology for transient synovitis of the hip, virologic cultures of the effusion have not identified organisms. Therefore viral is not the best answer. [32 p.667] **Answer D**

Slipped capital femoral epiphysis is associated with obese children. **Answer E**

Case 74-76

74. Answer B: This patient has gastroesophageal reflux disease. The typical symptom is heartburn; in this case the disease is refractory to antacids and famotidine. Reclining after eating, chocolate, coffee, caffeine, cigarettes, fatty meals, peppermint, and alcohol worsen the condition. [60 pp 599-600]

Dyspepsia is defined as pain or discomfort centered in the upper abdomen. Heartburn (retrosternal burning) should be distinguished from dyspepsia. Patients with dyspepsia often have heartburn as an additional complaint. When heartburn (pyrosis) coupled with regurgitation is the dominant complaint, gastroesophageal reflux disease is nearly always present and should be distinguished from dyspepsia. [60 p.571] **Answer A**

Epigastric pain (dyspepsia) is the hallmark of peptic ulcer disease, which is usually relieved by eating or antacids, with a recurrence of pain two to four hours later. [60 pp. 618-619] **Answer C**

Zollinger-Ellison syndrome is caused by gastrin-secreting neuroendocrine tumors (gastrinomas), which result in hypergastrinemia and acid secretion. Over 90% of patients with this syndrome develop peptic ulcers. In most cases, the two conditions are indistinguishable and present as peptic ulcer disease. [60 pp.626-627] **Answer D**

Mallory-Weiss syndrome is characterized by a non-penetrating mucosal tear at the gastroesophageal junction, which is associated with hematemesis. Answer E.

75. Answer C: Hypersympathetic activity from GERD will result in tissue texture changes at T2-T8 because these segments receive sympathetic innervation from the esophagus, so T3-T8 is the best choice.

C3-C6 have no sympathetic fibers associated with the esophagus. **Answer A**

T1-T4 receive sympathetic innervation from the head and neck. **Answer B**

T10-T11 receive sympathetic innervation from the middle GI tract. **Answer D**

L1-L2 have no sympathetic fibers associated with the esophagus. **Answer E**

76. Answer C: Chapman's reflex point for hyperacidity is located just lateral of the sternum at the interspace of ribs 5 and 6 on the left side. [56 p.1052] Overall, this is a very difficult question.

Just lateral of the sternum at the interspace of ribs 4 and 5 on the left side is the Chapman's reflex point for the left lower lung. [56 p.1053] **Answer A**

Just lateral to the sternum at the interspace of ribs 5 and 6 on the right side is the Chapman's reflex point for the liver. [56 p.1052] **Answer B**

Just lateral to the sternum at the interspace of ribs 6 and 7 on the right side is the Chapman's reflex point for the liver and gall bladder. [56 p.1052] **Answer D**

Just lateral to the sternum at the interspace of ribs 6 and 7 on the left side is the Chapman's reflex point for peristalsis of the stomach. [56 p.1052] Answer E

Case 77-78

77. Answer C: This is a description of ideal posture when viewing a patient from the side. [25 p.37]

Military posture, as viewed from the side (in relation to a plumb line) is described as: head tilted slightly posteriorly, cervical curve and thoracic curve normal, anterior cervical and posterior thoracic deviation from plumb line, anterior pelvic tilt, knees extended, ankles plantar flexed. **Answer A**. [25 p.38]

Swayback posture as viewed from the side (in relation to a plumb line) is described as: head forward, cervical spine lordotic, thoracic spine kyphotic, decreased lordosis of lumbar spine, posterior tilt of pelvis, hip and knee joints hyper-extended. [25 p.38] **Answer B**

Anterior postural deviation as viewed from the side (in relation to a plumb line) is described as: entire body leans forward, deviating anteriorly from plumb line, patient's weight supported by metatarsals. [25 p.38] **Answer E**

Flat back posture as viewed from the side (in relation to a plumb line) is described as: head forward, cervical spine has slightly increased lordosis, thoracic spine slightly kyphotic in upper portion then flattens in lower segments, lumbar lordosis flattened, and hips and knees extended. [25 p.38] **Answer D**

78. Answer D: Flat back posture as viewed from the side (in relation to a plumb line) is described as: head forward, cervical spine has slightly increased lordosis, thoracic spine slightly kyphotic in upper portion then flattens in lower segments, lumbar lordosis flattened, and hips and knees extended. [25 p.38]

Military posture, as viewed from the side (in relation to a plumb line) is described as: head tilted slightly posteriorly, cervical curve and thoracic curve normal, anterior cervical and posterior thoracic deviation from plumb line, anterior pelvic tilt, knees extended, ankles plantar flexed. [25 p.38] **Answer A**

Swayback posture as viewed from the side (in relation to a plumb line) is described as: head forward, cervical spine lordotic, thoracic spine kyphotic, decreased lordosis of lumbar spine, posterior tilt of pelvis, hip and knee joints hyper-extended. [25 p.38] **Answer B**

Posterior postural deviation as viewed from the side (in relation to a plumb line) is described as: entire body leans backward, deviating posteriorly, balance maintained by anterior thrust of pelvis and hips, and marked lordosis from mid-thoracic spine down. [25 p.38] **Answer C**

Anterior postural deviation as viewed from the side (in relation to a plumb line) is described as: entire body leans forward, deviating anteriorly from plumb line, patient's weight supported by metatarsals. [25 p.38] **Answer E**

Case 79-82

79. Answer E: The anterior scalene originates from the posterior tubercle of the transverse processes of C3-C6 and inserts onto rib 1.

Platysma attaches to the fascia and skin of the pectoralis major and the deltoid inferiorly. It attaches to the mandible superiorly. **Answer A**

Longus colli is found in three parts of the anterior surface of the vertebral column between the atlas and the body of C3. **Answer B**

The posterior scalene originates from the posterior tubercles of the transverse processes of C4-C6. Its insertion is the external border of the second rib. **Answer C**

The sternocleidomastoid muscle originates from the mastoid process and the lateral half of the nuchal line of the occipital bone; it inserts at the manubrium and the medial clavicle. **Answer D**

80. Answer D: The position describes the left seventh anterior cervical tenderpoint. This corresponds to the left sternocleidomastoid muscle (SCM) and it is considered a maverick point. The appropriate treatment position is to rotate away (right), and sidebend toward (left). [26 p.46]

All other answers would therefore be incorrect. **Answers A, B, C, and E**

81. Answer E: Torticollis results from a shortening of the sternocleidomastoid (SCM) muscle.

A first rib dysfunction or second rib elevation would not likely occur with spasm of the SCM since it does not attach to these structures. **Answers A and C**

The SCM rotates the head in the opposite direction, therefore it would cause right cervical rotation. **Answer B**

Spasm of the SCM is not associated with thoracic outlet syndrome. **Answer D**

82. Answer C: In a group exhalation dysfunction, the key rib is the uppermost rib; treatment is directed at this key rib. The posterior scalene muscle attaches to the second rib, and is used for a muscle energy treatment of an exhalation dysfunction.

The anterior and middle scalenes are used to treat an exhalation dysfunction of the 1st rib. **Answers A and B**

Pectoralis minor is used to treat an exhalation dysfunction of ribs 3-5. **Answer D**

Serratus anterior is used to treat an exhalation dysfunction of ribs 6-9. **Answer E**

Case 83-84

83. Answer A: A right on left sacral torsion would have an L5 that is non-neutral (meaning either flexed or extended), rotated left, sidebent left with a seated flexion test positive on the right (opposite the axis of the torsion). For a further explanation of how L5 influences sacral movement in sacral torsions, see Chapter 6 Sacrum and Innominates.

A non-neutral dysfunction of L5 that is rotated right and sidebent right and a positive seated flexion test on the left would be associated with a left on right sacral torsion. **Answer B**

A neutral dysfunction of L5 that is rotated right and sidebent left and a positive seated flexion test on the right would be associated with a left on left sacral torsion. **Answer C**

A neutral dysfunction of L5 that is rotated left and sidebent right and a positive seated flexion test on the left would be associated with a right on right sacral torsion. **Answer D**

A flexed dysfunction of L5 that is rotated right and sidebent right and a positive seated flexion test on the right could not be associated with any sacral torsion. **Answer E**

84. Answer C: Springing is present over the part of the sacrum that has freedom of motion anteriorly. [33] The left inferior lateral angle moves anterior (as the right sacral base moves posterior) and thus will spring freely in a right on left sacral torsion.

The left superior sulcus and the right inferior lateral angle will not spring freely because they are part of the left oblique axis of the torsion. As a general rule, motion (springing) over the parts of the oblique axis is restricted. [33] **Answers A and D**

The right sulcus is rotated posteriorly. Springing is restricted over the part of the sacrum that has moved posterior. **Answer B**

In order to perform the lumbosacral spring test, the physician will spring at the lumbosacral junction (this includes the sacral base). The lumbosacral spring test is positive (meaning it does not spring) in a backward sacral torsion. **Answer E**

Matching

85. Answer E: The liver pump is a lymphatic technique that involves patient cooperation (exhaling and inhaling) upon command, while the practitioner's hand leans on the thoracic cage applying a vibratory motion. This results in a pumping action in the liver. This is indicated in several conditions, such as congestive heart failure, congestion of the liver, etc. But it is contraindicated in acute hepatitis. [56 p.1070]

86. Answer B: The Galbreath Technique is a mandibular drainage technique that relaxes the medial pterygoid muscle, which enables the tensor veli palatini muscle to functionally open the eustachian tube. [35 p.17] This technique is useful in acute otitis media. [56 p.1241]

87. Answer A: The pedal (a.k.a. Dalrymple) pump is a venous and lymphatic drainage technique applied through the lower extremities. [56 p.1241] It is contraindicated in patients with deep venous thrombosis. [35 p.229]

88. Answer C: The thoracic pump is a technique that consists of intermittent compression of the thoracic cage, which is indicated for pneumonia and other pulmonary conditions. [56 p.1241]

89. Answer D: The splenic pump improves immune function and is indicated in infection and fever, however, it is contraindicated in splenomegaly. This is a common finding in infectious mononucleosis. [35 p.228]

90. Answer B: Relaxing the medial pterygoid muscle (see answer 86) helps decongest the rich medial pterygoid plexus. (Note: The COMLEX exam may use an answer more than once in a matching set.) [35 p.17]

COMLEX B EXAMINATION

COMLEX B EXAMINATION

1. A 47-year-old female presents to your office with low back pain. Upon inspection of the lumbar spine, you observe a left lateral convexity. Palpation reveals fullness in the left paraspinal musculature and L2 - L5 have transverse processes posterior on the left. Given the above information the somatic dysfunction is most consistent with:

    A) Type II mechanics with the lumbar spine sidebent left, rotated left
    B) Type II mechanics with the lumbar spine sidebent right, rotated right
    C) Type I mechanics with the lumbar spine sidebent right, rotated left
    D) Type I mechanics with the lumbar spine sidebent left, rotated right
    E) There is not enough information given to make a correct diagnosis

2. In a 41-year-old male with back pain, you observe that thoracic segments T8 - T12 have a convexity to the right. Which of the following is the best statement regarding this group somatic dysfunction?

    A) T9's right transverse process is more anterior
    B) T12 is limited in right rotation compared to L1
    C) T10's left transverse process is more caudad compared to its right
    D) Ribs 7 - 12 are limited in exhalation on the left
    E) T9 is rotated right, sidebent right

3. As a sports medicine physician you are consulted on a 23 year-old female with patello- femoral tracking syndrome. In addition to medication and osteopathic treatment you decide to facilitate the patient's recovery by recommending exercises to strengthen the vastus medialis. You inform her that while in the supine position with the knee fully extended, she should tighten her quadriceps, hold for 5 seconds then relax. Which of the following statements most accurately describes this type of exercise?

    A) Eccentric contraction in which there is no increase in vastus medialis tension.
    B) Concentric contraction in which there is an increase in vastus medialis tension.
    C) Isometric contraction in which there is an increase in vastus medialis tension.
    D) Eccentric contraction in which there is a shortening of the muscle.
    E) Isotonic contraction in which there is an increase is vastus medialis tension.

4. C3 is extended, sidebent left and rotated left. If you decide to use a direct muscle energy technique to correct this dysfunction how would you position C3?

    A) In flexion, sidebent right, rotated right
    B) In flexion, sidebent left, rotated right
    C) In extension, sidebent left, rotated left
    D) In extension, sidebent right, rotated right
    E) In extension, sidebent left, rotated right

5. An 81-year-old male with atherosclerotic heart disease was admitted to the hospital with an exacerbation of COPD. He eventually developed pneumonia and went into acute respiratory failure. He was intubated and received assisted mechanical ventilation for 2 weeks. He was extubated and transferred to a general medical floor where he spent two additional weeks. Today, he arrives at a skilled nursing facility where you are the covering house physician. On your admission history and physical exam, the patient complains of low back pain. On examination, you notice that this severely debilitated male has generalized muscle atrophy and requires maximal assistance with bed mobility. He is unable to tolerate sitting or standing. You conclude that his back pain is due to his prolonged bedridden state. Which of the following treatment protocols is best suited for this patient?

A) Low velocity moderate amplitude techniques followed by gentle isometric exercises to strengthen the lumbar spine
B) Myofascial release of the sacrum followed by isotonic exercises with low resistance to strengthen the lumbar spine
C) Rib raising to help with respiration followed by muscle energy to the pelvis and lumbar somatic dysfunctions
D) Indirect treatments to the lumbar fascia followed by direct gentle articulatory techniques
E) Myofascial release to the thoraco-lumbar junction followed by gentle high velocity low amplitude treatment

6. In a patient with a history of tension headaches, structural exam reveals the following: C5 resists lateral translation to the left. There is right-sided fullness at C2 and the right articular pillar of C2 resists anterior glide. Given the above information, what else is most likely true regarding physical examination?

A) C2 is flexed
B) C2 is rotated left
C) The atlanto-axial joint is rotated right
D) C5 is rotated left
E) The atlas is rotated left.

7. Which of the following is true regarding the cervical spine?

A) Hypertrophic changes at the C4/C5 facet joint and degenerative changes at the corresponding joint of Luschka may cause C4 nerve root entrapment
B) The synovium of the uncovertebral joint is continuous with that of the facet joint.
C) The main motion of the OA joint is rotation
D) The joints of Luschka play an important role in cervical sidebending
E) Restriction within the sternocleidomastoid will decrease neck rotation to the contralateral side

8. Which of the following biomechanical or structural abnormalities best explain why a patient with COPD has an increased AP diameter of his/her chest?

    A) Fibrotic changes within the diaphragm due to chronic hypoxia results in a flattened diaphragm and an increased total lung capacity.
    B) Continuous accessory muscle use will pull the ribs superiorly, resulting in an expanded thoracic cage.
    C) The destruction of elastic fibers and chronic air trapping results in permanent inhaled rib positions.
    D) Chronic deoxygenation of peripheral tissues results in a physiologic expansion of the thoracic cage as a compensatory mechanism.
    E) Exaggerated sympathetic input from visceral afferents causes broncho-aveolar expansion and results in an increased AP diameter.

9. With deep inspiration, ribs 6-10 increase the chest wall diameter:

    A) Anteriorly along an oblique plane
    B) Anteriorly around a transverse axis
    C) Laterally around an anterior-posterior axis
    D) Laterally around a transverse axis
    E) Laterally around a vertical axis

10. A 34-year-old male presents to your office with severe low back pain. The pain started yesterday while he was working on his car and is now radiating into his lower extremities. What additional information in this patient's history would most impact the immediate diagnosis and treatment?

    A) Absent unilateral superficial abdominal reflex
    B) Presence of incontinence
    C) Loss of Achilles reflex
    D) Down-going plantar response with Babinski's testing
    E) Unilateral loss of cremasteric reflex

11. A posterior fibular head dysfunction can cause direct compression on which of the following peripheral nerves?

    A) Common fibular
    B) Obturator
    C) Sciatic
    D) Tibial
    E) Sural

12. A 23-year-old medical student is complaining of left sided low back/sacroiliac pain. The pain started one week ago while studying for board exams. On examination, you notice he has a positive standing flexion test on the left, his left ASIS is inferior, the left PSIS is superior and the right sacral sulcus is freely mobile. Based on the information given, what is the most likely diagnosis?

  A) Left sacral rotation on a left oblique axis (L on L)
  B) Unilateral sacral flexion on the right (USF$_R$).
  C) Left posterior innominate.
  D) Left anterior innominate.
  E) Left superior innominate shear.

13. A 34-year-old male truck driver presents to you with a chief complaint of moderate to severe low back pain. He gives a history of falling onto his buttocks three days prior. With the patient standing, there is a noticeable absence of the lumbar lordosis. With the patient prone, the ILA's are equal in depth. Motion testing reveals no motion at the lumbosacral junction. Which of the following most correctly describes the sacral dysfunction?

  A) A bilaterally flexed sacrum that has rotated around its superior transverse axis.
  B) A bilaterally extended sacrum that has rotated around its superior transverse axis.
  C) A bilaterally flexed sacrum that has rotated around its middle transverse axis
  D) A bilaterally extended sacrum that has rotated around its middle transverse axis
  E) The axis for the sacral dysfunction cannot be specified.

14. In a patient with low back pain structural examination reveals: A deep sacral sulcus on the right. A posterior ILA on the left. A negative lumbosacral spring test. A positive seated flexion test on the right. Given these findings, which is the most likely diagnosis?

  A) Right sacral rotation on a right oblique axis
  B) Left sacral rotation on a left oblique axis
  C) Left sacral rotation on a right oblique axis
  D) Right sacral rotation on a left oblique axis
  E) Unilateral sacral flexion on the right

15. The rationale for having a positive seated flexion test in a patient with a left on left sacral torsion is:
  A) Posterior rotation of the right innominate produces right iliosacral dysfunction
  B) The anterior glide of the right sacral base produces right sacroilial dysfunction.
  C) Posterior glide of the left ILA produces left sacroilial dysfunction
  D) Anterior rotation of the right innominate produces sacroilial dysfunction
  E) Anterior glide of the left sacral sulcus produces left iliosacral dysfunction

16. Plexopathy involving the medial cord of the brachial plexus will have the greatest effect on which of the following movements?

  A) Elbow flexion
  B) Elbow extension
  C) Finger abduction
  D) Shoulder abduction
  E) Shoulder external rotation

17. A 19-year-old volleyball player dislocated her shoulder while spiking a volleyball several weeks ago. She immediately was taken to the ER where it was re-located. She was started in a rehabilitation program working with her trainer and team physician. Since the injury, her pain has diminished however she still has some persistent weakness with arm abduction. On examination, strength testing is 5/5 except for arm abduction, which is 2/5. Muscle stretch reflexes in the upper extremities are normal and symmetric. X-rays are normal. What is the most likely etiology of her persistent weakness?

    A) Injury to the dorsal scapular nerve
    B) Injury to the inferior gleno-humeral ligament
    C) Complete tear of the supraspinatus tendon
    D) Incomplete rupture of the deltoid at its insertion site
    E) Injury to the axillary nerve

18. In a patient with an anterior fibular head somatic dysfunction, which of the following statements is true?

    A) The above type of dysfunction does not easily respond to treatment
    B) The somatic dysfunction will increase the amount of passive plantar flexion
    C) It can result in foot drop
    D) The tibio-fibular synovial articulation will resist posterior glide
    E) It is often seen in common ankle sprains

19. An 18-year-old male suffered a closed head injury from a motor vehicle accident 21 days ago. He was recently admitted to a rehabilitation hospital where he has been making moderate progress until two days ago when he developed increasing confusion and urinary incontinence. Based on these symptoms, what craniosacral techniques would this patient most likely benefit from?

    A) Occipital condylar decompression to stimulate the reticular activating system
    B) Venous sinus technique to improve drainage and decrease any residual cranial edema
    C) CV4 technique to enhance arousal
    D) Sacral rocking to improve bladder control
    E) All cranial treatment is absolutely contraindicated in this patient.

20. When palpating the head for the cranial rhythmic impulse using the vault hold, the index fingers should be in contact with which structure?

    A) The frontal bone
    B) The sphenoid bone
    C) The parietal bone
    D) The temporal bone
    E) The occipital bone

21. A 56-year-old obese male is admitted to the hospital with severe right upper quadrant pain radiating to the tip of his right scapula. The pain started suddenly after eating a fatty meal. He has had one episode of vomiting. Examination demonstrates pain and guarding of the right upper quadrant. Lab values are as follows:

Alkaline Phosphatase	= 220U/L	Normal = 39 - 117U/L
Alanine aminotransferase	= 17U/L	Normal = 8-20U/L
Aspartate aminotransferase	= 20U/L	Normal = 8-20U/L
Lactate dehydrogenase =	250U/L	Normal = 45-90U/L
Bilirubin, serum		
Total	= 1.3mg/dl	Normal = 0.1 - 1.0mg/dl
Direct	= 0.7mg/dl	Normal = 0.0 - 0.3mg/dl

The tenderness that he is experiencing at the tip of his scapula could be most accurately described as:

A) Somatic-visceral reflex
B) Viscero-somatic reflex
C) Chapman's point
D) Trigger point
E) Counterstrain tenderpoint

22. Which of the following is true regarding goals of manipulation in a patient with asthma?

A) Bronchodilate by stimulating the parasympathetic nervous system.
B) Normalize the phrenic nerve with a CV4 technique.
C) Encourage perfusion of lung parenchyma by stimulating the sympathetic nervous system
D) Decrease the thoraco-abdominal pressure gradient by redoming the diaphragm
E) Improve ventilation and perfusion (V/Q) function of the lungs with rib raising

23. Head and neck lymphatic congestion and drying of the nasopharyngeal mucosa is most likely associated with increased autonomic activity originating from the pre-ganglionic nerve fibers of which structure?

A) Vagus nerve
B) Inferior cervical ganglia
C) Superior cervical ganglia
D) Intermediolateral cells of the spinal cord at T1 - T4
E) Intermediolateral cells of the spinal cord at T5 - T7

24. Which of the following is true regarding the sympathetic nervous innervation to the kidneys and ureters?

A) Sympathetic innervation arises from the cell bodies in the spinal cord at the level of T8 - T10.
B) Increased sympathetic tone causes vasoconstriction of afferent arterioles thus increasing the glomerular filtration rate.
C) Stimulating sympathetics will restore normal peristaltic waves in the ureters
D) Preganglionic fibers for the kidney and upper ureters synapse in the superior mesenteric ganglion.
E) Sympathetic stimulation contracts the detrusor and relaxes the trigone resulting in micturition.

25. A 67-year-old male with a history of congestive heart failure presents to the ER in a very anxious state with shortness of breath and bilateral lower extremity edema. After appropriate diuresis, the patient stabilizes. You decide to perform OMT to re-establish homeostasis and enhance lymphatic drainage. Which of the following describes the most appropriate and proper sequencing of treatment?

   A) Thoracic inlet release, rib raising, redome the diaphragm, pelvic diaphragm release, pedal pump.
   B) Pedal pump, pelvic diaphragm release, redome the diaphragm, thoracic inlet release, pectoral lift
   C) Pedal pump, pelvic diaphragm release, redome the diaphragm, rib raising
   D) Rib raising, CV4 technique, pectoral lift, pedal pump
   E) Redome the diaphragm, pelvic diaphragm release, pectoral lift

26. A 68-year-old man is brought to your office for a postural evaluation. The sagittal plane evaluation reveals that the patient's entire body leans anteriorly away from a plumb line that hangs from the ceiling to the floor in the exam room. The patient's weight is supported mainly by the metatarsals of his feet. Your postural assessment of this patient would be:

   A) Military posture
   B) Swayback posture
   C) Posterior postural deviation
   D) Flat back posture
   E) Anterior postural deviation

27. A patient with left shoulder pain has the following findings:
   The left clavicle at the sternum is more cephalad than the right.
   The right sternoclavicular head of the clavicle moves inferiorly when the patient shrugs his shoulders while the left does not.
   What is the most likely diagnosis?

   A) Left anterior rotation somatic dysfunction of the sternoclavicular joint
   B) Left anterior somatic dysfunction of the sternoclavicular joint
   C) Left inferior somatic dysfunction of the sternoclavicular joint
   D) Left superior somatic dysfunction of the sternoclavicular joint
   E) Left posterior somatic dysfunction of the sternoclavicular joint

28. A patient complains of epigastric pain that is relieved upon eating food and recurs about three hours after he eats. Upper endoscopy is performed and erosions are found in the gastric mucosa. At which spinal level would you expect to find palpatory changes related to a viscerosomatic reflex?

   A) C7
   B) T4
   C) T6
   D) T10
   E) T12

29. A 21 year old complains of a headache, severe facial pain, greenish purulent nasal discharge and nasal congestion. At what spinal levels would you expect to find the tissue texture changes related to a viscerosomatic reflex?
   A) T1-T3
   B) T4-T6
   C) T7-T9
   D) T10-T12
   E) T12-L2

30. What area of the thoracic vertebra is most commonly palpated for evaluation of a patient's thoracic somatic dysfunction?
   A) Spinous process
   B) Superior costal facet
   C) Pedicle
   D) Transverse costal facet
   E) Transverse processes

31. A patient in severe unrelenting pain from a recently herniated disc in the lumbar spine seeks treatment for his condition. The patient has a history of peptic ulcer disease and deep vein thrombosis. The patient is currently taking Coumadin (Warfarin) daily. What would be the most appropriate management of this patient?
   A) Non-steroidal anti-inflammatory agent, bed rest for 5 days, indirect techniques
   B) Non-steroidal anti-inflammatory, bed rest for 2 days, counterstrain
   C) Opioid analgesic, bed rest for 2 days, indirect techniques
   D) Acetaminophen, bed rest for 5 days, HVLA
   E) Opioid analgesic, bed rest for 5 days, muscle energy

32. A football player gets hit on the side of his right hip. The patient complains of right hip pain. Structural examination reveals no sacral dysfunction. The left ASIS is 6 inches from the midline, while the right ASIS is 5 inches from the midline. The left ASIS moves easily with posterior compression as compared to the right. What is the most likely diagnosis?

   A) A left anterior innominate rotation
   B) A right innominate inflare
   C) A left innominate outflare
   D) A right anterior innominate rotation
   E) A left superior innominate shear

33. A patient was in their car, turned to the left, and reached for the seat belt when a sharp pain was felt in the low back area. The patient has never had back pain before and has no radiating numbness or tingling in the lower extremities. The structural examination reveals no lumbar dysfunction. The right sulcus is deep and the left ILA is posterior. The left superior sulcus does not spring as compared to the right, and the left ILA does not spring. The most likely diagnosis is:

   A) Left unilateral sacral extension
   B) Left sacral margin posterior
   C) Right sacral margin posterior
   D) Bilateral sacral flexion
   E) Bilateral sacral extension

34. A patient was snowboarding and fell several times. The patient now complains of left arm pain. The findings of the structural exam are: a decreased carrying angle of the left arm, the olecranon process is restricted in medial glide, and the wrist and hand are abducted. The most likely diagnosis is?
    A) Posterior radial head dysfunction
    B) Adduction dysfunction of the ulna
    C) Abduction dysfunction of the ulna
    D) Anterior radial head dysfunction
    E) Cervical radiculopathy

35. A patient is diagnosed with a first-degree ankle sprain. What is the most likely injured ligament?
    A) Anterior talofibular
    B) Posterior talofibular
    C) Calcaneofibular
    D) Tibiocalcaneal
    E) Deltoid

36. A patient complains of hip pain for one day. Range of motion testing reveals:

	Left	Right
External rotation	60 degrees	60 degrees
Internal rotation	20 degrees	35 degrees

The most likely diagnosis is.
    A) Tight left external rotators
    B) Tight left internal rotators
    C) Lax left external rotators
    D) Tight right internal rotators
    E) Lax right internal rotators

37. A 54-year-old alcoholic male patient complains of tender bumps at the distal palmar crease of his hand. Physical exam reveals subcutaneous nodules and palmar fascia contracture of the ring finger. The most likely diagnosis is:

    A) DeQuervain's disease
    B) Heberden node
    C) Syphilis
    D) Bouchard's node
    E) Dupuytren's contracture

38. In a patient with lumbosacral pain, there is a positive seated flexion test on the left. The left sacral sulcus is deep and moves freely with anterior glide. The right ILA resists anterior glide. Based on the information given what is the most likely diagnosis?

    A) Unilateral sacral flexion on the right
    B) Right sacral torsion on a right oblique axis (R on R)
    C) Left sacral torsion on a left oblique axis (L on L)
    D) Left sacral torsion on a right oblique axis (L on R)
    E) Right sacral torsion on a left oblique axis (R on L)

Case 39-40

A patient comes to the emergency room complaining of wrist and elbow pain. Yesterday while at work, he fell forward on his outstretched arm hyper-extending his wrist. There is no history of direct trauma to the elbow. The wrist is warm, slightly edematous and there is significantly decreased range of motion of the wrist and forearm. Palpatory exam reveals severe pain on the volar aspect of the wrist at the ulna-carpal junction. Pulses are normal and sensation is intact. X-rays of the wrist show some soft tissue swelling surrounding the wrist but there is no evidence of fracture or carpal dislocation. X-rays of the elbow are negative.

39. Which of the following is the best statement regarding the initial management of this patient's injury?

   A) A bone scan should be ordered to rule out a scaphoid fracture.
   B) Since this patient is likely to have a fracture of the scaphoid bone, he should be treated empirically by casting his wrist and forearm for 4 - 6 weeks.
   C) Due to the likelihood of a non-displaced fracture of the scaphoid, this patient should be empirically treated with closed reduction and external fixation with percutaneous pinning.
   D) Due to the acute nature of this illness, the patient's wrist should be immobilized with a soft splint and a thoracic inlet release and pectoral lift can be done to reduce edema.
   E) Pain at the volar aspect of the wrist most likely represents an ulnar somatic dysfunction. This can easily be treated with muscle energy and HVLA to restore ulnar carpal glide.

40. Given the mechanism of injury, if the above patient suffered a radial head dysfunction, which of the following findings would you most likely expect to observe on physical examination?

   A) Decreased supination of the affected forearm
   B) Increased carrying angle of the affected elbow
   C) Increased adduction of the affected wrist
   D) Increased abduction of the affected wrist
   E) Decreased posterior glide of the radial head at the affected elbow.

Case 41-42

A 34-year-old male is complaining of severe right-sided low back pain radiating into the foot. The pain started yesterday and is associated with calf cramping. He describes a shooting pain into his right foot that is made worse with forward flexion of the lumbar spine. On examination, the pelvis is shifted to the left. There is an absence of lumbar lordosis. The lumbar spine is sidebent to the right. The sacrum has rotated right around a right oblique axis. There is a positive straight leg raising test.

41. Which of the following statements is true?

    A) This patient's injury would have been prevented if he had received frequent OMT.
    B) The primary cause of this patient's pain is due to a shortened psoas on the right side.
    C) This patient is likely to have asymmetry with hip drop testing
    D) This patient will eventually need surgery due to the natural progression of symptoms associated with his diagnosis
    E) Due to the severity of the pain, initial analgesia should consist of oral opioids.

42. After two weeks of conservative management, the patient in the above question comes to your office still having significant pain. Electromyography shows abnormal findings in the anterior tibialis and extensor hallucis longus. Based on the innervation of the muscles involved, which nerve root is most likely affected?

    A) L3
    B) L5
    C) S1
    D) S2
    E) There is not enough information given to specify an answer

Case 43-45

A 78-year-old male underwent abdominal aortic aneurysm repair with graft yesterday. He is currently in the intensive care unit. The operation was successful and postoperatively the patient is doing well.

Physical exam reveals:
   Patient appears to be in no acute distress
   Vital Signs:
   Temperature 99.5, Heart rate 72, Respiration 16 and shallow, Blood pressure 120/60, mild incision pain approximately 4/10 controlled with PCA pump.

Heart: Regular rate and rhythm. No murmurs, gallops or rubs.
Lungs: Decreased respiratory excursion throughout the lung fields. Few scattered bi-basilar crackles.
Abdomen: Hypoactive bowel sounds, incision clean and dry with no evidence of erythema.
Extremities: Strong peripheral pulses. There is trace edema in both lower extremities

43. What is the most likely etiology of the bi-basilar crackles in this patient?

   A) Pulmonary embolism
   B) Postoperative atelectasis
   C) Congestive heart failure
   D) Pneumonia
   E) Pericardial effusion

44. Which of the following is the most appropriate technique for treating the cause of the bi-basilar crackles?

   A) Rib raising
   B) Condylar decompression
   C) Pedal pump
   D) Liver pump
   E) Abdominal pump

45. Which of the following manipulative techniques would be contraindicated in this patient?

   A) Pedal pump
   B) Thoracic inlet release
   C) Rib raising
   D) CV4 bulb decompression
   E) Indirect myofascial release

COPYRIGHT 2009

Case 46-49

A 35-year-old man comes to your office with back pain. He has no previous history of back pain. He denies recent heavy lifting, however he remembers that he misjudged the distance when stepping off a curb two weeks ago. At first he states that walking "did not feel right", but now, he has developed moderate lower back pain. On examination, he has a positive standing and seated flexion tests on the left. His left ASIS and PSIS are superior when compared to the right. His left sacral sulcus is deep and his left ILA is slightly posterior and markedly inferior. Springing is restricted at the left ILA.

46. The most likely sacral diagnosis is:

   A) Right sacral rotation on a right oblique axis
   B) Left sacral rotation on a right oblique axis
   C) Left sacral rotation on a left oblique axis
   D) Unilateral sacral flexion on the left
   E) Unilateral sacral extension on the left

47. The most likely pelvic diagnosis is:

   A) Anterior rotated innominate
   B) Posterior rotated innominate
   C) Superior innominate shear
   D) Inferior innominate shear
   E) Superior pubic shear

48. With the patient in the prone position you passively flex the right knee. He is able to touch his right heel to his right buttock. However, when doing the same to the left leg, his left heel remains 6 inches away with maximal knee flexion and you notice that his left hip flexes slightly with this maneuver. Restriction is most likely present in which of the following muscles?

   A) Sartorius
   B) Rectus femoris
   C) Vastus medialis
   D) Gracilis
   E) Hamstrings

49. The delayed development of pain can best be explained by:

   A) No previous history of back pain
   B) The force imparted by the ground transmitting to the lumbar spine immediately causing local somatic dysfunction
   C) Postural compensatory mechanisms
   D) A somatoform disorder
   E) The patient has a high tolerance to pain

Case 50-51

A 47-year-old female comes in with low back and buttock pain. On structural examination she has a positive seated flexion test on the left. The right sulcus is deeper and the lumbosacral spring test is positive. Range of motion testing reveals left leg adduction to 35°, right leg adduction to 15°.

50. What is the most likely sacral diagnosis?

A) Right on right torsion
B) Left on right torsion
C) Right on left torsion
D) Left unilateral sacral flexion
E) Right unilateral sacral extension

51. Which of the following is true regarding this patient's hip musculature?

A) Right adductors are restricted
B) Left adductors are restricted
C) Right gluteus medius and tensor fascia lata are restricted
D) Left gluteus medius and tensor fascia lata are restricted
E) Right gluteus medius and tensor fascia lata have increased flexibility

Case 52-55

A 34-year-old female comes into your office complaining of mild left-sided thoracic pain. The pain started about a week after the patient began driving her new sports car that has very low riding seats. The pain is non-radiating and worsens with inhalation. X-rays and EKG reveal no abnormalities. Your structural exam reveals that ribs 3-5 on the left are more caudad and lag behind during inhalation. Tenderpoints are noted on ribs 3-5 in the left mid axillary line.

52. Which of the following most correctly describes the somatic dysfunction?

    A) Type I thoracic dysfunction
    B) Type II thoracic dysfunction
    C) Right sidebending thoracic dysfunction
    D) Left rib 3-5 inhalation dysfunction
    E) Left rib 3-5 exhalation dysfunction

53. In order to correct the somatic dysfunction, treatment should be directed at which rib?

    A) Rib 2
    B) Rib 3
    C) Rib 4
    D) Rib 5
    E) Rib 6

54. If a muscle energy technique is used to treat this dysfunction, which muscle should be recruited?

    A) Posterior scalene
    B) Teres major
    C) Pectoralis minor
    D) Pectoralis major
    E) Serratus anterior

55. Which of the following correctly describes counterstrain treatment for the above dysfunction?

    A) Minimal thoracic flexion, left rotation, right sidebending.
    B) Minimal thoracic flexion, left rotation, left sidebending.
    C) Marked thoracic flexion, left rotation, left sidebending.
    D) Neutral thoracic spine, right rotation, left sidebending.
    E) Neutral thoracic spine, left rotation, right sidebending.

Case 56-59

A 52-year-old male with atrial fibrillation comes to your office complaining of new onset right shoulder pain. The pain started 24 hours ago during his golf tournament. The patient recalls that the pain came about immediately following a golf swing. The pain, which is greatest at the tip of the right acromion does not radiate. He denies any numbness or tingling in his upper extremity. There is full passive range of motion. At rest, with his arm by his side, the patient has little pain. However, the pain becomes moderate to severe when he attempts to hold his arm above his head. X-rays of his shoulder show no fracture. His medications include Coumadin (Warfarin) and hydrochlorothiazide.

56. You instruct your patient to abduct his arms and then slowly lower them. When he attempts to comply, you notice that he is unable to slowly lower the right arm smoothly. What disorder does this suggest?

    A) Adhesive capsulitis
    B) Bicipital tendonitis
    C) Osteoarthritis of the glenohumeral joint
    D) Rotator cuff tear
    E) Thoracic outlet syndrome

57. Given the patient's history and physical findings, which of the following treatments would be inappropriate?

    A) Ultrasound to the shoulder
    B) Left upper extremity sling
    C) Ice to the shoulder region
    D) Fascial release of the shoulder
    E) Cervical HVLA

58. In addition to osteopathic treatment, the most appropriate oral medication to treat this patient's pain is:

    A) Ibuprofen
    B) Rofecoxib
    C) Indomethacin
    D) Depomedrol
    E) Hydrocodone

59. The patient returns in two weeks for follow-up. He states that the pain has not improved. AP and lateral x-rays in your office showed a decreased sub-acromial space with a high riding humerus. What is the best radiographic study to determine the extent of this patient's injury?

    A) Computed tomography
    B) Magnetic resonance imaging
    C) Bone scan
    D) Axillary view radiograph
    E) Pet Scan

Case 60-62

A 13-year-old male comes to the emergency room with right wrist and elbow pain following a fall. He states that he fell forward on his outstretched arm.

60. Based on the history, what is the most likely diagnosis at the elbow?

    A) Adducted ulna
    B) Posterior radial head
    C) Abducted ulna
    D) Cubital tunnel syndrome
    E) Medial epicondylitis

On examination, there is no evidence of deformity of the forearm or wrist. Upon palpation, he has exquisite pain between the extensor pollicis longus and abductor pollicis longus tendons at the radiocarpal joint. There is mild edema at the radiocarpal joint. He has decreased flexion and extension at the wrist as well as decreased forearm supination. There is a tender point located at the musculotendonous insertion of the lateral epicondyle. X-rays of the wrist and elbow are normal without evidence of fracture

61. Which of the following techniques is contraindicated in this patient?

    A) Muscle energy to the upper extremity to increase supination
    B) Counterstrain to the tenderpoint
    C) Thoracic inlet release
    D) HVLA to the right wrist to improve range of motion
    E) Posterior axillary fold technique

62. The patient's wrist is splinted and he is told to follow-up in three weeks. At the next follow-up visit, the patient's pain has not improved. Which of the following would be the appropriate course of action?

    A) Prescribe a more effective pain medication and have the child follow up in a week
    B) Order a bone scan
    C) Immobilize the wrist for 2 weeks with a cast
    D) Reassure the parent and the child that the inflammation and pain are typical of wrist sprains
    E) None of the above are correct

Case 63-68

A 48-year-old male complains of low back pain with radiation to the right knee for 3 days. The patient was shoveling snow for several hours, and then was unable to straighten up. The patient has no previous history of low back pain. Physical examination reveals the patient to be in a forward flexed and leaning to the left posture. There are no neurological deficits. X-rays of the lumbar spine are negative for fracture. The following findings were found:

L1 FR_LS_L L5 FR_LS_L	(+) Lumbosacral spring test
Pelvis shifted to the right	Tenderpoint 1 inch medial to the left ASIS
(+) standing flexion test on the right	Right ASIS lower than the left
Shallow sacral sulcus on the left	ILA posterior and slightly inferior on the left

63. The primary cause of this patient's low back pain is:
   A) Piriformis syndrome
   B) Spondylolysis
   C) Herniated nucleus pulposus
   D) Psoas syndrome
   E) Lumbar stenosis

64. Manipulation of which somatic dysfunction is considered essential for the patient's primary cause of low back pain?
   A) L1 FR_LS_L
   B) L5 FR_LS_L
   C) Sacrum
   D) Left innominate
   E) Right innominate

65. The sacral diagnosis is:
   A) Right rotation on a right oblique axis
   B) Right rotation on a left oblique axis
   C) Left rotation on a left oblique axis
   D) Left rotation on a right oblique axis
   E) Right unilateral sacral extension

66. Radiation of pain into this patient's right knee is most directly related to:
   A) Psoas spasm
   B) Spondylosis
   C) Disc herniation
   D) Spondylolisthesis
   E) Piriformis muscle spasm

67. The innominate diagnosis is:
   A) Left anterior rotation
   B) Right anterior rotation
   C) Left posterior rotation
   D) Right posterior rotation
   E) Indiscernible from the information given

Question #68 pertains to the case on the previous page

68. What would be the correct Jones counterstrain treatment position for this patient's tenderpoint?
    A) Patient supine, hips and knees flexed and sidebent to the right
    B) Patient prone, hips and knees extended and sidebent to the right
    C) Patient supine, hips and knees flexed and sidebent to the left
    D) Patient prone, hips and knees extended and sidebent to the left
    E) Patient supine, hips and knees extended and sidebent to the left

Case 69-71

A 17-year-old female complains of anterior knee pain that gets worse when she runs, jumps or climbs stairs. Physical exam reveals pain is reproducible on squatting and when the knee is flexed. There is point tenderness on the undersurface of the patella and there is some patellar crepitus.

69. The most likely diagnosis is:

    A) Osgood-Schlatter disease
    B) Baker's cyst
    C) Patellar tendon tendonitis
    D) Housemaid's knee
    E) Patello-femoral syndrome

70. The above patient's condition has been most closely associated with:

    A) Genu recurvatum
    B) Increased Q angle
    C) Decreased Q angle
    D) Coxa valgus
    E) Coxa varus

71. Decreasing myofascial restrictions in which muscle would most likely result in greatest reduction in this patient's symptoms?
    A) Vastus lateralis
    B) Semimembranosus
    C) Semitendinosus
    D) Vastus medialis
    E) Quadriceps

Case 72-73

A 34-year-old female complains of dyspnea, fatigue, weakness, weight loss, and increased appetite. On physical exam you note a goiter, warm sweaty skin, and hand tremor.

72. You would expect to find tissue texture changes due to a viscerosomatic reflex at which spinal level?

    A) C3-C5
    B) T1-T4
    C) T5-T9
    D) T9-T12
    E) L1-L2

73. To confirm your diagnosis you would find an anterior Chapman's point just lateral to the sternum at the interspace of:

    A) Ribs 1 and 2
    B) Ribs 2 and 3
    C) Ribs 3 and 4
    D) Ribs 4 and 5
    E) Ribs 5 and 6

Case 74-75

A patient complains of bloody diarrhea. A colonoscopy reveals the mucosa of the recto-sigmoid region is edematous, friable, and with numerous erosions.

74. At which spinal level would you expect to find palpatory changes related to a viscerosomatic reflex?

    A) C3-T5
    B) T1-T4
    C) T5-T9
    D) T10-T11
    E) T12-L2

75. The above patient would have a predictable reflex gangliform contraction located at:

    A) Right proximal area of the iliotibial tract
    B) Right distal area of the iliotibial tract
    C) Left proximal area of the iliotibial tract
    D) Left distal area of the iliotibial tract
    E) The superior rami of the pubis

Case 76-81

A patient complains of chest pain, especially when she exhales. The pain is localized to ribs 8-10 on the left.

76. These ribs are characterized as:
    A) Bifid ribs
    B) Atypical ribs
    C) True ribs
    D) Floating ribs
    E) False ribs

77. Upon further assessment of ribs 8 - 10 the lower edge of the rib shaft is more prominent and more elevated laterally than anteriorly. There was a failure of these ribs to move during exhalation. What is the most likely diagnosis?
    A) Ribs 8-10 exhalation dysfunction, pump handle predominant
    B) Ribs 8-10 exhalation dysfunction, bucket handle predominant
    C) Ribs 8-10 inhalation dysfunction, pump handle predominant
    D) Ribs 8-10 inhalation dysfunction, bucket handle predominant
    E) Ribs 8-10 inhalation dysfunction, caliper motion predominant

78. Evaluation of ribs 5-7 on the right reveal that the ribs are depressed anteriorly and the inferior edges of the posterior rib angles are more prominent. The ribs move caudally during exhalation but do not move cephalad upon inhalation. What is the most likely diagnosis?
    A) Ribs 5-7 inhalation dysfunction, pump handle predominant
    B) Ribs 5-7 inhalation dysfunction, bucket handle predominant
    C) Ribs 5-7 inhalation dysfunction, caliper motion predominant
    D) Ribs 5-7 exhalation dysfunction, bucket handle predominant
    E) Ribs 5-7 exhalation dysfunction, pump handle predominant

79. In this patient, which of the following choices is the most appropriate regarding treatment for the somatic dysfunction of ribs 5-7 using muscle energy?
    A) Treat rib 5 using the pectoralis minor muscle
    B) Treat rib 5 using the serratus anterior muscle
    C) Treat rib 6 using the pectoralis minor muscle
    D) Treat rib 7 using the serratus anterior muscle
    E) Treat rib 7 using the pectoralis minor muscle

80. Muscle energy treatment of the somatic dysfunction of ribs 5-7 was discontinued because the patient complained of pain. Using counterstrain, where would you locate the tenderpoint to direct your treatment for this group dysfunction?
    A) On the mid-axillary line on rib 5
    B) On the mid-axillary line on rib 6
    C) On the mid-axillary line on rib 7
    D) On the rib angle of rib 5
    E) On the rib angle of rib 7

81. It is recommended that the above tenderpoint is treated for:
    A) 15 seconds
    B) 30 seconds
    C) 60 seconds
    D) 90 seconds
    E) 2 minutes

Directions: For each numbered item (patient characteristic) select the one lettered heading (gait) most closely associated with it. Each lettered heading may be selected once, more than once, or not at all.

  A. High steppage gait
  B. Ataxic gait
  C. Shuffling (festinating) gait
  D. Waddling gait
  E. Hemiplegic gait
  F. Elevated pelvis gait
  G. Antalgic gait
  H. Gluteus medius gait
  I. Scissor gait

82. A 70-year-old-male with rigidity, resting tremor, bradykinesia has a slow walking speed and his feet do not clear the ground.

83. A 56-year-old-male is observed to shift his body to the right side when he walks. The patient has a positive Trendelenberg sign when standing on the right foot.

84. A patient with a history of muscular dystrophy has weakness of the pelvic-girdle muscles, increased lordosis, pot-bellied posture and appears to roll from side to side when he walks.

85. A 63-year-old-male with a right peroneal compression neuropathy has a complete foot drop. When he ambulates he flexes his right hip more than his left in order to clear his right toes.

86. A 16-year-old-female with spastic diplegic cerebral palsy walks with her legs adducted, crossing alternately in front of one another.

87. A patient with a left-sided paresis from a stroke ambulates by leaning to the right side, advancing the left leg in a circumduction pattern while the left foot drags on the floor.

88. A patient has a severely painful bunion in his right foot that results in a short stance phase on the right and a rapidly executed swing phase of the left leg.

COMLEX B
ANSWERS

COMLEX B Answers

1. Answer C: The patient has a left lateral convexity. In other words, the lumbar spine is sidebent to the right. You also note on palpation that there is left paraspinal fullness and L2 - L5 have transverse processes posterior on the left (i.e. L2 - L5 is rotated to the left). When the spine sidebends and rotates in opposite directions, we call this type I mechanics. Type I mechanics occur when the spine is in the neutral position (no flexion or extension) and are typical of group dysfunctions. Type II mechanics occur when the spine is either flexed or extended, in this case sidebending and rotation would be in the same direction. Type II mechanics are typical of single vertebral dysfunctions.

2. Answer C: If T8 - T12 have a convexity to the right, there is a group dysfunction that is sidebent left and rotated right. Remember group dysfunctions occur in the neutral plane and in such a case they sidebend and rotate to opposite sides. If T10 is sidebent left, then its left transverse process will be more caudad than its right transverse process.

If T9 is rotated to the right, then its right transverse process would be more posterior. **Answer A**

If T12 is rotated right, it will be limited in left rotation. **Answer B**

A thoracic dysfunction does not always preclude a rib dysfunction. There is not sufficient information given to determine if a rib dysfunction is present. **Answer D**

The question is describing a neutral dysfunction that is rotated right, sidebent left. Therefore T9 cannot be rotated right and sidebent right. **Answer E**

3. Answer C: The patient in the above question is performing a type of isometric contraction. The definition of an isometric contraction is a muscle contraction that results in an increase in tension without a change in length.

Concentric and eccentric contractions are contractions in which there is an approximation (concentric) or lengthening (eccentric) of muscular origin and insertion. Tension is not related to these type of contractions. **Answers A, B and D**

An isotonic contraction is one in which there is an approximation of the muscle's origin and insertion without an increase in muscle tension. The difference between concentric and isotonic contractions is that concentric contractions can have variable tensions. **Answer E**

4. Answer A: Direct muscle energy treatment would reverse all three planes of C3 (i.e. C3 would be placed in such a way that the segment is against its restrictive barrier in all three planes). In order to correctly perform typical muscle energy the segment must be flexed, sidebent right, and rotated right.

Flexing, sidebending left and rotating right would not reverses all 3 planes of motion. **Answer B**

Extending, sidebending left, and rotating left will place C3 away from the restrictive barrier. This position would be used for an indirect treatment. **Answer C**

Extending would not place the segment against its restrictive barrier. **Answers D and E**

5. Answer D: The elderly patient in the above question is recovering from severe pulmonary complications from his COPD. He has been bedridden for several weeks and he has coronary disease. As noted in the Foundations of Osteopathic Medicine elderly patients and hospitalized patients typically respond better with indirect techniques or gentle direct techniques, such as rib raising.

This patient could not tolerate isometric exercise due to his low vitality. **Answer A**

The patient will not be able to tolerate isotonic exercises with low resistance, even though myofascial release of the sacrum may help this patient. **Answer B**

Although rib raising will help the patient's respiratory status, this patient will not be able to tolerate muscle energy because of his low vitality. **Answer C**

Although this patient may tolerate myofascial release, he has been bedridden for several weeks. Thus, his bone mineral density may be decreased to the level of osteoporosis. High velocity low amplitude techniques are thus contraindicated. **Answer E**

6. Answer D: If C5 resists lateral translation to the left. This indicates that C5 resists right sidebending. If it resists right sidebending, it is sidebent left. If it is sidebent left, it must be rotated left (C5 follows the rules of type II mechanics).

Since the question did not test C2 in flexion and extension, we do not know whether C2 is flexed, extended or neutral. **Answer A**

A common way to test for rotation in the cervical spine is to push anterior on the articular pillar of the cervical spine at each segment. If there is resistance on one side compared to the other then the segment is rotated toward that side. In order to test rotation at C2 the practitioner would push anterior on each articular pillar. The above patient has paraspinal fullness on the right and the right articular pillar resists anterior glide, this indicates that C2 is rotated to the right. **Answer B**

The above question does not describe the direction of the atlanto-axial joint (C1 on C2). **Answers C and E**

7. Answer D: The joints of Luschka (also called the uncovertebral joints) are only located in the cervical spine. Most authors agree that they are not true synovial joints, however they play an important role in cervical motion, especially sidebending. They also serve to protect nerve roots from disc herniation.

Since the C5 nerve root exits between the C4 and C5 vertebrae, degenerative changes of the joint of Luschka and hypertrophy of the facet joint may cause C5 nerve root entrapment, not the C4 nerve root. **Answer A**

If the uncovertebral joint (a.k.a. the joint of Luschka) was a true synovial joint (again most authors think that it is not) its synovium would not be continuous with that of the facet joint. This is because the facet joints and uncovertebral joints are located on opposite sides of the intervertebral foramen. **Answer B**

The main motion of the OA joint is flexion and extension. Approximately half of the flexion and extension of the C-spine stems from the OA joint. **Answer C**

263

Restriction within the sternocleidomastoid muscle will decrease rotation to the ipsilateral side. **Answer E**

8. Answer C: Destruction of elastic fibers results from years of smoking. (an emphysema type of COPD). Irritation of the lung parenchyma may result in an overproduction of mucus causing obstruction and air trapping (chronic bronchitis and asthma type of COPD). These two factors expand the chest cavity and can result in an increased lung capacity, thus permanently positioning the ribs in inhalation.

Patients with COPD will have impaired oxygenation, however it will not result in a fibrosis and flattening of the diaphragm. If this were true all skeletal muscles in the body would be fibrosed. **Answer A**

Most accessory muscles will help elevate the ribs into inhalation, however these muscles are not strong enough to overcome the natural recoil of the lungs. **Answer B**

Chronic deoxygenation will result in a change in minute ventilation, rather than a permanent expansion of the thoracic cage. **Answer D**

Increased sympathetic tone from visceral afferents results in bronchodilation and consequently broncho-avelolar expansion. However, this is not the primary reason for an increased AP diameter in a person with COPD. **Answer E**

9. Answer C: Ribs 6-10 primarily move in a bucket-handle motion. Movement is around an AP axis, therefore, inhalation will increase the transverse diameter of the chest wall. [28 p.226]

Physiologic rib motion does not occur along an oblique plane. **Answer A**

Pump-handle ribs will increase the chest wall anteriorly around a transverse axis. **Answer B**

Rib movement around a transverse axis could not expand the ribcage laterally. **Answer D**

Ribs do not move around a vertical axis. **Answer E**

10. Answer B: A patient with low back pain radiating into BOTH lower extremities may be of neurogenic or musculoskeletal origin. Of all the neurogenic or musculoskeletal possibilities the most important entity to rule out is Cauda Equina Syndrome (CES). CES is an entrapment of terminal nerve roots of the spinal cord. This can be due to a central disc herniation. If S2-S4 nerve roots are involved incontinence can result. If this occurs, immediate surgical decompression is indicated. If decompression is delayed, this may result in irreversible incontinence.

Unilateral loss of the superficial abdominal reflex indicates a lower motor neuron lesion from T7 - L2, depending on where the absence is noted. If a lower motor neuron lesion was suspected, such as a herniated disc, it may impact his diagnosis, but his treatment is still likely to be conservative management. **Answer A**

If the patient had an absent Achilles reflex, this would indicate a lower motor neuron lesion at S1. If this were present, the treatment would still likely be conservative. **Answer C**

A downgoing plantar response when trying to elicit a Babinski reflex is a normal adult response. In other words, there is no Babinski reflex. Therefore, there is no suspected upper motor neuron lesion.

However, the patient may still have a lower motor neuron lesion present. **Answer D**

A unilateral loss of the cremasteric reflex suggests a lower motor neuron lesion between L1 and L2. This finding may impact diagnosis and treatment, however it would not impact the diagnosis and treatment as much as it would if it were cauda equina syndrome. **Answer E**

11. Answer A: The common fibular nerve (a.k.a. common peroneal nerve) courses behind (posterior to) the fibular head. A posterior fibular head dysfunction can exert pressure directly on the common fibular nerve resulting in foot drop.

Fibular head dysfunction will not directly compress the obturator or sciatic nerves. **Answers B and C**

The tibial nerve courses through the popliteal fossa, it is not affected by a fibular head dysfunction. **Answer D**

The sural nerve is made up of fibers from the common peroneal and tibial. It would not be compressed in fibular head dysfunction since these branches arise proximal to the fibular head. **Answer E**

12. Answer D: A positive standing flexion test indicates that the patient has a somatic dysfunction of the pelvis. In this case the positive standing flexion test is on the left side, therefore the dysfunction is on the left side. An inferior ASIS and a superior PSIS on the ipsilateral side indicates an anterior innominate.

With a unilateral sacral flexion on the right (USF$_R$) and a left sacral rotation on a left oblique axis (L on L), the right sulcus is freely mobile. However the question does not mention that it is deep, nor does the question state that there is a positive seated flexion test. Therefore you cannot assume sacral dysfunction in the above question. **Answer A and B**

With a left posterior innominate the left ASIS would be superior, and the left PSIS would be inferior. **Answer C**

With a superior innominate shear (upslip innominate or superior innominate subluxation) both the left ASIS and the PSIS would be superior. **Answer E**

13. Answer D: A noticeable absence in the lumbar lordosis, no motion of the lumbosacral junction and symmetrical ILA's indicate a bilaterally extended sacrum. A bilateral sacral extension (a.k.a. sacral base extension or extended sacral base) somatic dysfunction occurs about a middle transverse axis. [28] [p.402] For more details see Chapter 6 Sacrum and Innominates

In a patient with a bilaterally flexed sacrum, the lumbosacral junction will spring easily and the patient is likely to have an increased lumbar lordosis. In addition, respiration and craniosacral motion occur about the superior transverse axis. **Answers A, B, and C**

A bilaterally flexed or extended sacrum will have rotated around the middle transverse axis; therefore, the axis can be specified. [28 p.402] **Answer E**

14. Answer B: Left sacral rotation on a left oblique axis.

The patient has a positive seated flexion test on the right. In sacral rotation on an oblique axis, the seated flexion test is positive on the opposite side of the axis. Therefore we can eliminate right rotation on a right oblique axis. **Answer A**

The patient has a negative lumbosacral spring test. A lumbosacral spring test will be positive (no spring at the lumbosacral junction) if part of or the entire sacral base has moved posteriorly. The sacral base will move posterior a with backward sacral torsion (a right rotation on a left oblique axis or left rotation on a right oblique axis. **Answers C and D**

In a unilateral sacral flexion on the right the patient will have a posterior and inferior ILA on the right (not the left). **Answer E**

15. **Answer B**: The seated flexion test assesses sacral motion on the ilium. In other words, it assesses sacroilial motion. If there is an alteration (dysfunction) of sacral motion on the ilium, then there is sacroilial dysfunction. In a left on left sacral torsion, the right sacral base of the sacrum (sacral sulcus) will move anteriorly. This will produce an alteration of sacral motion in the right SI joint (right SI joint dysfunction).

Posterior rotation of the right innominate produces right iliosacral dysfunction and thus will produce a positive standing flexion test on the right. Iliosacral dysfunction is movement of the innominate on the sacrum. **Answer A**

Posterior glide of the left ILA does not produce left sacroilial dysfunction. Remember the seated flexion test is positive on the opposite side of the oblique axis in a sacral torsion. **Answer C**

Anterior rotation of the right innominate produces right iliosacral dysfunction and thus will produce a positive standing flexion test on the right. **Answer D**

In a left on left torsion the left sacral sulcus does not glide anteriorly (the right glides anteriorly). **Answer E**

16. **Answer C**: Injury to the medial cord of the brachial plexus is likely to affect C8, T1 and muscles innervated by the median and ulnar nerves. The interossi muscles of the hand are responsible for finger abduction. The ulnar nerve innervates the interossi.

The musculocutaneous nerve is responsible for elbow flexion. This nerve originates from the lateral cord. **Answer A**

The radial nerve is responsible for elbow extension. This nerve originates from the posterior cord. **Answer B**

The axillary nerve is primarily responsible for shoulder abduction. This nerve originates from the posterior cord. **Answer D**

The teres major (axillary nerve) and infraspinatus (suprascapular nerve) are responsible for shoulder external rotation. These nerves originate from the posterior and lateral cords respectively. **Answer E**

17. **Answer E**: The axillary nerve courses around the posterior aspect of the humeral head. The anterior/inferior dislocation can stretch the axillary nerve thus injuring it. Approximately 10% - 18% of shoulder dislocations will result in injury to the axillary nerve. [54] Typical muscle stretch reflexes (deep tendon reflexes) that are tested in the upper extremity are biceps, triceps and brachioradialis reflexes. Injury to the axillary nerve will not affect these reflexes.

The dorsal scapular nerve innervates the rhomboids and is not susceptible to injury with shoulder dislocation. **Answer A**

Although anterior/inferior shoulder dislocations typically disrupt the inferior glenohumeral ligament, it is not the most likely cause of arm abduction weakness. **Answer B**

Although complete tears of the supraspinatus tendon may lead to arm abduction weakness, shoulder dislocations do not typically result in complete supraspinatus tears. **Answer C**

Shoulder dislocations are not likely to rupture the deltoid muscle. **Answer D**

18. Answer D: There are 2 tibio-fibular articulations. The proximal articulation is synovial and the distal articulation is syndesmotic. In an anterior fibular head dysfunction, the proximal tibio-fibular articulation will be displaced anteriorly and will resist posterior glide.

A fibular head somatic dysfunction responds well to manipulative treatments. [37] HVLA, muscle energy and Indirect methods are commonly used techniques. **Answer A**

A fibular head anterior is associated with an externally rotated talus causing the foot to appear more dorsiflexed and everted. Increased motion in these planes is seen as a result. **Answer B**

The common peroneal nerve courses posteriorly to the fibular head. Posterior fibular head dysfunction can result in compression of this nerve causing foot drop. **Answer C**

The most common ankle sprain occurs with the foot in supination (plantar flexion, inversion and internal rotation). These ankle sprains are associated with posterior fibular head somatic dysfunctions. **Answer E**

19. Answer E: The above patient has developed symptoms of a post-traumatic hydrocephalus (PTH). PTH may present as dementia, ataxia and urinary incontinence. Craniosacral therapy is absolutely contraindicated in situations with increased intracranial pressure. Craniosacral therapy is relatively contraindicated in patients who have had a traumatic brain injury.

20. Answer B: The purpose of the vault hold is to address strains at the SBS. The index fingers contact the greater wings of the sphenoid. [25 p.410]

Fingers do not contact the frontal bone in a vault hold. **Answer A**

The middle fingers contact the zygomatic processes of the temporal bones. [1 p.539] **Answer C**

The ring fingers contact the mastoid processes of the temporal bones. [1 p.539] **Answer D**

The little fingers contact the squamous portions of the occiput. [1 p.539, 25 p.410] **Answer E**

21. **Answer B:** A viscero-somatic reflex occurs when localized visceral stimuli (in this case, from the gallbladder) produce patterns of reflex response in segmentally related somatic structures (in this case, at the tip of the scapula).

A somato-visceral reflex occurs when abnormal somatic stimuli enters the spinal cord and results in altered function of the visceral structure. **Answer A**

Although a Chapman's reflex point does represent a viscero-somatic reflex, it typically is described as a smooth firm, discretely palpable nodule approximately 2 -3 mm in diameter located within the deep fascia or on the periostium of the bone. It is not typically described as generalized tenderness. In addition, the posterior Chapman's point for the gallbladder is located at the T6 spinous or transverse process on the right. **Answer C**

A trigger point is "a hypersensitive focus, usually within a taut band of skeletal muscle or in the muscle fascia". Again the above question does not describe discrete tenderness, therefore it cannot be assumed that the patient has a trigger point. **Answer D**

A Jones tenderpoint is a small, tense area usually in the belly of a muscle that is used to diagnose and treat somatic dysfunctions. The question does not describe a discrete tense area, therefore, it cannot be assumed that this patient has a counterstrain tenderpoint **Answer E**

22. **Answer E:** Rib raising will increase costal wall motion thus increasing ventilation. It will also normalize sympathetic tone thus increasing tissue perfusion.

Stimulating the sympathetic nervous system would cause bronchodilation; stimulating the parasympathetic nervous system would cause bronchoconstriction. **Answer A**

Cranial manipulation may normalize the vagus nerve, not the phrenic nerve. **Answer B**

Decreasing the sympathetic nervous system will encourage perfusion of the lung parenchyma. **Answer C**

Redoming the diaphragm will increase the thoraco-abdominal pressure gradient and improve lymphatic return. **Answer D**

23. **Answer D:** Hypersympathetic activity to the head and neck structures will lead to vasoconstriction producing lymphatic congestion. [35 p.3] It will also inhibit secretion from the nasopharyngeal mucous membranes that produces dryness. [35 p.3] Sympathetic nerve fibers arise from the intermediolateral cells of the spinal cord. Although it has nothing to do with this question, hypersympathetic activity to the respiratory epithelium (lungs) will lead to increased secretion via increased goblet cell production.

The parasympathetic fibers (from the vagus nerve) will not lead to nasal and pharyngeal dryness or lymphatic congestion. **Answer A**

Postganglionic fibers that supply the head and neck structures stem from the cervical chain ganglia, however pre-ganglionic fibers originate from the intermediolateral cell column in the spinal cord. **Answers B and C**

The autonomic nervous system that supplies the head and neck do not originate from T5 - T7. **Answer E**

24. Answer D: Preganglionic fibers for the kidney and upper ureters synapse in the superior mesenteric ganglion, while fibers for the lower ureter synapse on the inferior mesenteric ganglion.

Sympathetic innervation arises from the cell bodies in the spinal cord at the level of T10 - L1. **Answer A**

Sympathetic stimulation causes vasoconstriction of afferent arterioles thus decreasing the glomerular filtration rate. **Answer B**

The parasympathetics will maintain normal peristaltic waves in the ureters, whereas sympathetic stimulation could cause ureterospasm. **Answer C**

Sympathetic stimulation contracts the trigone (sphincter), relaxes the detrusor (bladder wall) resulting in urinary retention. **Answer E**

25. Answer A: Treatment to improve lymphatic return should start with removal of all central restrictions (release the diaphragm and rib raising), followed by release of the periphery (lymphatic pumps). The basic lymphatic treatment program includes: [1 p.947]
   1) Releasing the diaphragms: Restrictions within the thoracic inlet will obstruct lymph drainage from anywhere in the body. Redoming the diaphragm will produce effective pressure gradients and enhance lymph return. Restrictions within the pelvic diaphragm will decrease lower extremity lymphatic drainage.
   2) Rib raising to reduce hypersympathetic activity (larger lymph channels receive sympathetic innervation and mobilizing ribs will also enhance respiration).
   3) Lymphatic pumps: A pedal pump will promote further lymph return.

There is a lot of debate about which diaphragm to release first; most say release the thoracic inlet first, but this answer is not fully established. What you should remember for the boards is to release the diaphragm and perform rib raising before starting lymphatic pumps.

As a general rule, diaphragms are first released before applying lymphatic techniques. This ensures the least amount of lymphatic resistance and maximizes the performance of the lymphatic technique (in this case pedal pump). **Answers B and C**

Although rib raising, pectoral lift and pedal pumps will enhance lymphatic drainage, this answer does not list any diaphragm releases and therefore it is not the best answer. **Answer D**

Answer E is not the best answer because it does not address the lower extremity edema. **Answer E**

26. Answer E: Anterior postural deviation as viewed from the sagittal plane (in relation to a plumb line) is described as: entire body leans forward, deviating anteriorly from plumb line, patient's weight supported by metatarsals. [25 p.38]

Military posture, as viewed from the sagittal plane (in relation to a plumb line) is described as: head tilted slightly posteriorly, cervical curve and thoracic curve normal, anterior cervical and posterior thoracic deviation from plumb line, anterior pelvic tilt, knees extended, ankles plantar flexed. [25 p.38] **Answer A**

Swayback posture as viewed from the sagittal plane (in relation to a plumb line) is described as: head forward, cervical spine lordotic, thoracic spine kyphotic, decreased lordosis of lumbar spine, posterior tilt of pelvis, hip and knee joints hyperextended. [25 p.38] **Answer B**

Posterior postural deviation as viewed from the sagittal plane (in relation to a plumb line) is described as: entire body leans backward, deviating posteriorly, balance maintained by anterior thrust of pelvis and hips, and marked lordosis from mid-thoracic spine down. [25 p.38] **Answer C**

Flat back posture as viewed from the sagittal plane (in relation to a plumb line) is described as: head forward, cervical spine has slightly increased lordosis, thoracic spine slightly kyphotic in upper portion then flattens in lower segments, lumbar lordosis flattened, and hips and knees extended. [25 p.38] **Answer D**

27. Answer D: The clavicle moves in three different directions. First, it moves superior and inferior with shrugging and depressing the shoulder. Second, it moves anterior and posterior with retraction and protraction of the shoulder. Third, it rotates anteriorly and posteriorly with internal and external rotation of the arm when it is abducted at 90°. [28 p.163] Shrugging the shoulder will cause the lateral end of the clavicle to move superior; this will cause the medial end to move inferior. If it does not, this indicates that a somatic dysfunction is present. Since you name somatic dysfunctions in the direction of freer motion, the clavicle has a superior somatic dysfunction at the sternum.

28. Answer C: This patient has peptic ulcer disease. The gastric ulcer would cause viscerosomatic changes to occur at the T6 spinal level.

C7 is not associated with viscerosomatic changes related to peptic ulcer disease. **Answer A**

T4 receives sympathetic innervation from the head and neck, heart, esophagus and lungs. **Answer B**

T10 and T12 receive sympathetic innervation from the middle and lower GI tract. **Answers D and E**

29. Answer A: This patient most likely has sinusitis, and would have viscerosomatic reflex changes at T1-T3 spinal levels.

T4-T6 spinal levels are associated with the viscerosomatic reflexes from the lungs and esophagus. **Answer B**

T7-T9 spinal levels are associated with the viscerosomatic reflexes from the upper GI tract. **Answer C**

T10-T12 spinal levels are associated with the viscerosomatic reflexes from the middle GI tract and the gonads. **Answer D**

T12-L2 spinal levels are associated with the lower GI tract. **Answer E**

30. Answer E: The most accepted area of the thoracic vertebra for palpatory evaluation of the thoracic spine is the transverse process.

The spinous process could be used, but convention dictates that it is the transverse processes. **Answer A**

Answers B, C, and D would be ineffective for diagnosis and are not readily palpable.

31. Answer C: This patient is in severe pain. Usually, first line medications are non-steroidal anti-inflammatory agents. However in this case, they are contraindicated because the patient is at high risk for a GI bleed (a history of peptic ulcer disease complicated by the fact that he is on Coumadin [Warfarin]). Therefore given his level of pain, an opiod is indicated. Deyo and colleagues [31] demonstrated that bed rest for two days helped patients return to work quicker and did not worsen their back pain. In addition, prolonged bed rest in the above patient may predispose him to forming another DVT. A patient with this level of pain is well suited for gentle techniques such as indirect techniques.

NSAIDS are contraindicated in this patient due to the high risk of GI bleed. **Answers A and B**

Five days of bed rest would not benefit the patient any more than 2 days and HVLA may injure the patient. **Answer D**

Deyo and collegues [31] demonstrated that bed rest for two days did not worsen patient's back pain and helped patients return to work quicker. Therefore this is not the best answer. **Answer E**

32. Answer B: This patient has a right inflared innominate caused by the hit to the lateral side of the hip. The laterality of the dysfunction was determined by the ASIS compression test. A positive test occurs if one ASIS resists posterior compression, indicating the side of the dysfunction. The static findings indicate that the distance from the right ASIS to the umbilicus is shorter than the left. This indicates an innominate inflare.

Left anterior innominate rotation, a left innominate outflare and a left superior innominate shear would have a positive ASIS compression test on the left, not the right. **Answers A, C, and E**

A right anterior innominate rotation would have a positive ASIS compression test on the right. The static findings would show that the ASIS on the right is inferior and the right PSIS is higher on the right compared to the left. The distance from the ASIS to the umbilicus would be equal. **Answer D**

33. Answer B: A left sacral margin posterior is the diagnosis. The left sulcus and the left ILA would be posterior and will resist springing.

A left unilateral sacral extension would have the static findings of a shallow left sulcus, a superior and slightly anterior left ILA and a positive left seated flexion test. **Answer A**

In a right sacral margin posterior both the right sulcus and the right ILA would be posterior and resist springing. **Answer C**

A bilateral sacral flexion has equally deep right and left sulci with equally shallow ILA's that resist springing. **Answer D**

A bilateral sacral extension has equally shallow right and left sulci, which resist springing and has equally deep ILA's. **Answer E**

34. Answer B: An adducted dysfunction of the ulna would have a decreased carrying angle, the hand and wrist would be abducted and the olecranon process would prefer lateral glide.

271

A posterior radial head dysfunction would cause the forearm to prefer pronation, and the radial head would resist anterior glide. Falling on a pronated forearm causes this dysfunction. The carrying angle is not affected in radial head dysfunctions. **Answer A**

An abducted ulna would have a increased carrying angle; the olecranon process would be restricted in medial glide, and the wrist and hand would be adducted. **Answer C**

An anterior radial head dysfunction would cause the forearm to prefer supination and the radial head would resist posterior glide. Falling backward on a supinated forearm can cause this dysfunction. The carrying angle is not affected in radial head dysfunctions. **Answer D**

Cervical radiculopathy is nerve root compression. It can occur with trauma, usually to the neck, not to the upper extremity and typically numbness and tingling in the extremity would be present. **Answer E**

35. **Answer A**: The most injured ligament of the foot is the anterior talofibular ligament.

The posterior talofibular and calcaneofibular ligaments are less frequently injured and are associated with a grade II and III ankle sprains. **Answers B and C**

The tibiocalcaneal ligament is a portion of the deltoid ligament. It is rarely injured. **Answer D**

Since the ankle is stable in dorsiflexion and the deltoid ligament very strong, injury to this ligament is rare. **Answer E**

36. **Answer A**: Normal values for range of motion varies due to age, gender and flexibility. Therefore it is more important to focus on asymmetry. The patient in the question has asymmetry of her internal rotators. The patient could have a problem on the right or left, however out of the answers given the only one that is possible is tight left external rotators. Tight left external rotators would decrease left internal rotation. Another possible answer is lax right external rotators. Lax right external rotators will increase right internal rotation, however this choice is not given.

Tight left internal rotators would decrease left external rotation. **Answer B**

Lax left external rotators would increase left internal rotation. **Answer C**

Tight right internal rotators will decrease right external rotation. **Answer D**

Lax right internal rotators will increase right external rotation. **Answer E**

37. **Answer E**: This patient has Dupuytren's contracture. This condition is characterized by contracture of the palmar fascia and nodule formation. There appears to be a genetic predisposition and is frequently found in alcoholics. [25 p. 294]

DeQuervain's disease is a tendonitis of the abductor pollicis longus, extensor pollicis longus or extensor pollicis brevis tendons. **Answer A**

Herberden's nodes are cartilaginous and bony enlargements of the distal interphalangeal joints of the fingers in degenerative joint diseases. It is most commonly seen in osteoarthritis. [25 p. 294] **Answer B**

Secondary stage of syphilis presents with a rash on the palms of the hands and feet, however, this patient has nodules, not a rash. **Answer C**

Bouchard's nodes are cartilaginous and bony enlargements of the proximal interphalangeal joints of the fingers in degenerative joint diseases. It is most commonly seen in rheumatoid arthritis. **Answer D**

38. Answer B: Right sacral torsion on a right oblique axis. In a sacral torsion, the seated flexion test (the test that checks for sacral dysfunction) is positive on the opposite side of the axis. A left deep sulcus that moves freely with anterior glide (springing) and a right ILA that resists springing indicates right rotation.

In a left sacral torsion on a left oblique axis, a right sacral torsion on a left oblique axis and in a unilateral sacral flexion on the right, the seated flexion test would be positive on the right. **Answers A, C and E**

In a left sacral torsion on a right oblique axis, the left sacral sulcus would be posterior (shallow) and it would resist anterior glide. In addition the right ILA would be anterior and move freely with anterior glide. **Answer D**

Case 39-40

39. Answer D: The above patient is likely to have suffered a severe wrist sprain. Initial management should include edema reduction along with immobilization until pain free range of motion can be restored.

Although 10-20% of patients with a scaphoid fracture will have negative x-rays, pain is usually present in the anatomic snuffbox, since the scaphoid is located on the radial side of the wrist. The above patient has pain located on the volar aspect at the ulnar-carpal joint. This is not typical of a scaphoid fracture. **Answers A, B and C**

There is no evidence in the osteopathic literature that specifies pain at the volar aspect of the wrist most likely represents an ulnar somatic dysfunction. In addition, muscle energy and HVLA are contraindicated in acute strains and sprains. **Answer E**

40. Answer A: Falling forward on an outstretched (pronated) arm typically causes a posterior radial head somatic dysfunction. This will result in decreased supination of the forearm, pain at the radial head and decreased (or restricted) anterior glide of the radial head at the elbow.

Increased carrying angle and increased wrist adduction is associated with an abducted ulnar somatic dysfunction. **Answers B and C**

Increased wrist abduction is associated with an adducted ulnar somatic dysfunction. **Answer D**

Decreased posterior glide of the radial head is associated with an anterior radial head somatic dysfunction. Falling backward on an outstretched (supinated) arm typically causes an anterior radial head somatic dysfunction. **Answer E**

Case 41-42

41. Answer C: The above patient most likely has an acute herniated disk and subsequently has a lumbar sidebending dysfunction. Asymmetry will be present with hip drop testing with a lumbar sidebending dysfunction.

Currently there is no literature suggesting frequent OMT prevents herniated discs. **Answer A**

Although the pelvis can be shifted to the left in a right psoas syndrome, a pelvic shift is also a common finding in a person with a herniated disc. In addition, psoas syndrome is not associated with a positive straight leg raising test and radiation of pain into the foot. **Answer B**

Most herniated discs do not require surgery (approximately 95% can be treated conservatively). Answer D

According to the World Health Organization, non-malignant pain should be initially treated with non-narcotic analgesia. If this fails, narcotics can then be initiated. **Answer E**

42. Answer B: The anterior tibialis is innervated by the L4 and L5 nerve roots. [3 p.445] The extensor hallucis longus is innervated by the L5 and S1 nerve roots. [3 p.445] L5 is the only nerve root listed above that shares these two muscles, therefore this is the nerve root that is most likely to be affected in the above patient.

Case 43-45

43. Answer B: This patient recently underwent major abdominal surgery. It is common for a post-operative patient to have limited chest wall motion. This typically leads to atalectasis. Atalectasis is the most common etiology of bi-basilar crackles in any post-surgical patient.

A pulmonary embolus is an acute event that will result in respiratory distress due to hypoxia. This patient does not have a pulmonary embolus. **Answer A**

Although congestive heart failure could lead to bi-basilar crackles, the patient has a normal respiratory rate and is not complaining of dyspnea or orthopnea. In addition, typically a patient in CHF will have an S3 gallop on auscultation of the heart. **Answer C**

Atalectasis could lead to pneumonia, however this would be more likely if the patient had a fever or cough. **Answer D**

This patient is not likely to have a pericardial effusion since the surgery was local to the abdominal cavity. **Answer E**

44. Answer A: The bi-basilar crackles are due to limited chest wall motion. This patient has recently undergone a major surgery. Deep breathing is likely to cause him abdominal pain and pain medication may limit respiratory effort. Therefore, any manipulative treatment that will enhance respiration will be beneficial to this patient. Rib raising will increase chest wall motion, enhance diaphragmatic excursion and enhance lymphatic return. In addition, rib raising will help normalize sympathetic influence to the viscera.

Condylar decompression may influence the vagus nerve, but this will not increase chest wall motion to remove the bi-basilar crackles. **Answer B**

The pedal pump, abdominal pump and liver pump are contraindicated in patients where there is a nearby incision or who have had recent abdominal surgery. **Answers C, D and E**

45. **Answer A**: The pedal pump utilizes the intermittent movement of the abdominal contents up against the diaphragm. [35 p.218] This movement may disrupt recent abdominal surgery and therefore it is contraindicated. [35 p.220]

Thoracic inlet release would be indicated in this patient to improve lymphatic return from the lower extremities and the lungs. **Answer B**

Rib raising is also indicated in this patient as described above. Rib raising is contraindicated in recent spinal surgery and rib or spinal fractures. **Answer C**

Craniosacral techniques as well as indirect myofascial release techniques are typically well tolerated in the post-operative patient, and therefore not contraindicated in this scenario. **Answers D and E**

Case 46-49

46. **Answer D**: The patient has a unilateral sacral flexion on the left. The findings for this dysfunction are: left sulcus deeper, left ILA significantly inferior, left ILA slightly posterior. Positive seated flexion test on the left. Motion (springing) at the left sulcus is present. Motion (springing) at the left ILA is restricted.

In a right sacral rotation on a right oblique axis, the right ILA would be posterior and slightly inferior. **Answer A**

In a left sacral rotation on a right oblique axis, the left sulcus would be shallow. **Answer B**

In a left sacral rotation on a left oblique axis, the right sulcus would be deep. **Answer C**

In a unilateral sacral extension on the left, the left sulcus is shallow and the left ILA is significantly superior and slightly anterior. **Answer E**

47. **Answer C**: The patient has a superior innominate shear. The findings in this dysfunction are: the ASIS & PSIS are more superior ipsilaterally. There is a shorter leg ipsilaterally and there is a positive standing flexion test ipsilaterally.

In an anterior rotated innominate, the ASIS is more inferior ipsilaterally and the PSIS is more superior ipsilaterally. **Answer A**

In a posterior rotated innominate, the ASIS is more superior ipsilaterally and the PSIS is more inferior ipsilaterally. **Answer B**

In an inferior innominate shear the ASIS and PSIS are more inferior ipsilaterally. **Answer D**

In a superior pubic shear, the ASIS's and PSIS's appear to be level and the pubic bone is superior ipsilaterally. **Answer E**

48. **Answer B:** The rectus femoris originates from the AIIS and inserts onto the quadriceps tendon. This muscle (along with the quadriceps) extends the knee. In addition, since it does attach above the hip it will also flex the hip to a small extent. To test restriction in this muscle the knee is passively flexed when the patient is in the prone position; if the knee cannot touch the buttocks and the hip starts to flex, the test is positive. This test is called Ely's test.

Although the Sartorius muscle flexes the hip, it inserts with the gracilis and semitendinosus via the pes anserine tendon and flexes the knee. **Answer A**

Stretching the vastus medialis will not flex the hip since it does not attach above the hip. **Answer C**

The gracilis muscle adducts and flexes the knee. **Answer D**

The hamstrings flex the knee and extend the hip. **Answer E**

49. Answer C: When somatic dysfunction occurs due to a short leg syndrome, the lumbar paraspinal musculature compensates so that the spine may remain straight and the eyes level. The lower back pain could have developed due to the overuse of these compensating dorsal muscles.

There is no temporal relation to the onset of back pain after minor trauma and previous history of back pain. **Answer A**

Although the force imparted by the ground probably did result in somatic dysfunction, this does not explain why it took two weeks for the pain to develop. The length of time from onset and the identification of a primary mechanism strongly suggest that the patient's back pain is the result of a secondary process. **Answer B**

Although somatoform disorder (psychogenic etiology) is possible, given a primary offending cause, this is not the most likely cause of this patient's pain. **Answer D**

If the patient has a high tolerance to pain, there is no reason why he would be experiencing pain now if the intensity of the pain is the same as it were two weeks ago. **Answer E**

Case 50-51

50. Answer B: The above patient has a left on right torsion. In sacral torsions, the seated flexion test is positive on the opposite side of the axis. In this case, the patient has a positive seated flexion test on the left, which this implies a right oblique axis. The lumbosacral spring test is positive; therefore the sacrum has rotated backward. This will also make the right sulcus deeper.

In a right on right torsion, the lumbosacral spring test is negative and the left sulcus is deeper. **Answer A**

In a right on left torsion, the seated flexion test would be positive on the right and the left sulcus is deeper. **Answer C**

In a left unilateral sacral flexion the left sulcus would be deeper, and the lumbosacral spring test would be negative. **Answer D**

In a right unilateral sacral extension, the left sulcus would be deeper. **Answer E**

51. Answer C: The patient's right leg is limited in adduction indicating that the right abductors (gluteus medius and tensor fascia lata) are restricted.

If the right adductors were restricted, right leg abduction would be decreased. **Answer A**

If the left adductors were restricted, left leg abduction would be decreased. **Answer B**

If the left abductors were restricted, left leg adduction would be decreased. **Answer D**

If the right abductors had increased flexibility, the right leg would have increased adduction. **Answer E**

Case 52-55

52. Answer E: Exhalation dysfunctions are characterized by one or a group of ribs held down. These ribs typically lag behind in inhalation. Pain usually increases with inhalation. Also anterior rib tenderpoints (in the mid axillary line) are often associated with anteriorly depressed ribs.

Although most rib dysfunctions are due to thoracic dysfunctions, the case does not include a thoracic dysfunction, therefore it cannot be assumed that the patient has one. **Answers A, B and C**

Inhalation dysfunctions are characterized by one or a group of ribs held up. These ribs typically lag behind in exhalation. Pain usually increases with exhalation. Also, posterior rib tenderpoints are often associated with posteriorly depressed ribs. **Answer D**

53. Answer B: In a group dysfunction usually one "key" rib is responsible in causing the dysfunction. In exhalation dysfunctions the "key" rib is the uppermost rib of the dysfunction, in this case rib 3.

If the patient were to have an inhalation dysfunction, treatment would be directed at rib 5. **Answer D**

54. Answer C: Ribs 3-5 are held down in exhalation. The pectoralis minor muscle originates from the coracoid process and inserts on ribs 3-5. Activation of this muscle with muscle energy would pull the shaft of the ribs superior, correcting the dysfunction.

The posterior scalene is used to treat a somatic dysfunction of rib 2. **Answer A**

The teres major and pectoralis major are not muscles used to treat rib dysfunctions. **Answers B and D**

The serratus anterior is used to treat a somatic dysfunction of ribs 6-9. **Answer E**

55. Answer B: The anterior tenderpoints for ribs 3-6 are all treated by sidebending and rotating toward the side of the tenderpoint and encouraging slight flexion. As a general rule, rib tenderpoints are treated for 2 minutes as opposed to 90 seconds. Dr. Jones felt that the positioning for rib dysfunctions could be uncomfortable for the patient and an extra 30 seconds were needed for the patient to relax.

Case 56-59

56. Answer D: The question describes a positive drop arm test. A rotator cuff tear is often associated with trauma and will result in sharp pain at the tip of the acromion, pain with active abduction and a positive drop arm test.

Restricted passive and active range of motion is characteristic of adhesive capsulitis. **Answer A**

Bicipital tendonitis will result in pain at the bicipital grove and increased pain with shoulder and elbow flexion. **Answer B**

Osteoarthritis is characterized by a gradual onset of pain and limited passive range of motion. Answer C

Thoracic outlet syndrome is due to compression of the neurovascular bundle. This typically results in pain radiating into the upper extremity. **Answer E**

57. **Answer A:** Ultrasound, which is a form of deep heat, increases the inflammatory response and will worsen the patient's edema.

Ice will help decrease edema following a musculoskeletal injury. It is indicated for the initial management of the injury. **Answer B**

Although it is not recommended that the patient wear a sling for more than a week, it can be used initially to provide relative rest depending on the severity of the injury and patient's activities of daily living. **Answer C**

A fascial release of the shoulder may be attempted to decrease myofascial restrictions and improve lymphatic return to reduce edema and promote healing. **Answer D**

HVLA to the cervical spine is not contraindicated in this patient. It will not directly affect the glenohumeral joint. **Answer E**

58. **Answer B:** Rofecoxib is a non-steroidal anti-inflammatory agent that achieves its effects by inhibiting cyclooxygenase 2 (COX-2). By selectively inhibiting COX-2 it is less likely to cause a GI bleed. Since the patient is on Coumadin (Warfarin) the patient will be at a greater risk if a GI bleed develops. Another medicine that would be indicated for this patient is acetaminophen.

Ibuprofen and indomethacin are NSAID's that would put the patient at an increased risk for GI bleed. **Answers A and C**

Rotator cuff tears are not treated with oral steroids due to the numerous adverse effects of this class of medications. The same beneficial effects can be achieved with non-steroidal anti-inflammatory agents. **Answer D**

Narcotics are reserved for pain that does not respond to non-narcotic medication. **Answer E**

59. **Answer B:** A decreased sub-acromial space and a high riding humerus raises the likelihood of a complete rotator cuff tear. An MRI is the best imaging study to identify the extent of the injury.

A CT scan (computed tomography scan) does not show the detail of soft tissue as would an MRI. **Answer A**

A bone scan and PET scan would show general inflammation in the area of the shoulder but would not identify the extent of soft tissue injury. **Answers C and E**

An axillary radiograph is the best view to determine if there is a shoulder dislocation. It will not identify a rotator cuff tear. **Answer D**

Case 60-62

60. **Answer B:** A posterior radial head may present as a sharp pain at the wrist or elbow and may result from a fall on an outstretched arm. On examination, the posterior radial head will resist anterior glide at the elbow and the forearm will be restricted with supination.

The other answers listed are possible, however none are associated specifically with a fall on an outstretched arm. **Answers A, C, D and E**

61. **Answer D**: The anatomic snuff box is located at the radiocarpal joint and is bordered by the extensor pollicis longus and abductor pollicis longus tendons. Since the patient has pain at the anatomic snuff box with some edema and decreased range of motion at the wrist, he may have a fracture of the scaphoid bone. HVLA is contraindicated in areas of the fracture.

Muscle energy to the upper extremity to increase supination is not contraindicated because this technique can be modified so that no stress is applied to the radiocarpal joint. A cross extensor reflex muscle energy could also be used. This would require treating the left upper extremity in order to achieve a therapeutic effect in the right upper extremity. **Answer A**

Counterstrain is not contraindicated because this technique can also be modified so that no stress is applied to the radiocarpal joint. **Answer B**

Thoracic inlet release and posterior axillary fold techniques are indicated in this scenario because both techniques will help open lymphatic channels and help decrease the edema in this person's right upper extremity. **Answers C and E**

62. **Answer B**: Since the patient had pain at the anatomic snuff box and symptoms have not improved in 3 weeks time, the diagnosis of fracture should be considered. Although the X-rays of the wrist are normal, the patient may still have a small non-displaced scaphoid fracture. The scaphoid bone is the most common bone fractured in the wrist and often presents with pain in the anatomic snuffbox. X-rays may be normal for a week or longer. [29 p.467] If a fracture is suspected, the practitioner may obtain a second set of x-rays, or a bone scan can be ordered. A bone scan will accurately identify a fractured scaphoid. [57 p.73]

Putting the child on a pain medication without immobilizing the wrist is ill advised, especially with the likelihood of a fracture. **Answer A**

Appropriate management for a scaphoid wrist fracture is immobilization of the wrist for 3 months. Due to the lack of a rich blood supply, the healing of a fractured scaphoid is characteristically slow. Immobilizing the wrist for two weeks will not allow the fracture to fully heal. **Answer C**

Wrist sprains typically improve within a week's time. If the swelling and pain are increased, the diagnosis of a fracture should be considered. Answer D

Case 63-68

63. **Answer D**: This is a classic presentation of psoas syndrome. Typical signs and symptoms include: a high lumbar somatic dysfunction, pelvic shift to the opposite side of the psoas spasm and a contralateral piriformis spasm. The contralateral piriformis muscle spasm may irritate the sciatic nerve causing radiation of pain down the thigh, but not usually past the knee. [56 p.748]

Piriformis syndrome is a peripheral neuritis of the sciatic nerve usually due to an irritation or inflammation of the piriformis muscle. [25 p. 446] **Answer A**

COPYRIGHT 2009

Spondylolysis is a fracture of the pars interarticularis without anterior displacement. This typically is seen as a "collar" on the scotty dog in oblique views of the lumbar spine. **Answer B**

A herniated nucleus pulposus would likely cause a radiating pain below the knee and into the foot. **Answer C**

Lumbar stenosis is usually characterized as back pain with radiation into the lower leg or legs. It can be accompanied with paresthesias and pain worsens with lumbar extension. **Answer E**

64. **Answer A:** The key somatic dysfunction is usually found at L1 or L2. Treatment of this "key" somatic dysfunction is essential for the patient's comfort and for effective, long lasting effects. [56 p.748]

Although treatment of other somatic dysfunctions may restore symmetry, these dysfunctions are not considered the key somatic dysfunction. **Answers B, C, D, E**

65. **Answer D:** A positive lumbosacral spring test limits the choices to a backward sacral torsion and unilateral sacral extension. The left ILA is posterior and slightly inferior and the left sacral sulcus is shallow, indicating left rotation on a right oblique axis.

Right rotation on a right oblique axis and left rotation on a left oblique axis would have negative lumbosacral spring tests. **Answers A and C**

In a right rotation on a left oblique axis, the right sulcus would be shallow and the left ILA would be anterior and slightly superior. **Answer B**

In a right unilateral sacral extension, the right sulcus would be shallow. **Answer E**

66. **Answer E:** Psoas syndrome could result in a contralateral piriformis muscle spasm. This may irritate the sciatic nerve and may radiate pain to the knee. [56 p.748]

Although the patient certainly does have psoas syndrome on the left side, it is not most directly related to the pain radiating into the right knee. **Answer A**

Since the x-ray findings are normal, the patient is not likely to have spondylolysis, therefore it is not likely the cause of his pain. **Answer B**

Although disc herniation will typically cause radiation of pain, this is not likely in this patient because herniated discs usually result in a neurologic deficit. **Answer C**

Since the lumbar x-rays are negative, this patient does not have spondylolisthesis. **Answer D**

67. **Answer B:** A right anterior innominate rotation has a lower right ASIS than the left, a right PSIS higher than the left, and a positive standing flexion test on the right.

A left anterior and left posterior innominate rotation would have positive standing flexion tests on the left. **Answers A and C**

A right posterior rotation would have the same standing flexion test, but would have a higher ASIS on the right than the left, and the right PSIS would be lower than the left. **Answer D**

68. **Answer C:** The psoas muscle is primarily a hip flexor, so the patient should be in the supine position, not prone (Answers B and D), with the hip and knees flexed, not extended (**Answer E**) and sidebent toward the affected muscle, not away (**Answer A**)

Case 69-71

69. Answer E: Patello-femoral syndrome (also known as lateral femoral patella tracking syndrome) is among the most common causes of knee complaints in primary care medicine, particularly among adolescents and young adults. The patient's chief complaint is anterior knee pain that is exacerbated with running, jumping and climbing stairs. [32 p.361]

Osgood-Schlotter's is a traction apophysitis of the tibial tubercle. **Answer A.** Pain and inflammation are located at the tibial tubercle. Housemaid's knee, Answer D, also has enlargement and pain at the tibial tuberosity, which is caused by constant kneeling on hard surfaces. Both of these conditions are responsible for anterior knee pain, but at a very localized area, and do not account for the point tenderness on the posterior aspect of the patella or the patellar crepitus.

Baker's cyst is usually found in the popliteal fossa of the knee and does not result in anterior knee pain. These cysts can be associated with degeneration of the posterior horn of the medial meniscus. [32 p.327] **Answer B**

Patellar tendonitis is an inflammation of the patellar tendon usually caused by overuse. It results in pain at the insertion into the patella. Patellar crepitus is not an associated finding. **Answer C** [32 p.356]

70. Answer B: An increased Q angle has a major effect on the tracking of the patella. As the Q angle increases, the patient's knees become more knock-kneed (genu valgus), causing an abnormal tracking of the patella, predisposing the patella to irregular or accelerated wear. The patella may even sublux laterally with these biomechanical forces, especially with dysfunction or weakness of the vastus medialis muscle. [1 p.627]

Genu recurvatum is a hyperextension of the knee due to ligament laxity, also called back knee, and has not been associated with patello-femoral syndrome. [49] **Answer A**

A decreased Q-angle is not associated with patello-femoral syndrome; see explanation for answer B. **Answer C**

Coxa valgus occurs when the angle between the neck and shaft of the femur is greater than 135 degrees. This has no association with patello-femoral syndrome. **Answer D**

Coxa vara has not been associated with patello-femoral syndrome. **Answer E**

71. Answer A: Patello-femoral syndrome is caused by a mal-tracking of the patella. Typically the patella tracks too far laterally, this is usually due to a weak vastus medialis and a tight vastus lateralis. Decreasing myofascial restrictions in the vastus lateralis would have the greatest effect on this patient's symptoms. Surgical treatment for patello-femoral syndrome consists of a lateral patella release.

Decreasing myofascial restrictions in the vastus medialis could theoretically worsen this condition. **Answer D**

Decreasing myofascial restrictions in other muscles may help, but considering the biomechanics of the problem, it will not have the greatest effect. **Answers B, C and E**

Case 72-73

72. **Answer B:** This patient has signs and symptoms consistent with hyperthyroidism. T1-T4 receives sympathetic innervation from the thyroid. [35 p.192]

Although C3-C5 may have tissue texture changes from local effects, it is less likely to be involved in a viscerosomatic reflex since the sympathetic nervous system stems from T1 - L2. **Answer A**

T5-T9 receives sympathetic innervation from the upper GI tract. **Answer C**

T9-T12 and L1 - L2 receive sympathetic innervation from below the diaphragm. **Answers D and E**

73. **Answer B:** The patient has hyperthyroidism, and the Chapman's reflex point associated with thyroid dysfunction is found at both interspaces of ribs 2 and 3, just lateral to the sternum. [56 p.1053]

Next to the sternum at the interspace of ribs 1 and 2 is the Chapman's point for the tonsils. [56 p.1053]
Answer A

Next to the sternum at the interspace of ribs 3 and 4 is the Chapman's point for the upper lung. [56 p.1053]
Answer C

Next to the sternum at the interspace of ribs 4 and 5 is the Chapman's point for the lower lung. [56 p.1053]
Answer D

Next to the sternum at the interspace of ribs 5 and 6 on the left is the Chapman's point for stomach acidity, and on the right is the Chapman's point for the liver. [56 p.1053] **Answer E**

Case 74-75

74. **Answer E:** Pathology in the recto-sigmoid area would cause a viscerosomatic change at the T12-L2 spinal level.

C3 - C5 spinal segments are not involved in a viscero-somatic reflex in the recto-sigmoid region.
Answer A

T1-T4 receives sympathetic innervation from the head and neck. **Answer B**

T5-T9 receives sympathetic innervation from the upper GI tract. **Answer C**

T10-T12 receives sympathetic innervation from the middle GI tract. **Answer D**

75. **Answer C:** The term "gangliform contraction" is the original term Frank Chapman used for his reflex points. It was not until much later that these "gangliform contractions" became "Chapman's points". The Chapman's point for the recto-sigmoid colon is located on the left proximal femur at the greater trochanter in the iliotibial tract.

The Chapman's point for the iliocecal area is located on the right proximal femur at the greater trochanter within the iliotibial tract. **Answer A**

The Chapman's point for the right half of the transverse colon is located on the right distal femur in the iliotibial tract. **Answer B**

The Chapman's point for the left half of the transverse colon is located on the left distal femur in the iliotibial tract. **Answer D**

The Chapman's point for the ovaries and urethra is located on the superior rami of the pubis. **Answer E**

Case 76-81

76. Answer E: Ribs 8-10 are classified as false ribs. False ribs are those ribs that do not directly attach to the sternum.

Bifid ribs occur in 1-2% of the population, but this abnormality is present in 8.4% of Somoans. The condition is usually unilateral, and appears as an 8th true rib. **Answer A**

The atypical ribs are 1, 2, 11, and 12. Sometimes rib 10 is considered atypical. **Answer B**

True ribs directly attach to the sternum. The true ribs are ribs 1-7. **Answer C**

The floating ribs are ribs 11 and 12. **Answer D**

77. Answer D: Bucket handle ribs 8-10 that have an inhalation dysfunction do not move caudally in exhalation and may cause pain during the exhalation phase of respiration. Upon static assessment, the lower edge of the rib shaft is more prominent and elevated laterally.

Answers A and B are incorrect because the ribs are not in exhalation dysfunction.

If the ribs had a pump-handle dysfunction, they would be elevated anteriorly. **Answer C**

Laterally elevated ribs are more closely associated to bucket-handle dysfunctions, not caliper dysfunctions. **Answer E**

78. Answer E: In exhalation dysfunctions, the rib moves caudad on expiration and is restricted on inspiration. In pump-handle dysfunctions the findings are concentrated on the anterior part of the rib in the mid-clavicular line and the rib angle.

In inhalation dysfunctions, the rib moves cephalad on inspiration and it is restricted on expiration. **Answers A, B, and C**

In bucket handle dysfunctions the findings are concentrated on the lateral part of the rib in the mid-axillary line. **Answers B and D**

79. Answer A: In a group exhalation dysfunction the key rib is the top most rib of the group, which is rib 5. The correct muscle to use for a muscle energy treatment of rib 5 is the pectoralis minor muscle.

Rib 5 is the key rib, but it is not treated with the serratus anterior muscle. **Answer B**

Ribs 6 and 7 are not the key ribs, therefore these answers can be easily eliminated. **Answers C, D, and E**

80. Answer A: In a group exhalation dysfunction the key rib is the top most rib of the group, which is rib 5. Anterior tenderpoints are associated with depressed ribs (exhalation dysfunctions). [56 p.1011] The tenderpoint for rib 5 is located in the mid-axillary line.

Ribs 6 and 7 should not be treated because neither are the key rib. **Answers B, C and E**

Posterior tenderpoints are associated with elevated ribs (inhalation dysfunctions). [56 p.1011] **Answers D and E**

81. **Answer E:** In order to allow extra time for the patient to relax, it is recommended that rib tenderpoints be treated for 2 minutes.

All other body counterstrain points are typically treated for 90 seconds. **Answer D**

There are no other intervals of time used for counterstrain. **Answers A, B, and C**

Matching

82. **Answer C:** This is typically described as short, flat-footed shuffling steps in which the foot does not clear the ground. In Parkinsonism, rigidity, tremor, paucity of movement, shuffling with haste, and difficulty in starting, stopping, or turning are also seen. [25 p. 243]

83. **Answer H:** This gait is characterized by a shift of the body toward the side of the weak gluteus medius. In this case the person's right gluteus medius muscle is weak. He compensates by shifting his body weight toward the weak side. By doing this he prevents the left side of his pelvis from dropping. [25 p. 243]

84. **Answer D**: A waddling gait can be described as rolling from side to side. The pelvic rotation and pelvic tilt are increased. This has been described as a penguin walk. Muscular dystrophy with weakness of hips, exaggerated lordosis, and pot-bellied posture can produce this gait. [25 p. 243]

85. **Answer A**: A high steppage gait will typically result from a foot drop. In this case the effected side is raised higher (hip is flexed more) in order to clear the foot.

86. **Answer I**: In scissor gait the legs are adducted, crossing alternately in front of one another. Both adductors typically have spasticity. This is a common type of gait in children with cerebral palsy. [25 p. 243]

87. **Answer E**: In this type of gait, the leg is extended at the knee with plantar flexion at the ankle. The patient leans to the stronger side (in this case the right side) and advances the leg by curcumducting it. Since the ankle is plantar flexed the foot tends to drag against the floor. [25 p. 242]

88. **Answer G**: Antalgic gait is characterized by a short stance phase while the patient is standing on the painful extremity. During this short stance phase there is a rapidly executed swing phase of the opposite leg. The patient tries to avoid standing on a painful extremity. [25 p. 243]

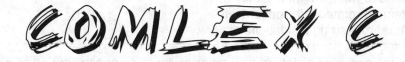

COMLEX C
EXAMINATION

COMLEX C EXAMINATION

1. Which of the following statements concerning treatment of rib dysfunctions is true?

   A) If a thoracic dysfunctions is present it should be treated before rib dysfunctions
   B) Exhalation dysfunctions cannot be treated with HVLA
   C) In general, posterior tenderpoints are treated by rotating and sidebending the thorax toward the dysfunction
   D) Muscle energy techniques are contraindicated in elderly patients with COPD
   E) An inhalation dysfunction of ribs 6-9 can be corrected by contracting the serratus anterior muscle

2. A patient is found to have a posterior transverse process on the right at L2. Flexion of the lumbar spine increases the asymmetry at this segment, whereas extension restores symmetry. Which of the following is the correct muscle energy (direct) treatment position.

   A) Flexed rotated left sidebent left
   B) Flexed rotated right sidebent right
   C) Extended rotated right sidebent right
   D) Extended rotated left sidebent left
   E) Neutral rotated right sidebent left

3. A 19-year-old male with no history of past medical illness comes to your office with neck pain. Active neck range of motion reveals painful right rotation to 45 degrees, and painless left rotation to 90 degrees. Which of the following statements is true regarding this patient's range of motion.

   A) Since the patient has limited right rotation he likely has limited left sidebending
   B) Since the patient has limited right rotation he likely has limited right sidebending
   C) This patient is likely to have decreased passive range of motion to the right.
   D) The patient is likely to have full passive range of motion with right rotation to the physiologic barrier.
   E) This patient demonstrated that he has full left rotation to the anatomic barrier.

4. A 21-year-old male is in the intensive care unit following a motor vehicle accident. He has sustained bilateral tibia/fibula fractures and several rib fractures. He underwent closed reduction/external fixation of his tib/fib fractures 24 hours ago. He has been extubated since the surgery and is complaining of severe pain at the surgical site as well as at the chest wall. Ultrasound on the lower extremities is negative for deep venous thrombosis. Which one of the following is the best statement regarding osteopathic treatment for this patient?

   A) This patient should receive osteopathic manipulation daily until he is transferred out of the unit.
   B) This patient should receive direct active forms of treatment such as muscle energy.
   C) This patient should receive one extensive session of osteopathic treatment then followed-up in two weeks.
   D) Osteopathic treatment is contraindicated in this patient due to the acute nature of the illness.
   E) This patient should receive indirect myofascial release and diaphragm release to improve lymphatic return.

5. In a patient with low back pain, L5 is flexed and sidebent right. Which of the following is true?

   A) You would expect L5 to rotate easily to the left, based on the laws of type II spinal mechanics.
   B) You would expect L5 to sidebend easily to the right, based on the laws of type I spinal mechanics
   C) You would expect L5 to resist right rotation in the flexed position.
   D) You would expect the right transverse process of L5 to become more posterior as the spine moves from flexion to extension.
   E) You would expect the sacrum to be rotated forward on a left oblique axis if a torsion was present.

6. You are asked to evaluate a 20-year-old male with severe unrelenting low back pain. He is unable to move without excruciating pain and rates the pain 10 out of 10. The pain is localized and there is no numbness or tingling in the lower extremities. On examination, there are no neurological deficits. Straight leg raising test is negative. X-rays are negative for fracture, but demonstrates a straightening of the lumbar lordosis. Structural examination reveals an anterior rotated innominate on the right; a left on left sacral torsion and L2 is FRRSR. Tenderpoints are noted one inch medial to the right ASIS. The paraspinal tissues are edematous, erythematous, and boggy with increased moisture and hypertonic muscles. Given the above information, what osteopathic treatment is best suited for this patient initially to improve his symptoms?

   A) Muscle energy to the innominates.
   B) Counterstrain to iliopsoas tenderpoints.
   C) Muscle energy to sacrum.
   D) High-velocity low amplitude techniques to the lumbar spine.
   E) All osteopathic treatment is contraindicated due to the acute nature of his injury.

7. In a patient with neck pain, the second cervical segment is found to resist translation to the left with the head in the flexed position. The segment translates equally to the left and right in the extended position. Given the above diagnosis, which is the correct muscle energy (direct) technique?

   A) C2 should be placed in flexion, right sidebending and right rotation and the patient would be asked to rotate his head to the left against resistance.
   B) C2 should be placed in flexion, left sidebending and left rotation and the patient would be asked to rotate his head to the right against resistance.
   C) C2 should be placed in extension, right sidebending and right rotation and the patient would be asked to rotate his head to the left against resistance.
   D) C2 should be placed in extension, left sidebending and left rotation and the patient would be asked to rotate his head to the right against resistance.
   E) C2 should be placed in extension, left sidebending and left rotation and the patient would be asked to rotate his head to the left against resistance.

8. Which of the following is true regarding the anatomy and biomechanics of the thoracic region?

   A) When a patient is standing with their arms at their side, the medial border of the spine of the scapula is immediately lateral to the spinous process of T1.
   B) The spinous processes of the thoracic region point increasing downward, such that T1's spinous process is approximately at the level of the transverse process of T2.
   C) Restriction within Sibson's fascia is likely to limit lymphatic drainage from the left lower extremity.
   D) The main motion of the thoracic cage is about a transverse axis.
   E) At quiet breathing the diaphragm bears 80 - 90% of the workload.

9. Which of the following best explains the role of the quadratus lumborum.

   A) Inhalation causes relaxation of the quadratus lumborum and permits cephalad movement of rib 12.
   B) Contraction will result in posterior translation of ribs 11 and 12.
   C) It is the 1st structure to react to stress in the lumbosacral area.
   D) Contraction will increase lumbar lordosis and increase the intercostal space between the 11th and 12th ribs.
   E) It plays little role in lymphatic drainage

10. Which of the following is the best statement regarding anatomy and biomechanics of the lumbar spine?

    A) The lumbar spine moves easiest about a sagittal axis
    B) Lumbarization increased the flexibility of the lumbosacral unit thus decreasing the likelihood of degenerative joint disease.
    C) The S1 nerve root will exit between the L5 and S1 vertebrae.
    D) Central disc herniations are more common than posterior-lateral disc herniations.
    E) Radicular symptoms from a herniated disc will often worsen when the lumbar spine is flexed.

11. A 72-year-old male comes to your office with chronic low back pain. He has a 20+year history of diabetes and was recently diagnosed with prostate cancer. His back pain is a dull ache that radiates into the right buttock and thigh. The pain is made worse with standing or walking. Pain is relieved with sitting. On examination, pulses are strong in the lower extremities and capillary refill is adequate. Range of motion of his lumbar spine is decreased. Sensation is decreased in both feet in a stocking like distribution. Muscle testing is 5/5 in both lower extremities. Reflex testing is 2+ at the patella bilaterally, and absent at the Achilles bilaterally. Considering this patient's symptoms, what is the most likely finding this patient will have on radiological studies?

    A) A herniated nucleus pulposus on magnetic resonance imaging
    B) Lytic lesions involving the lumbar vertebrae
    C) Spondylolisthesis of L5 on S1.
    D) Spondylosis of the lumbar spine
    E) Compression fracture of the lumbar vertebrae.

12. In a patient with lowback/gluteal pain physical examination shows the following:
Positive seated flexion test on the right, left ILA posterior/inferior, and right sacral base is anterior.
   Lumbosacral spring test is negative and lumbar curve is convex to the right. Assuming the
   patient has a sacral torsion what would be the expected L5 dysfunction?

   A) L5 FR$_L$S$_L$
   B) L5 FR$_R$S$_R$
   C) L5 ER$_R$S$_R$
   D) L5 NS$_L$R$_R$
   E) L5 NS$_R$R$_L$

13. Which of the following is the best answer regarding pelvic biomechanics?

   A) During ambulation, weight bearing on the left leg will induce sacral rotation around a
      right oblique axis.
   B) The stance phase of gait is associated with anterior rotation of the innominate.
   C) As a person inhales the lumbosacral angle increases
   D) The sacrum nutates with craniosacral flexion
   E) A positive seated flexion test on the right will always indicate sacral dysfunction on a left
      oblique axis.

14. Evaluation of a patient with hip and groin pain reveals a positive standing and seated flexion
   test on the right. The left ASIS appears more caudad and the left PSIS is more cephalad when
   compared to the right. The lumbosacral junction springs freely. The right sacral base is more
   anterior when compared to the left. What of the following is the best answer?

   A) This patient has a posterior rotated innominate on the left
   B) The above patient is likely to have tight quadriceps on the right
   C) This patient has a right shortened psoas
   D) ASIS compression of the pelvis on the right will demonstrate adequate resiliency
   E) This patient is likely to have an apparent short leg on the right

15. 52-year-old man comes to your office with low back pain of acute onset. Examination reveals a
   positive standing flexion test on the left. The right anterior superior iliac spine (ASIS) is more
   anterior and inferior than the left. The most likely diagnosis is:

   A) Right superior pubic shear
   B) Right posterior innominate
   C) Right anterior innominate
   D) Left posterior innominate
   E) Left anterior innominate

16. Which of the following anatomic sacral somatic dysfunctions is often seen in the post-partum
   patient?

   A) Bilateral sacral extension
   B) Bilateral sacral flexion
   C) Forward sacral torsion
   D) Backward sacral torsion
   E) Unilateral sacral flexion

17. Injury to the C5 and C6 nerve roots of the brachial plexus is most likely to produce which of the following effects?

    A) Waiters tip deformity
    B) Wrist drop
    C) Claw hand
    D) Benediction sign
    E) Klumpke's palsy

18. Which of the following is typically seen in golfers elbow.

    A) A history of overuse of the wrist extensor muscles.
    B) Pain with resisted wrist flexion
    C) Positive Tinel's sign at the cubital tunnel
    D) Posterior radial head dysfunction.
    E) Pain at the olecranon process of the ulna.

19. The most common injured ligament in the ankle is:
    A) Spring ligament
    B) Anterior talofibular ligament
    C) Posterior talofibular ligament
    D) Deltoid ligament
    E) Calcaneofibular ligament

20. Craniosacral flexion is associated with:

    A) Counternutation of the sacrum around a middle transverse axis
    B) Caudad motion of the spinal dura
    C) External rotation of the frontal bone
    D) Increased AP diameter of the cranium
    E) Nausea

21. A patient has a CRI of 8 cycles/min with severely decreased excursion of the flexion and extension mechanism. The technique that will most effectively restore normal amplitude of the CRI is?

    A) Temporal rocking
    B) CV4 decompression
    C) V-spread
    D) Venous sinus technique
    E) Frontal lift

22. Which structures/locations are least likely to be influenced in a patient with cardiac dysfunction?

    A) The intercostal space between rib 2 and 3 at the sternal junction
    B) The cranial base
    C) The second cervical vertebrae
    D) The second thoracic vertebrae
    E) The seventh thoracic vertebrae

23. You approach your osteopathic professor one day with a very serious question. "A friend of yours" is having difficulty with premature ejaculation. As a concerned friend you ask the professor if there are any specific OMT techniques that may help this type of ejaculatory dysfunction. The professor explains that OMT may help alter visceral input from facilitated segments. Based on your knowledge of the autonomic nervous system and visceral innervation, you come to the conclusion that treatment of which structure(s) may help "your friends" premature ejaculation?

   A) Occipito-atlantal joint
   B) Sacrum
   C) T4 - T6
   D) T8 - T10
   E) T12 - L2

24. Abnormal visceral afferent input from cardiac muscle is most likely to manifest somatic changes in paraspinal musculature adjacent to which vertebral level.

   A) C5 - C7
   B) T3 - T4
   C) T7 - T9
   D) T9 - T12
   E) L1 - L3

25. A patient with diverticulosis is likely to have chronic changes related to a Chapman's point in which of the following areas?

   A) Periumbilically
   B) Iliotibial band on the left
   C) Paraspinal muscles at T9
   D) Spinous process of T11
   E) Paraspinal muscles at L4

26. Manipulation of which spinal segments may decrease blood pressure by decreasing fluid retention?

   A) C3-C4
   B) C5-C7
   C) T5-T9
   D) T10-T11
   E) T12 - L1

27. A patient with back pain received osteopathic manipulative treatment. The following was done:
    HVLA to C3, C5, T4, L1, L5 and right innominate
    Muscle energy to the sacrum,
    Counterstrain to the piriformis muscle

Based on the above information what is the maximum number of treated areas that should be filled
   out on the Osteopathic Soap Note Form?

   A) 1-2 areas
   B) 3-4areas
   C) 5-6 areas
   D) 7-8 areas
   E) 9-10 areas

28. During your evaluation of a patient complaining of neck pain you find a decrease in flexion and
    extension. What structure typically has the greatest movement in flexion and extension?

   A) Occipital condyles
   B) Atlanto-axial joint
   C) C3
   D) C5
   E) C7

29. A patient with renal failure for 8 months would be expected to have:

   A) Acute tissue texture changes at T7
   B) Chronic tissue texture changes at T9
   C) Acute tissue texture changes at T11
   D) Chronic tissue texture changes at T11
   E) Acute tissue texture changes at T9

30. A 68-year-old male complains of a headache and blurred vision for several months.
Physical examination reveals an abnormal opthalmotonometry. At what spinal levels would you
   expect to find the tissue texture changes related to a viscerosomatic reflex?

   A) T1-T3
   B) T5-T6
   C) T7-T9
   D) T10-T12
   E) T12-L2

31. A patient complains of mid-thoracic back pain for three days. While evaluating T5 you find that
    your right thumb is more anterior than your left, and symmetry is not restored after flexion or
    extension. What is the diagnosis for this somatic dysfunction?

   A) T5 FR_RS_R
   B) T5 ER_LS_L
   C) T5 NR_LS_R
   D) T5 NR_RS_L
   E) T5 ER_RS_R

32. A patient comes to your office after "his back went out" earlier that morning. Standing postural x-rays determine that there is significant sacral base unleveling. Which ligament is thought to be the first ligament to become painful in lumbosacral decompensation?

   A) Sacrotuberous
   B) Anterior sacroiliac
   C) Iliolumbar
   D) Posterior sacroiliac
   E) Sacrospinous

33. A patient comes to your office after sustaining a fall. Structural exam reveals a negative seated flexion test and a positive standing flexion test. The left ASIS is 5 inches from midline and the right is 4 inches from midline. AP compression of the right ASIS demonstrates adequate resiliency, whereas the left side is restricted. What is the most likely diagnosis?

   A) A left anterior innominate rotation
   B) A right innominate inflare
   C) A left innominate outflare
   D) A right superior innominate shear
   E) A left superior innominate shear

34. A female patient underwent a right-sided radical mastectomy 3 years ago for breast cancer. As a result, she has residual swelling in her right upper extremity. The patient completed a course of chemotherapy and was informed last year that she is cancer free. The patient wishes to have osteopathic treatment to decrease her edema. The physical exam reveals pitting edema in the right upper extremity. Which of the following is the most accurate statement regarding lymphatic treatment?

   A) Proper lymphatic treatment includes, opening the thoracic duct, then releasing the thoracoabdominal diaphragm then applying the posterior axillary fold technique
   B) Proper lymphatic treatment includes, a thoraco-abdominal diaphragm release, posterior axillary fold technique and pedal pump
   C) Lymphatic treatment is absolutely contraindicated in this patient because of the history of cancer.
   D) Lymphatic techniques will be of no use since the anatomy has been altered.
   E) Lymphatic treatment should be postponed until re-occurrence of cancer is ruled out.

35. A patient tripped and fell backward on an outstretched right hand. The patient complains of pain on the lateral side of his right elbow. The physical exam reveals the right forearm prefers supination and the radial head is tender to palpation and restricted in posterior glide. The most likely diagnosis is:

   A) Lateral epicondylitis
   B) Posterior radial head
   C) Anterior radial head
   D) Adduction dysfunction of the ulna
   E) Abduction dysfunction of the ulna

36. A patient in a car accident, who was not wearing a seat belt, hit his forehead on the steering wheel and the back of his head on the head rest. The patient went to the emergency room and was discharged. X-ray and CT scan were negative. The patient has a constant dull headache. Cranial sacral examination reveals decreased amplitude to the point where it is barely detectable. The most likely craniosacral strain pattern is:

A) Torsion
B) Sidebending and rotation
C) Vertical strain
D) Lateral strain
E) Compression

37. A 35-year-old female who is obese complains of left foot pain. The pain is worse in the morning when she gets out of bed or if she stands at work for a long period of time. The pain is located on the bottom of her foot at the anterior-medial aspect of the calcaneus. The most likely diagnosis is:

A) Pes planus
B) Pes cavus
C) Tarsal tunnel syndrome
D) Plantar fasciitis
E) Morton neuroma

Case 38-39

An 81-year-old male comes to your clinic with a complaint of right shoulder pain. He injured his shoulder while playing golf three months ago. He went to the emergency room, where the doctor told him he most likely tore his rotator cuff. He was given a sling and discharged. He has been using the sling for three months. His pain is mostly resolved, however he still has some pain with shoulder movement. On examination, inspection of the shoulder is normal without atrophy. There is tenderness at the tip of the acromion, however shoulder impingement signs are negative. Active and passive range of motion testing reveals: 60° of glenohumeral abduction, 60° of forward flexion, 10° of external rotation, 20° of internal rotation of the left, extension is normal. Pain is present at the end of range of motion in all planes. Range of motion testing of the left shoulder is normal. X-rays are normal and there is no evidence of a high riding humeral head.

38. Which of the following statements best explains this patient's decreased range of motion.

   A) The patient suffered a partial tear in his rotator cuff resulting in pain and thus limiting his range of motion.
   B) The patient suffered a complete tear in his rotator cuff resulting in limited range of motion
   C) Chronic Impingement has resulted in inflammation of the rotator cuff tendons thus causing limited range of motion.
   D) Prolonged immobility of the shoulder has resulted in fibrosis of the joint capsule causing decreased range of motion.
   E) A tear in the anterior glenoid labrum resulted in decreased range of motion in the stated planes and preserved range of motion with extension.

39. Which of the following statements accurately describes the best course of treatment?

   A) Weekly muscle energy to the scapula stabilizers and continued use of the shoulder sling.
   B) Avoiding overhead activities and myofascial release to the shoulder musculature.
   C) Referral to a surgical specialist for evaluation of a rotator cuff tear.
   D) This patient should begin progressive resistive exercises to strengthen his rotator cuff
   E) This patient may benefit from Spencer techniques to free up restrictions in the glenohumeral joint followed by gentle strengthening of the rotator cuff.

Case 40-43

A 33-year-old female comes to your office with a three-day history of a severe headache. The pain originates from the base of the occiput and radiates into the right temporal region. The patient reports that she started experiencing nausea, vomiting and vertigo today. Pain intensifies in brightly lit rooms. She smokes one pack of cigarettes a day. Her allergies include ragweed. Osteopathic structural examination reveals tenderness in the right trapezius and right temporalis muscles. Palpation of these tender areas does not refer pain. There is a tenderpoint at the articular pillar of C2 on the right.

40. Which of the following is true regarding her headache?

    A) It is likely due to an alteration of the intracranial blood supply
    B) It is likely due to hypertonicity of the trapezius muscle.
    C) Treatment may consist of myofascial stretch using vapocoolant spray
    D) Pain will resolve with counterstrain to the temporalis muscle
    E) It is likely due to degeneration of the joints of Luschka in the lower cervical spine.

41. What is the rationale for using rib raising on this patient?

    A) It will increase sympathetic tone thus promoting cranial vasoconstriction
    B) It will decrease sympathetic tone thus promoting cranial vasoconstriction
    C) It will increase sympathetic tone thus limiting cranial vasoconstriction
    D) It will decrease sympathetic tone thus limiting cranial vasoconstriction
    E) It will be of no benefit to this patient

42. Which of the following medications is most appropriate for initial treatment of this patient's headache?

    A) Butalbital
    B) Valproic acid
    C) Sumatriptan
    D) Propranolol
    E) Atenolol

43. The patient returns to your office for follow-up in three days. She reports that her headache has resolved and she was able to get some rest after your OMT treatment. Which of the following best indicates follow-up care?

    A) Since symptoms have resolved, there is no reason to examine the patient and no need for further OMT.
    B) Re-evaluate your patient today and determine if further intervention is necessary.
    C) Repeat the same OMT treatment today and have the patient return in one week if her symptoms return.
    D) Repeat the same OMT treatment two more times to insure adequate resolution of somatic dysfunction.
    E) Refer to physical therapy for initiating ultrasound therapy to the trapezius.

Case 44-46

A 17-year-old lacrosse player comes to the athletic trainer's office with low back pain. As the team physician he asks to see you. The athlete states that the pain started several weeks ago, it is localized to the lumbosacral spine and worsens with backward bending. Pain was mild at first, now it is severe enough that he can no longer play. On examination, there is tenderness of the lumbar paraspinals. The spinous processes of the lumbar vertebrae do not appear prominent unlike the L5 vertebra and sacrum. Examination of the lower extremities reveals normal muscle strength and sensation. On structural examination of the lumbo-sacral region, there is a positive seated flexion test on the right, a deep sacral sulcus on the left, and L5 is rotated to the left. The L5 findings are exaggerated upon backward bending, symmetry is restored with forward flexion. The sacrum does not spring at the lumbosacral junction.

44. The most likely etiology of this patient's acute low back pain is?

    A) Herniated nucleus pulposus
    B) Spondylolisthesis
    C) Osteoarthritis of the lumbar spine.
    D) Spinal stenosis
    E) Facet tropism

45. Given the above finding what is the diagnosis at L5?

    A) Flexed, rotated left, sidebent left
    B) Extended, rotated left sidebent left
    C) Extended, rotated right, sidebent right
    D) Neutral, rotated right, sidebent left
    E) Neutral, rotated left sidebent right

46. Given the above findings, what is the sacral diagnosis?

    A) Left sacral rotation on a right oblique axis
    B) Left sacral rotation of a left oblique axis
    C) Right sacral torsion on a left oblique axis
    D) Right sacral torsion on a right oblique axis
    E) Bilateral sacral extension

Case 47-50

A 17-year-old high school gymnast comes to your office for a high school physical. Throughout her school career she has been having intermittent back pain. The back pain is localized to the right thoraco-lumbar region and worsens with spinal extension. On examination, her right shoulder is lower than her left, and her right iliac crest is higher. Her right leg is 1.2cm shorter than the left. L2 is flexed, rotated right and sidebent right. Her lumbar spine appears to be sidebent to the right and L5 is rotated left. She has full range of motion and reverses her scoliotic curve on spinal motion testing. Pelvis shifts easily to the left and resistance is present with right pelvic shift. There is a tenderpoints in the center of her left buttocks. On standing postural x-ray of the spine and pelvis the scoliotic curve measures 140 and the left femoral head is 12mm caudad compared to the right. A spina bifida occulta is noted on x-rays without evidence of spondylolysis or spondylolisthesis.

47. Which of the following most accurately describes this patient's scoliosis?
    A) A functional dextroscoliosis
    B) A structural dextroscoliosis
    C) A structural levoscoliosis
    D) A structural kyphoscoliosis
    E) A functional levoscoliosis

48. What is the most likely cause of this patient's scoliosis?
    A) Idiopathic scoliosis
    B) Central spasticity
    C) Psoas syndrome
    D) Spina bifida
    E) Muscle weakness

49. Which of the following is the best treatment for this patient's scoliosis?
    A) Only OMT would be needed to completely straighten the scoliotic curve
    B) Physical therapy, OMT and Konstancin exercises
    C) Physical therapy, OMT, Konstancin exercises, and spinal bracing
    D) Physical therapy, OMT, Konstancin exercises, spinal bracing and botulinum toxin A injections into the paraspinals
    E) Neurosurgical referral

50. You decide that this patient may benefit further from a heel lift. Which statement best describes an appropriate heel lift therapy protocol?
    A) A 1/8" heel lift should be placed under the right foot and increased 1/8" every two weeks until a total height of 3/4" is achieved.
    B) A 1/8" heel lift should be placed under the right foot and increased 1/16" every two weeks until a total height of 3/8" is achieved.
    C) A 1/8" heel lift should be placed under the right foot and increased 1/8" in two weeks for a total height of ½".
    D) A 1/8" heel lift should be placed under the right foot and increased 1/8" in two weeks for a total height of ¼".
    E) A ½" heel lift should be placed under the right foot and the patient should return in two weeks for follow-up heel lift evaluation.

Case 51-54

During the evaluation of a patient's upper back pain, you notice that your right thumb is more posterior upon palpation of the transverse processes of T4. T4 returns to neutral position with flexion of the thoracic spine, whereas extension of the thoracic spine increases the asymmetry.

51. Which of the following is the most correct assessment of T4?

   A) Sidebent left, rotated left
   B) Sidebent right, rotated right
   C) Sidebent right, rotated left
   D) Sidebent left, rotated right
   E) Rotated left, no sidebending component

52. If treating this patient with HVLA in a supine position, which of the following is correct regarding hand placement and direction of force?

   A) The thenar eminence is placed under the right transverse process of T5, force is perpendicular to the table
   B) The thenar eminence is placed under the right transverse process of T4, force is perpendicular to the table
   C) The thenar eminence is placed under the right transverse process of T3, force is 45° caudad
   D) The thenar eminence is placed under the right transverse process of T4, force is 45° cephalad
   E) The thenar eminence is placed under the right transverse process of T5, force is 45° cephalad

53. Which of the following correctly describes the treatment position when treating the above somatic dysfunction with facilitated positional release?

   A) Marked extension of the thoracic spine, right rotation, right sidebending
   B) Marked flexion of the thoracic spine, right rotation, right sidebending
   C) Flattened thoracic kyphosis, right rotation, right sidebending
   D) Marked flexion of the thoracic spine, left rotation left sidebending
   E) Marked extension of the thoracic spine, left rotation, left sidebending.

54. Which of the following organs would be LEAST affected by an autonomic imbalance at T4?

   A) Heart
   B) Esophagus
   C) Stomach
   D) Lungs
   E) Tongue

Case 55-58

A 53-year-old male comes to the emergency department complaining of low back pain. He states that the pain he is experiencing now is similar to his back pain that he had when he herniated a disc two years ago. He brings in x-rays and an MRI from two years ago. X-rays show spondylosis at L5/S1. The MRI demonstrated a left posterior lateral herniated disc at this level. The back pain radiates from the lumbar spine into his left foot.

55. Which of the following maneuvers would be expected to decrease this patient's pain?

    A) Active lumbar flexion in a standing position
    B) Passive lumbar extension in the prone position
    C) Valsalva maneuver
    D) Straight leg raising
    E) Ambulation

56. Which of the following physical signs may be observed in the above patient if there was compression of the S1 nerve root?

    A) Decreased ability for the patient to walk on his toes
    B) Decreased ability for the patient to walk on his heels
    C) Absent patellar tendon reflex
    D) Decreased sensation on the dorsum of the foot
    E) Sustained clonus with ankle dorsiflexion

57. The x-ray finding in the above patient is most consistent with?

    A) Anterior slippage of the L5 vertebrae on the sacrum
    B) A defect in the pars interarticularis
    C) Degenerative changes and osteophytic lipping
    D) Compression fracture of L5
    E) Ankylosing spondylitis

58. Which of the following organs would be least affected by an autonomic imbalance of the upper lumbar spine?

    A) Ureters
    B) Urinary bladder
    C) Descending colon
    D) Penis
    E) Adrenal medulla

Case 59-63

You are assessing a newborn in the hospital nursery. The child was born yesterday, delivered at 41 weeks by spontaneous vaginal delivery complicated by shoulder dystocia. At birth the child was 10lbs 2oz. in weight and measured 21inches from head to toe. The Apgars were 9 and 10. The mother has been attempting to breast-feed, however the child is having difficulty latching on to the breast. On examination, the infant appears to be nervous and irritable. Flexing and abducting the hips while exerting pressure on the greater trochanters demonstrates that the child has a right hip click.

59. What is the most likely cause of the shoulder dystocia?

    A) Gynecoid pelvic shape
    B) The child was macrosomic
    C) The mother did not receive prenatal care
    D) The obstetrician probably used forceps during delivery
    E) Premature rupture of membranes

60. Which of the following is the most serious neurologic complication that has been associated with shoulder dystocia?

    A) Amblyopia
    B) Klumpke's palsy
    C) Erb-Duchenne's palsy
    D) Bell's palsy
    E) Cerebral palsy

61. Which osteopathic treatment is indicated to treat this newborns suckling problem?

    A) Rib raising
    B) CV4 technique
    C) Condylar decompression
    D) Sphenopalatine ganglion release
    E) Temporal rocking

62. Which of the following somatic dysfunctions has been linked with suckling difficulties in the newborn?

    A) Upper thoracic dysfunction
    B) Hyperparasympathetic tone
    C) Maxillae dysfunction
    D) Cranial nerve dysfunction
    E) TMJ dysfunction

63. Which of the following best explains the most appropriate course of action for this patient's hip click?
    A) Weekly osteopathic manipulation to decrease myofascial restrictions and optimize femoral head position in the acetabulum.
    B) Monthly radiographs to determine the position of the femur in the acetabulum.
    C) Monthly ultrasounds of the hip to determine the position of the femoral head in the acetabulum
    D) Pavlik harness with follow-up CT scan to determine the adequacy of reduction and position.
    E) Rigid casting with the hips in frog leg position.

Case 64-67

A 42-year-old cachectic cancer patient is complaining of buttock pain that radiates to the left calf. The patient is a computer programmer who is working a lot of overtime. The patient has lost 50 lbs, which he attributes to adverse effects of chemotherapy. His referred pain is worsened with prolonged sitting. Physical exam reveals no neurologic deficits in the lower extremities. There is a tenderpoint located in the middle of the left buttock. The lumbar spine is symmetric and has full range of motion without pain.

64. The most likely diagnosis is:
    A) Psoas syndrome
    B) Posterior facet syndrome
    C) Cauda equina syndrome
    D) Piriformis syndrome
    E) Sacroiliac joint syndrome

65. Treatment should be directed at one which of the following:

    A) Psoas muscle
    B) Posterior facet capsule
    C) Sacroiliac joint
    D) Piriformis muscle
    E) Surgical decompression of the lumbar spine

66. The most appropriate osteopathic treatment for this patient's tenderness is:

    A) HVLA
    B) Sacral rocking
    C) Still technique
    D) Cranial sacral
    E) Counterstrain

67. This condition could be prevented by which of the following?

    A) Gain weight, cushion on chair, frequent breaks
    B) Lose weight, hard chair, sit straight
    C) Gain weight, cushion on chair, no breaks
    D) Lose weight, cushion on chair, frequent breaks
    E) Gain weight, hard chair, frequent breaks

Case 68-71

A 24-year-old is complaining of buttock pain, proctalgia fugax, and dyspareunia. The patient remembers that the problem began after the birth of her 3-year-old son. The pain has been getting progressively worse. The patient feels her marriage is good and she still loves her husband, however she admits that she is often sad and cries a lot. The physical examination reveals external hemorrhoids, tenderness at the tip of the coccyx, and a tenderpoint ½ way between the inferior lateral angle of the sacrum and the greater trochanter in the right buttocks.

68. The most likely diagnosis is:
    A) Post partum depression
    B) Piriformis syndrome
    C) Cauda equina syndrome
    D) Sacroiliac joint syndrome
    E) Coccygodynla

69. The most appropriate management of the patient would be:
    A) GI consultation
    B) Psychiatric consultation
    C) Immediate surgical consultation
    D) SI joint injection
    E) Sacrococcygeal joint mobilization

70. The patient's tender point is from spasm of which muscle?
    A) Psoas
    B) Gluteus maximus
    C) Gluteus medius
    D) Gluteus minimus
    E) Piriformis

71. What would be the typical counterstrain treatment position for the patient's tenderpoint?

    A. Supine, lower extremity flexed, abducted and internally rotated
    B. Prone, lower extremity flexed, abducted and externally rotated
    C. Supine, lower extremity flexed, adducted and externally rotated
    D. Prone, lower extremity extended, abducted and internally rotated
    E. Supine, lower extremity extended, adducted and externally rotated

Case 72-73

A 6-month-old male presents with 101-degree fever, runny nose, vomiting, and diarrhea. Physical exam reveals decreased cone of light and erythema of the right tympanic membrane. Chest x-ray is negative for infiltrates, urinalysis is negative for infection, blood and cultures are negative.

72. Which of the following lymphatic techniques would be the most effective adjunctive therapy?

    A) Liver pump
    B) Spleen pump
    C) Abdominal pump
    D) Thoracic pump
    E) Galbreath Technique

73. Treatment of which cranial bone would most effectively improve this patient's symptoms?

    A) Frontal
    B) Occipital
    C) Parietal
    D) Temporal
    E) Maxilla

Case 74-75

A 35-year-old female comes to your office with an insidious onset of vague abdominal discomfort. She reports a loss of appetite and a 15-pound weight loss. She denies any melena or hematochezia. On physical exam no abdominal masses are palpable and bowel sounds are present in all quadrants. Stool guiac testing is negative for blood. No axillary or inguinal lymph nodes are palpable, however she does have a palpable lymph node at the periumbilical region.

74. The most likely diagnosis is:

    A) Peritonitis
    B) Pancreatitis
    C) Ectopic pregnancy
    D) Rectosigmoid cancer
    E) Gastric adenocarcinoma

75. At which spinal level would you expect to find palpatory changes related to a viscerosomatic reflex?

    A) T4
    B) T6
    C) T10
    D) T12
    E) L2

Case 76-77

A 46 year-old female comes to your office after she injured her back at work. Physical exam reveals tight lumbar paraspinals and tight hamstrings bilaterally. Lumbar spine X-ray reveals L5 is displaced 40% anteriorly on S1.

76. The most likely diagnosis is:

A) Grade 1 spondylolisthesis
B) Grade 2 spondylolisthesis
C) Grade 3 spondylolisthesis
D) Grade 4 spondylolisthesis
E) Grade 5 spondylolisthesis

77. Which of the following diagnostic studies will determine that the patient's pain is generated from the spondylolisthesis?

A) Magnetic resonance imaging
B) Bone Scan
C) CT scan
D) Lateral lumbar x-rays
E) Electromyography

Matching 78-82

Directions: For each numbered item (characteristic) select the one lettered heading (treatment type) most closely associated with it. Each lettered heading may be selected once, more than once, or not at all.

A. Counterstrain
B. Direct muscle energy
C. HVLA
D. Articulatory
E. Direct myofascial release

78. A treatment of tissues that involves a constant force toward a restrictive barrier to affect a change.
79. A treatment that considers the dysfunction to be a continuing, inappropriate strain reflex, which is inhibited by applying a position of mild strain in the direction exactly opposite to that of the false strain reflex.
80. A treatment that takes a joint through it's full motion with the goal of increased freedom in its range of movement.
81. A treatment that utilizes impulse mobilization of a joint to achieve its therapeutic effects.
82. A patient activated treatment from a precisely controlled position toward the restrictive barrier.

COMLEX C ANSWERS

COMLEX C ANSWERS

1. Answer A: Thoracic dysfunctions should be treated before rib dysfunctions. Rib dysfunctions may be caused by corresponding thoracic dysfunctions. If a thoracic dysfunction is present treat the thoracic spine before treating the specific rib dysfunction. [56 p.577]

Rib exhalation dysfunctions can be treated using the Kirksville Krunch technique. The technique is the same except that the thenar eminence is placed under the corresponding rib angle. **Answer B**

In general, posterior rib tenderpoints are treated by rotating and sidebending the thorax away from the dysfunction. **Answer C**

Although muscle energy techniques should not be performed on patients with low vitality who could be compromised by adding muscular exertion, elderly patients with COPD can typically manage active muscular contraction without exacerbating their COPD. **Answer D**

An exhalation dysfunction of ribs 6-9 can be corrected with muscle energy by contracting the serratus anterior. **Answer E**

2. Answer A: The above patient has a posterior transverse process on the right at L2. Symmetry is restored in extension. Therefore the somatic dysfunction is extended rotated right, sidebent right (ER_RS_R). A muscle energy treatment is a direct treatment that entails positioning the segment against its restrictive barrier (i.e. reversing all planes of motion). Thus, the correct treatment position in the above patient is flexed, rotated left and sidebent left (FR_LS_L).

3. Answer C: When you ask a patient to actively move a joint to it's end points you are asking the patient to demonstrate active range of motion. Passive range of motion is when a physician (or any other person for that matter) ranges a joint. Any person can actively move his/her joint to its physiologic barrier (if there is no somatic dysfunction present). Any other person can move someone else's joint to its anatomic barrier (if there is no somatic dysfunction present). When there is somatic dysfunction present, that person or physician can only move the joint to the restrictive barrier. Thus, all motion is lost beyond the restrictive barrier.

The question does not state which segment (or segments) is (are) restricting motion. Therefore, it cannot be determined if the dysfunctional segment follows type I or type II mechanics. **Answers A and B**

All motion (active or passive) is lost beyond the restrictive barrier. **Answer D**

The patient demonstrated full left rotation to the physiologic barrier, not the anatomic barrier. **Answer E**

4. Answer E: Diaphragm release techniques are not contraindicated in this patient. In addition, this patient could also tolerate some indirect myofascial release techniques.

Due to the severity of this person's illness he would not be able to tolerate daily OMT, nor would he be able to tolerate direct active forms of OMT. **Answers A and B**

Osteopathic treatment for those individuals in the intensive care unit should also be limited in dosage.

Usually these individuals cannot tolerate extensive osteopathic treatment sessions. **Answer C**

Although this patient is in critical condition he would be able to tolerate some mild forms of OMT. **Answer D**

5. Answer D: In the above patient L5 is flexed sidebent right and rotated right. Upon palpation of L5 transverse process, in the neutral position the right transverse process should be posterior. With flexion the asymmetry should resolve. With extension however the asymmetry will re-appear.

You would expect L5 to rotate easily to the right, based on the laws of type II spinal mechanics. **Answer A**

Since L5 is sidebent and rotated to the right, it will follow the laws governed by Type II spinal mechanics. **Answer B**

Since L5 is sidebent and rotated to the right, there should be an ease of right rotation with the segment in the flexed position. **Answer C**

If a sacral torsion was present, the sacrum would be rotated left on a right oblique axis (backward sacral torsion). **Answer E**

6. Answer B: The above patient has an acute lumbar strain. The patient has no evidence of neurologic impingement. According to the Foundations of Osteopathic Medicine, second edition, acute strains/sprains are often better treated with indirect techniques to prevent further strain. Counterstrain is an indirect passive treatment that will allow the patient's musculature to relax.

The patient will unlikely tolerate the positioning for muscle energy due to his severe pain. **Answers A and C**

HVLA may actually worsen the patient's pain if it is done initially, given the acute nature of his injury. **Answer D**

Osteopathic treatment is not contraindicated in acute lumbar strains. **Answer E**

7. Answer A: In the above question, C2 resists translation to the left with the head in the flexed position. Left translation induces right sidebending. Therefore, the cervical spine resists right sidebending. If it resists right sidebending then it must be sidebent left. Due to facet orientation, C2 always sidebends and rotates to the same side (type II mechanics). Therefore, if it is sidebent left, it must be rotated left. This resistance is worse when the head is in the flexed position, and eases with the head in the extended position. Since you name the dysfunction for where the segment wants to go C2 must be extended, sidebent left and rotated left. The correct muscle energy technique calls for a reversal of all planes of motion, therefore the segment should be placed in flexion, right rotation, right sidebending. And the patient would then be asked to rotate his head to the left. For further instruction on how to perform this technique see Foundations of Osteopathic Medicine, Second Edition. [56 p.890]

8. Answer C: Sibson's fascia forms the functional cervico-thoracic diaphragm (thoracic inlet) and is especially involved in the mechanics of fluid homeostasis in the entire body. [28 p.236] The thoracic duct, which drains the left upper extremity and bilateral lower extremities, passes through the thoracic inlet.

Therefore restriction within the thoracic inlet is likely to limit lymphatic drainage of the left lower extremity.

When a patient is standing with their arms at their side, the medial spine of the scapula is immediately lateral to the spinous process of T3, not T1. **Answer A**

Although the spinous processes point increasingly downward, the rule of three's dictates that the spinous process of T1 is located equal to the transverse processes of T1. **Answer B**

The main motion of the thoracic spine is rotation. Rotation moves about a vertical axis. **Answer D**

At quiet breathing the diaphragm bears 100% of the workload. [28 p.226] During exercise the diaphragm bears 60% of the workload; and the secondary muscles of respiration are responsible for 40% of the workload during exercise. **Answer E**

9. Answer D: Contraction of the quadratus will extend, and sidebend the lumbar spine as well as pull rib 12 down (caudad) thus increasing the 11th and 12th intercostal space.

Inhalation results in an eccentric contraction of the quadratus lumborum resulting in cephalad movement of rib 12. The latissimus dorsi also plays an important role in the movement of rib 12. **Answer A**

The quadratus lumborum does not attach to rib 11. **Answer B**

Although the quadratus lumborum tenderpoints have been referred as the most often overlooked cause of low back pain, it is thought that the iliolumbar ligament is one of the first structures to react to stress in the lumbosacral spine. [28 p.344] **Answer C**

Treatment of the diaphragm as well as the quadratus lumborum has proven successful in helping to promote lymphatic drainage. [28 p.373] **Answer E**

10. Answer E: Lumbar flexion will push the nucleus pulposus posterior and stretch the nerve roots. This will usually worsen radicular symptoms.

The lumbar spine moves easiest through flexion and extension. This is motion about a transverse axis and in a sagittal plane. **Answer A**

Lumbarization will alter the structure-function relationship of the lumbosacral junction, leading to early disc degeneration. **Answer B**

In the thoracic and lumbar regions the nerve root will exit the intervertebral foramina below its corresponding segment. For example the L5 nerve root will exit between L5 and S1. **Answer C**

The posterior longitudinal ligament narrows as it approaches the sacrum. This results in a posterio-lateral weakness making disc herniations more common in this area. Large central disc herniations that impinge S2-S4 can result in cauda equina syndrome, but this is uncommon. **Answer D**

11. Answer D: The patient's aggravating factors and alleviating factors along with the physical findings should indicate to the test taker that this patient most likely has lumbar spinal stenosis. Lumbar stenosis is narrowing of the spinal canal and/or intervertebral foramina. As the patient extends his lumbar spine (by standing or walking) the intervertebral foramen physiologically becomes more narrowed. If a patient has narrowing of this area neural impingement can occur. Patient's symptoms will usually improve with flexion of the lumbar spine (sitting). Radiographically, degenerative changes are present in patients with spinal stenosis. Spondylosis is a radiographic term for general degenerative changes. It is virtually a universal finding in elderly patients (even patients without spinal stenosis). Therefore out of the choices given, this is the most likely finding.

A herniated disc is possible, however it is less likely because the pain is made better with lumbar flexion (sitting). The absent Achilles reflexes is likely due to diabetic peripheral neuropathy. **Answer A**

Although we do not know the extent of this patient's prostate cancer, the likelihood of him having vertebral metastasis (usually seen as lytic lesions) is far less than the likelihood of spondylosis. **Answer B**

Spondylolisthesis is a much less frequent a finding than spondylosis in the elderly population. **Answer C**

Compression fractures of the lumbar spine are far less common than spondylosis. In addition, spondyltic changes are usually seen with and often occur before compression fractures. **Answer E**

12. Answer D: The above patient has a left sacral rotation on a left oblique axis (L on L). A positive seated flexion test indicates that the oblique axis would be on the left. A shallow (posterior) ILA on the left and right anterior sacral base (a deep sulcus on the right) indicates left rotation. The lumbosacral spring test will be negative with a forward torsion. In sacral torsions, L5 will follow a certain set of rules. These are:

Rule #1: When L5 is sidebent, a sacral oblique axis is engaged on the same side as the sidebending. Working backwards - if we have a left oblique sacral axis then we must have L5 sidebent left.

Rule #2: When L5 is rotated, the sacrum rotates in the opposite direction. Again working backwards - we have left rotation of the sacrum then L5 must be rotated right.

Now using Fryette's law, if L5 is sidebent left and rotated right (i.e. opposite directions) then it must be in the neutral plane (i.e. L5 NS$_L$R$_R$).

13. Answer B: There are two main phases of gait. 1) The swing phase and 2) the stance phase. The swing phase starts at toe off and terminates at heel strike. The stance phase starts at heel strike and terminates at toe off. In the swing phase the innominate rotates posteriorly around the inferior transverse axis of the sacrum. In the stance phase the innominate rotates anteriorly around the inferior axis of the sacrum.

When a person is ambulating the innominates rotate about a transverse axis (as above) while the sacrum rotates about two oblique axes. Weight bearing on the left leg will cause a left oblique axis to be engaged, and the opposite is true for the right leg. Sacral rotation will then occur about these two axes. **Answer A**

As a person inhales the diaphragm pushes downward, decreasing the lumbar lordosis causing the sacral base to move posterior. This motion will decrease the lumbosacral angle. **Answer C**

Nutation and counternutation are terms used for motion at the sacral base associated with craniosacral motion. Flexion of the cranial bones will cause the sacral base to extend (move posterior). This is called counternutation. Extension of the cranial bones will cause the sacral base to flex (move anterior). This is called nutation. **Answer D**

Sacral dysfunction on a left oblique axis will yield a positive seated flexion test on the right, however other sacral dysfunctions are also seen with a positive seated flexion test on the right (e.g. right unilateral sacral flexion or extension). Therefore a positive seated flexion test on the right will not always indicate a sacral dysfunction on a left oblique axis. **Answer E**

14. Answer E: The patient in the above question has positive standing and seated flexion tests (SFT & SeFT) on the right (i.e. the patient has a pelvic somatic dysfunction on the right). Since the left ASIS is caudad and the left PSIS is cephalad, the left innominate has rotated anteriorly. However, since the SFT indicates a somatic dysfunction on the right, the right innominate must have rotated posteriorly. This typically results in a shorter leg ipsilaterally (on the right).

See above paragraph. **Answer A**

Tight quadriceps is associated with an anteriorly rotated innominate. Tight hamstrings is associated with a posteriorly rotated innominate. **Answer B**

Although innominate dysfunctions can be associated with a shortened psoas (psoas syndrome), not all innominate dysfunctions are caused by a shortened psoas. In addition, findings that are common in psoas syndrome are a tenderpoint medial to the ASIS, high lumbar somatic dysfunction and a positive Thomas test. **Answer C**

The ASIS compression test identifies somatic dysfunction in the SI joint. Please see chapter 18 Special Tests on how to perform this test and it's interpretation. Since there is somatic dysfunction in the right SI joint, there will be resisted compression at the right ASIS. If there was no SI dysfunction on the right, there will be adequate compression (adequate resiliency) on this side. **Answer D**

15. Answer D: The above patient has a positive standing flexion test (SFT) on the left (i.e., the patient has a pelvic somatic dysfunction on the left). Since the right ASIS is more anterior and inferior than the left, the right innominate has rotated anterior when compared to the left. However, since the SFT indicates a somatic dysfunction on the left, the left innominate must have rotated posteriorly.

Since the patient has a positive standing flexion test on the left, he could not have a right innominate dysfunction. **Answers A, B and C**

If the patient had a left anterior innominate the left ASIS will appear anterior and inferior. Answer E

16. Answer B: Bilateral sacral flexion is a common dysfunction in the post-partum patient. [56 p.781, 35 p.158] The progression of the infant through the birth canal during delivery causes an anterior sacral base somatic dysfunction. An anterior sacral base in the post-partum patient has been associated with fatigue, depression and low energy. [35 p.158] Early treatment of this somatic dysfunction can avoid these symptoms.

Other somatic dysfunctions listed are not specifically seen in the post-partum patient. **Answers A, C, D and E**

17. Answer A: Erb-Duchenne's palsy is an injury to the upper portion of the brachial plexus. This often involves the C5, C6 nerve roots, but can extend in some cases to involve the C7 nerve root. Classically Erb's palsy will result in a waiters tip deformity.

Wrist drop is due to injury to the radial nerve usually distal to the brachial plexus (C6, C7 &C8 nerve roots). **Answer B**

Claw hand is due to injury to the median and ulnar nerves. **Answer C**

Benediction sign (also known as bishops deformity) typically results from injury to the ulnar nerve distal to the brachial plexus (C8). **Answer D**

Klumpe's palsy is due to injury to the lower brachial plexus. This typically involves the T1 and C8 nerve roots but may extend to include C7. **Answer E**

18. Answer B: Golfers elbow (a.k.a. medial epicondylitis) can be due to an overuse injury of the forearm pronators and wrist flexors. Patients typically have pain with resisted wrist flexion.

The patient with medial epicondylitis usually has a history of overuse of the wrist flexors muscles, not wrist extensors. **Answer A**

The ulnar nerve runs through the cubital tunnel. Entrapment of this nerve at this location can result in a positive Tinel's sign. It is not associated with medial epicondylitis. **Answer C**

Radial head dysfunction has not been linked to epicondylitis. **Answer D**

Pain at the olecranon process may been seen in triceps tendonitis or olecranon bursitis. **Answer E**

19. Answer B: The most common injured ligament in the foot is the Anterior TaloFibular (ATF) ligament. Why? Because it Always Tears First.

The spring ligament (calcaneonavicular ligament) is the main support of the medial longitudinal arch of the foot. [3p.495] It is not often injured, however it may become stretched and result in pes planus ("flat feet"). **Answer A**

The posterior talofibular and calcaneofibular ligament are thick and fairly strong. They are not injured as often as the anterior talofibular ligament. **Answers C and E**

The deltoid ligament is thick and strong, if it is injured it is usually associated with a fracture of the medial malleolus. **Answer D**

20. Answer C: Craniosacral flexion is associated with flexion of the midline bones and external rotation of the paired bones. The frontal bone is considered a paired bone because of the metopic suture.

Craniosacral flexion is associated with counternutation or sacral extension about the superior transverse axis. **Answer A**

Craniosacral extension is associated with caudad motion of the dura. **Answer B**

Increased AP diameter of the cranium is associated with craniosacral extension. **Answer D**

Physiologic motion of the cranium is not associated with nausea. **Answer E**

21. Answer B: The purpose of the CV4 decompression technique is to enhance the amplitude of the CRI. [14 p.170] This is accomplished by inducing a "still point" then allowing restoration of normal flexion and extension.

Temporal rocking can help eliminate restrictions in the temporal bone or nearby areas; it does not have as a significant effect on the amplitude of the CRI. **Answer A**

The V-spread is used to free restrictions of impacted sutures. It is not specifically designed to restore normal amplitude of the CRI. **Answer C**

The goal of the venous sinus technique is to enhance venous drainage through the jugular foramen. **Answer D**

The frontal lift aids in the balance of frontal bone membranous tension. **Answer E**

22. Answer E: Of the above choices, the seventh thoracic vertebra is least likely to be influenced in a patient with cardiac dysfunction.

The anterior Chapman's point for the myocardium is located at the intercostal space between rib 2 and 3 at the sternal junction. **Answer A**

Palpatory changes at the cranial base and C2 have been associated with vagal hyperactivity in patients with inferior wall infarctions. [35 p.60] **Answers B and C**

Palpatory changes at the second thoracic vertebrae (as well as T3) on the left have been associated with sympatheicotonia (increased sympathetic tone) in patients with anterior wall infarctions. [35 p.60] **Answer D**

23. Answer E: Ejaculation is a sympathetically mediated response. This event is activated by T11 - L2 (some authors [35] list L1 - L2). OMT (specifically to reduce sympathetic activity) to this area may help a patient who is having premature ejaculation.

Manipulation to the sacrum may help parasympathetic events (erection). **Answer B**

24. Answer B: Abnormal visceral stimuli from cardiac autonomic afferents are most likely to cause paraspinal musculature changes at T1 - T5.

Although the heart does receive fibers from the cervical chain ganglia,[35 p.54] abnormal visceral input is less likely to produce C5 - C7 paraspinal changes. Musculoskeletal changes due to vagal hypertonicity can be seen at C2 and the cranial base. **Answer A**

Paraspinal musculoskeletal changes from T7 - L2 typically will occur from visceral dysfunction below the diaphragm. **Answers C, D and E**

25. Answer B: Chapman's reflexes are predictable tissue texture abnormalities assumed to be a reflection of visceral dysfunction or pathology. The Chapman's point for the colon is along the femur within the iliotibial band.

The anterior Chapman's point for the adrenals and kidneys are located in the periumbilical region. **Answer A**

Changes in the paraspinals of T9 are too cephalad to represent a viscerosomatic from diverticulosis. **Answer C**

The posterior Chapman's point for the adrenals is located at the spinous process of T11. **Answer D**

The spinal cord ends at L2. There are no reported viscerosomatic changes occurring from L3 - L5. **Answer E**

26. Answer D: Experiments show that hypersympathetic tone to the kidneys for several weeks causes renal retention of fluid resulting in chronically elevated arterial pressure. Therefore, treatment toward the kidneys (T10 - T11) may decrease fluid retention and decrease arterial pressure. [35 p.125]

Manipulation of cervical segments will not decrease hypersympathetic tone in the kidneys. **Answers A and B**

T5-T9 receives sympathetic innervation from the upper GI tract. **Answer D**

Manipulation of T12 - L1 will not decrease hypersympathetic tone in the kidneys. It may alter the sympathetic tone to the ureters, however this is not the problem. **Answer E**

27. Answer C: The osteopathic SOAP note form is a standardized form that has been adopted by osteopathic schools. Senior medical students and interns should be familiar with this form. On the form there are ten regions of the body for examination and treatment

Area	Areas treated		Total
1. Cranium	none	=	0
2. Cervical	C3, C5	=	1
3. Thoracic	T4	=	1
4. Ribs	none	=	0
5. Abdomen	none	=	0
6. Lumbar	L1, L5	=	1
7. Sacrum	Sacrum	=	1
8. Pelvis	Right innominate	=	1
9. Upper extremity	none	=	0
10. Lower extremity	Piriformis	=	1
			6

There were six regions treated. Treatment of more than one dysfunction in a region only counts as one region. The piriformis muscle has its origin on the sacrum, and its insertion on the femur. It is considered primarily an external rotator of the lower extremity. Treatment of this muscle involves using the lower extremity and can therefore be considered the sixth region. [56 p.658]

28. Answer A: Most of the flexion and extension at the cervical spine stems from the occipito-atlantal (OA) joint. Specifically, it is the movement of the occipital condyles on the atlas. Approximately 50% of all the flexion and extension in the cervical spine stems from this joint.

The atlanto-axial (AA) joint's primary motion is rotation. **Answer B**

The lower cervical division C2 - C7 has varying degrees of all directions, however there is less flexion and extension at these joints compared to the OA joint. **Answers C, D and E**

29. **Answer D:** It is generally thought that chronic tissue texture changes occur after approximately 6 months of dysfunction. Acute renal failure is defined as reversible, and chronic renal failure is defined as irreversible renal failure. [43] This will cause chronic tissue changes at the T11 segment.

Answers A, C, and E are incorrect because it is a chronic condition, not acute, and they are at the wrong spinal level.

Chronic changes at T9 would be associated with chronic disease of the upper or middle GI tract. **Answer B**

30. **Answer A:** This patient most likely has glaucoma, and would have viscerosomatic changes at the T1-T4 spinal level.

T5-T6 spinal level is associated with the viscerosomatic reflex from the lungs and the esophagus. **Answer B**

T7-T9 spinal level is associated with the viscerosomatic reflex from the upper GI tract. **Answer C**

T10-T12 spinal level is associated with the viscerosomatic reflex from the middle GI tract and the gonads. **Answer D**

T12-L2 spinal level is associated with the lower GI tract. **Answer E**

31. **Answer C**: T5 Neutral, rotated left, sidebent right is the correct diagnosis. On the board exams it may be abbreviated as NR_LS_R. When your right thumb is more anterior, this implies that your left thumb is more posterior. This is a left rotation. Testing in flexion and extension did not restore symmetry to T5, so it is neutral in the sagittal plane. By Fryette's first law, when the segment is in the neutral plane (not flexed or extended) sidebending occurs to the opposite side of the rotation, therefore T5 NR_LS_R is the correct diagnosis.

In a segment that is FR_RS_R (Flexed rotated right, sidebent right) your left thumb would be posterior and symmetry would be restored in flexion. **Answers A**

In a ER_LS_L, (extended rotated left, sidebent left) symmetry would be restored in extension. **Answer B**

In a NR_RS_L (neutral, rotated right sidebent left) your right thumb would be posterior. **Answer D**

In a ER_RS_R (extended rotated right, sidebent right) symmetry would be restored in extension. **Answer E**

32. Answer C: The iliolumbar ligament is often the first ligament to become painful in lumbosacral decompensation. *28 p.407. 56p.746*

Sacrospinous, sacrotuberous and sacroiliac ligament may become painful in lumbosacral decompensation, however they is not the first. **Answers A, B, D, and E**

33. Answer C: This patient has a left outflared innominate. Although the patient has a positive SFT, the side of the SFT is not specified; therefore the side of the dysfunction was determined by the ASIS compression test. A positive test occurs if one ASIS resists posterior compression, this indicates the side of the dysfunction. In this case the right side demonstrates adequate resiliency (meaning that it is not restricted), however the left side is restricted. Therefore the somatic dysfunction is on the left. The static findings indicate that the distance from the right ASIS to the umbilicus is shorter than the left. This indicates a left innominate outflare.

A left anterior rotation would have an inferior ASIS and a superior PSIS on the left. The distance from the ASIS to the umbilicus would be equal. **Answer A**

A right inflared innominate and a right superior innominate shear would have an ASIS compression test positive on the right. **Answers B and D**

A left superior innominate shear would have a superior ASIS and PSIS on the left. The distance from the ASIS to the umbilicus would be equal. **Answer E**

34. Answer A: Proper lymphatic treatment includes, opening the thoracic duct, then releasing the thoracoabdominal diaphragm then applying the posterior axillary fold technique

Although variations in treatments vary, this is not the best choice because the patient should have her thoracic inlet released. The lymph from the right upper extremity will drain into the right lymphatic duct, which traverses the thoracic inlet. **Answer B**

Lymphatic treatment is not absolutely contraindicated in a patient with a history of cancer. **Answer C**

Lymphatic techniques have been shown to help in patients with post-surgical edema. **Answer D**

Residual limb edema following radical mastectomy is not uncommon. As long as the edema did not develop recently or there was no increase in her current edema, the chance of cancer re-occurance of cancer is low. Therefore the practitioner can proceed with lymphatic treatment. **Answer E**

35. Answer C: An anterior radial head dysfunction would cause the forearm to prefer supination and the radial head would resist posterior glide. Falling backward on a supinated forearm can cause this dysfunction.

Lateral epicondylitis is a strain of the extensor muscles of the forearm near the lateral epicondyle. It is usually due to overuse of the wrist extensors and not typically associated with trauma. **Answer A**

A posterior radial head dysfunction would cause the forearm to prefer pronation, and the radial head would resist anterior glide. Falling on a pronated forearm causes this dysfunction. **Answer B**

An adducted dysfunction of the ulna would have a decreased carrying angle, the hand and wrist would be adducted, and the olecranon process would prefer lateral glide. **Answer D**

An abducted ulna causes a decreased carrying angle of the arm; the olecranon process would be restricted in medial glide, and the wrist and hand would be abducted. **Answer E**

36. Answer E: A compression strain can be cause by a force to the back of the head, to the front of the head, or from a circumferential compression such as childbirth. [56 p.993]   It results in a little to no palpable C.R.I.

37. Answer D: The most common cause of foot pain in outpatient medicine is plantar fasciitis, which results from constant strain on the plantar fascia at its insertion into the medial tubercle of the calcaneus. The most common causes are obesity, prolonged standing, and improper footwear. The pain is worse in the morning, but usually subsides after a few minutes of ambulation. Diagnosis is confirmed by palpation over the plantar fascia on the medial heel. [32 p.464]

Pes planus is a flattened longitudinal arch; it is not typically associated with pain. **Answer A** [25 p. 336]

Pes cavus is an exaggerated height of the longitudinal arch; it also is not typically associated with pain. [49] **Answer B**

Tarsal tunnel syndrome is a complex of symptoms resulting from compression of the posterior tibial nerve or the plantar nerve in the tarsal tunnel. Symptoms include pain and paresthesias of the sole of the foot. [49] **Answer C**

Morton's neuroma is a fibroneuromatous reaction between the heads of the third and fourth metatarsals. [25 p. 336] Pain is present at the forefoot at the site of the neuroma [32 p.455] **Answer E**

Case 38-39

38. Answer D: Although the patient may have suffered a rotator cuff tear, it was the prolonged immobility that resulted in subsequent adhesive capsulitis. The hallmark feature of adhesive capsulitis is decreased range of motion with end range pain. Typically, adhesive capsulitis does not produce a decrease in extension range of motion.

A rotator cuff tear usually does produce shoulder pain and decreased active range of motion, however usually passive range of motion will be preserved. Classically, the prolonged immobilization will result in some degree of adhesive capsulitis and this will result in decreased passive range of motion. In addition, in a complete rotator cuff tear there will be a high riding humeral head (i.e. the superior portion of the humeral head will approximate the inferior surface of the acromion) **Answers A and B**

Chronic impingement can result in inflammation of the rotator cuff tendons, however this usually does not directly affect both passive and active range of motion. **Answer C**

A tear in the glenoid labrum is not necessarily associated with decreased range of motion with end range pain. In addition, a torn glenoid in a particular area does not decrease range of motion in one plane and preserve motion in another plane. **Answer E**

39. Answer E: The patient in the above question may have suffered a rotator cuff tear and now has subsequent adhesive capsulitis. The best treatment for this is gentle strengthening of the rotator cuff and stretching of the joint capsule. Stretching the joint capsule is easily done with Spencer techniques.

Continued immobilization of the shoulder with use of a sling may actually worsen this patient's condition. **Answer A**

Since this patient does not have any evidence of impingement of the shoulder, he would be cleared to do overhead activities. Overhead activities would be encouraged in this case to help stretch the joint capsule. **Answer B**

This patient most likely does not have a complete rotator cuff tear since x-rays are negative for a high riding humeral head, thus conservative management is preferred. In addition, based on this patient's age conservative management may be considered even in a complete tear. **Answer C**

Progressive resistive exercises are usually started after the patient has achieved full range of motion. **Answer D**

Case 40-43

40. Answer A: Classic migraines are thought to be caused by a vasoconstriction and vasodilatation of the blood supply to the cranium. [56 p.679] Symptoms of a classic migraine includes photophobia. Nausea and vomiting are not uncommon. These symptoms can be preceded by an aura.

Tension type headaches can be due to tension in the upper back or cervical spine musculature. Tension headaches are not usually associated with nausea and vomiting. Pain is often worse at the end of a workday due to muscle fatigue. **Answer B**

Trigger points are taut myofascial bands that refer pain when compressed. They can be treated with "spray and stretch" technique using vapocoolant spray. The above patient does not have any trigger points. **Answer C**

Counterstrain alone will not likely completely resolve the pain. Other treatments that would be useful would include techniques to reduce sympathetic tone to the head and neck structures to limit vasoconstriction. [56 p.679] **Answer D**

Degeneration of the joints of Luschka will likely result in axial cervical pain, or if there is compression of a nerve root, pain will likely radiate into the upper extremity. **Answer E**

41. Answer D: Increased sympathetic tone to innervated blood vessels of the cranium will cause vasoconstriction. The purpose of rib raising is to reduce hypersympathetic tone thus limiting vasoconstriction. Other somatic dysfunctions, such as cranial dysfunctions and axial dysfunctions may produce fascial strains that are transmitted to the head and may play a role in the origin of a migraine. [56 p.680]

Since classic migraines are thought to be caused by a vasoconstriction of innervated blood vessels and a vasodilatation of non-innervated blood vessels, techniques aimed at reducing sympathetic tone will decrease initial vasoconstriction. [56 p.679] **Answer E**

42. Answer C: Sumatriptan (Imatrex) can be used to treat acute migranes

Tension headaches are typically treated with butalbital in combination with acetominophen. Butalbital is a barbituate. **Answer A**

Valproic acid (depakote) atenolol (tenormin) and propranolol (Inderal) can be used for migrane prophylaxis. **Answers B, D and E**

43. Answer B: Although the patient's symptoms have resolved, the patient still may have some somatic dysfunction. Somatic dysfunctions, such as cranial dysfunctions and axial dysfunctions may produce fascial strains that are transmitted to the head and may play a role in the origin of a migraine. [56 p.680] If somatic dysfunction is found, treatment may prevent further headaches. Therefore, it is best to evaluate this patient again.

Although the patient's symptoms have resolved, the patient still may have some trapezius tenderness and some somatic dysfunction, therefore the patient should be examined. **Answer A**

All OMT treatments should be individualized to the patient's findings. Therefore it is recommended that the patient be examined and OMT should be directed specifically toward her dysfunction. It would be a disservice to the patient just to repeat the same treatment. **Answers C and D**

Although ultrasound is a form of deep heat and can help loosen tight muscles, this is not the best choice for two reasons. Ultrasound was not used initially; therefore you do not know if it the patient will benefit from it. Second, ultrasound should be used in addition to cervical stretching and strengthening in physical therapy. **Answer E**

Case 44-46
44. Answer B: This patient most likely has spondylolisthesis. This is not an uncommon cause of back pain for young athletes; especially those athletes that are involved with extension based athletic activities, such as lacrosse players. Pain is usually localized to the lumbo-sacral spine. Neurological examination is normal. There may be a positive "step-off sign" (upon palpating the spinous processes there is an obvious forward displacement at the area of the listhesis). In this case the spinous process of L5 is prominent, whereas the spinous processes of remainder of the lumbar spine are not.

Since the neurologic examination is normal, this patient is not likely to have a herniated disc. **Answer A**

Osteoarthritis of the lumbar spine and spinal stenosis is uncommon for a 17 year old. Typically pain arising from these conditions start after the 5th decade, unless there is a predisposing factor such as ankylosing spondylitis. **Answers C and D**

Although facet tropism is the most common anatomic anomaly of the lumbar spine and can lead to degenerative changes in the lumbar spine, alone it is not the primary cause of low back pain in the above patient. **Answer E**

45. Answer A: The patient in the above question is has a L5 somatic dysfunction that is rotated to the left. The findings are exaggerated upon backward bending (extension) and symmetry is restored with flexion. Therefore, L5 is flexed and rotated left. Since the segment is in the non-neutral position, rotation and sidebending must be towards the same side. Therefore, the segment is flexed rotated left and sidebent left.

46. Answer C: Since there is a positive seated flexion test on the right, the left sacral sulcus is deep, and the lumbo-sacral junction does not spring freely upon compression. The sacrum has rotated right on a left oblique axis. Since L5 has rotated left (and the sacrum has rotated right) the correct diagnosis is a right sacral torsion on a left oblique axis.

In a left sacral rotation on a right oblique axis, the seated flexion test would be positive on the left and the right sulcus would be deep compared to the left sulcus. **Answer A**

In a left sacral rotation on a left oblique axis, the lumbo-sacral junction would spring easily. **Answer B**

In a right sacral rotation on a right oblique axis, the lumbo-sacral junction would spring easily. **Answer D**

In a bilateral sacral extension, the sacral sulci would be symmetric and the seated flexion test would not demonstrate asymmetry. **Answer E**

Case 47-50

47. **Answer E:** The lumbar spine is sidebent to the right, therefore the patient has a levoscoliosis (for clarification see fig 5.1). Since the patient is able to reverse her scoliosis on range of motion testing, she has a functional scoliotic curve.

A dextroscoliosis describes a spine that is sidebent to the left. **Answers A and B**

A structural curve is a spinal curve that is relatively fixed and inflexible. A structural curve will not correct with sidebending in the opposite direction. **Answers B, C and D**

A kyphoscoliosis is a scoliosis that has resulted in an increase in kyphosis. **Answer D**

48. **Answer C:** The patient has some symptoms of right psoas syndrome (high lumbar dysfunction, pelvic shift to the left and left piriformis tenderpoint). Psoas syndrome can be a cause of scoliosis.

Although idiopathic scoliosis accounts for most cases (80%), in this case there is a musculoskeletal cause. **Answer A**

Central spasticity indicates an upper motor neuron origin, thus unless there was a history of cerebral or spinal cord injury this would not be the correct answer. **Answer B**

Spina bifida occulta has not been associated with scoliosis. **Answer D**

This patient has no history of muscle weakness. **Answer E**

49. **Answer B:** Mild scoliosis (Cobb angle of 5 - 150) is typically treated with conservative measures. This includes: physical therapy, Konstancin exercises and OMT. Konstancin exercises are a series of specific exercises that has been proven to improve the patient with scoliotic postural decompensation. [28] p.339

OMT is not intended to completely straighten scoliotic curves. [56 p.622] **Answer A**

Conservative therapy and spinal bracing are indicated in patients with moderate scoliotic curves (20 - 450). [56 p.622] **Answer C**

Botulinum toxin A (BOTOX) injections along with conservative management and bracing have been proven to be helpful in some small pilot studies in patients with moderate scoliosis. However, it is not considered the standard of care. **Answer D**

Neurosurgical referral is indicated for patients with severe scoliosis. [56 p.622] **Answer E**

50. Answer D: For a detailed explanation please see Chapter 5 - Short leg syndrome: section V). The "flexible" (i.e. not elderly or "fragile") patient should begin with 1/8" (~3.2mm) heel lift and increase 1/8" every two weeks. The final lift height should be ½ - ¾ of the measured leg length discrepancy, unless there was a recent sudden cause of the discrepancy (i.e. hip fracture or hip prosthesis). Since, the initial discrepancy was 12mm, an acceptable value for the final height would be 6.4mm (1/4") to 9mm (~3/8"). [56 p.616-617]

¾" is approximately 19.2mm which is much higher than the original height. **Answer A**

Although 3/8" is an acceptable final height, since the patient is not considered "fragile", the lift should be increased 1/8" every 2 weeks, after ¼" is achieved additional height should be added to the outside of the shoe. **Answer B**

Since the maximum heel lift should be ½ to ¾ of the total height, ½" (12.8mm) is too high. In addition, a maximum of ¼" may be applied to the inside of the shoe. If > ¼" is needed, then this must be applied to the outside of the shoe. **Answer C**

Since there was not a sudden cause of the leg length discrepancy (i.e. hip fracture or hip prosthesis, the final lift height should be ½ - ¾ of the measured leg length discrepancy. **Answer E**

Case 51-54

51. Answer B: If your right thumb is posterior, this indicates right rotation. Flexion returns T4 to the neutral position indicating a flexed type II somatic dysfunction. Fryette's principles state that in a non-neutral (flexed in this case) dysfunction sidebending and rotation are to the same side. If a segment is rotated right, then it is also sidebent right. Type II vertebral dysfunctions are typical of single vertebral dysfunctions.

52. Answer B: The thenar eminence is placed under the right transverse process of T4, force is directed perpendicular into the table. Using the Kirksville Krunch technique, to reverse all planes of a T4 FR_RS_R the physician's thenar eminence is placed under the right transverse process of T4 (to induce left rotation of the spine). The downward projection of the spinous process at T4 will induce extension at this joint when HVLA thrust is applied.

When treating a flexed somatic dysfunction the thrust is directed at the dysfunctional segment, not the one below. **Answer A**

Treating T3 will not have the greatest effect on the somatic dysfunction at T4. **Answer C**

When treating an extended somatic dysfunction of the thoracic spine, the thrust is directed at the segment below the dysfunctional segment at a 45° angle cephalad. Please see chapter 16 HVLA for specific details of treatment. The downward projection of the spinous processes of the thoracic spine will automatically produce an extension moment with an HVLA thrust. In extended somatic dysfunctions, the ideal thrust would be toward flexion. By treating the segment below, an extension moment is induced at this segment, thus producing relative flexion of the segment above (the dysfunctional segment). Although most clinical osteopathic practitioners do not necessarily treat the segment below in extended somatic dysfunctions, it is explained here because this is the way it is explained in the Foundations for Osteopathic Medicine, Second Edition pages 861-862.

53. **Answer C**: Although facilitated positional release is an indirect technique, somatic dysfunctions of the spine are treated with the spine in the neutral position. This entails flattening the thoracic kyphosis, and flattening the lordosis of the lumbar and cervical spine. The segment is then positioned away from the restrictive barrier. In this case sidebent and rotated right.

54. **Answer C:** The stomach generally receives autonomic innervation from T5-T9. Although there is some overlap, out of the other answers T4 is least likely to affect the stomach.

The heart receives autonomic innervation from T1 - T5. **Answer A**

The esophagus receives autonomic innervation from T2 - T8. **Answer B**

The respiratory system receives autonomic innervation from T2 - T7. [56 p.103] **Answer D**

The tongue is a head structure and will receive autonomic innervation from T1 - T4. **Answer E**

Case 55-58

55. **Answer B**: Symptoms from a herniated disc typically improve with lumbar extension. Therapeutic exercises called the McKenzie program has been specifically designed to reduce low back pain caused by herniated discs. Most of the McKenzie exercises are extension-based maneuvers. The theory behind these extension techniques is that lumbar extension draws the nucleus back into the center of the intervertebral disc.

Active lumbar flexion will push the disc posteriorly, this typically worsens the patient's pain. **Answer A**

Valsalva maneuvers will typically increase pain associated with a herniated disc. **Answer C**

Straight leg raising test will stretch the sciatic nerve, this typically causes the nerve to be pulled over the herniated disc, thus causing pain. **Answer D**

Ambulation increases axial load and compresses the intervertebral disc resulting in increased pain. **Answer E**

56. **Answer A:** Decreased ability of the patient to walk on their toes. Although the S1 nerve root innervates several parts of the lower extremity, it is intimately involved in plantar flexion of the foot.

Heel walking tests the strength of the main ankle dorsiflexor, which is the anterior tibialis. This muscle is innervated by L4 and L5 nerve roots. **Answer B**

An absent patella reflex may indicate pathology of the L4 nerve root. **Answers C**

Sensation at the dorsum of the foot is supplied by L5. **Answer D**

Sustained ankle clonus is associated with an upper motor neuron lesion; a herniated disc at L5-S1 would result in nerve root (lower motor neuron) compression. **Answer E**

57. Answer C: Spondylolysis is a radiological term for degenerative changes in the intervertebral discs and anklyosing of the adjacent vertebral bodies.

Anterior slippage of the L5 vertebrae on the sacrum is spondylolisthesis, not spondylosis. **Answer A**

A defect in the pars interarticularis is spondylolysis, not spondylosis. **Answer B**

Spondylosis is not associated with compression fractures. **Answer D**

Ankylosing spondylitis is a systemic disease that results in ankylosing of several vertebrae starting at the lumbosacral spine and proceeding cephalad. Although spondylosis can include ankylosing of adjacent vertebral bodies, a 53-year-old male with ankylosing spondylitis would have several joints involved, not just at L5/S1. **Answer E**

58. Answer E: Adrenal medulla. The adrenal medulla receives sympathetic innervation from T10.

The ureters receive sympathetic innervation from T10-L2. **Answer A**

The urinary bladder receives sympathetic innervation from T11-L2. **Answer B**

The descending colon receives sympathetic innervation from T12-L2. **Answer C**

The penis receives sympathetic innervation from T11-L2. **Answer D**

Case 59-63

59. Answer B: Shoulder dystocia is the inability of the child's shoulders to fit comfortable through the mother's pelvis. Shoulder dystocia is often associated with macrosomia. Any neonate weighing over 4000g is considered macrosomic.

The gynecoid pelvis typically has adequate space along the birth canal when compared to other pelvic types. Therefore it is less likely cause of shoulder dystocia. **Answer A**

Maternal prenatal care and forceps delivery are not associated with shoulder dystocia. **Answers C and D**

Premature rupture of membranes is not associated with shoulder dystocia. **Answer E**

60. Answer C: Erb-Duchenne's palsy is often due to excessive traction placed on the head and neck while the shoulder is depressed. This can occur when the fetus' shoulders are having difficulty exiting the pelvis.

Shoulder dystocia is not associated with amblyopia. **Answer A**

Klumpke's palsy is any injury to the lower brachial plexus. It can be due to extreme abduction and extension of the shoulder. It is not associated with shoulder dystocia. **Answer B**

Bell's palsy results in an injury to the facial nerve and is not associated with childbirth. **Answer D**

Cerebral palsy is primarily a disorder of movement and posture that is due to a non-progressive lesion to an immature brain. It is not associated with shoulder dystocia. **Answer E**

61. Answer C: Suckling dysfunction can be associated with condylar compression. The treatment of choice is condylar decompression.

62. Answer D: Suckling difficulties have been associated with condylar compression and/or restrictions at the jugular foramen. Condylar compression causes cranial nerve XII dysfunction. Other possible causes of suckling dysfunctions have been associated with restrictions at the jugular foramen causing cranial nerve IX and X dysfunction.

63. Answer D: The patient in the above case has a positive Ortolani's sign. This is indicative of congenital dysplasia of the hip. Treatment for this involves the application of a fundamental osteopathic prooopt: growth and maturation of the skeleton follows function. [25 p. 480] Many orthopedists today use the Pavlik harness to hold a dislocatable hip in place. This brace allows the child to flex the hip and kick while the hip in a physiologic position. For a more detailed explanation of treatment of developmental dysplasia of the hip refer to Foundations of Osteopathic Medicine, Second Edition, pages 479-482.

Osteopathic treatment may be used in addition to the above treatment. However, alone it is not considered to be the most appropriate course of action. **Answer A**

Monthly radiological testing and observation is not an adequate course of action. As the child gets older, especially as the child begins to ambulate, it becomes more difficult to obtain adequate reduction without surgery. **Answers B and C**

Rigid casting is an older form of treatment. Placing the hips in the "frog" position may put added stress on the hip while it is reduced and is generally not considered to be the optimal position. **Answer E**

Case 64-67

64. Answer D: Piriformis syndrome is a peripheral neuritis of the sciatic nerve. Symptoms are easily confused with those of a herniated lumbar disk or facet joint pathology. The patient often complains of hip and buttock pain radiating down the posterior thigh, possibly to the calf or foot. On physical exam there is an absence of neurologic deficits, and a characteristically exquisite tenderpoint anywhere along the piriformis muscle. Factors causing this syndrome are irritation or inflammation of the sciatic nerve, including piriformis muscle spasm, local trauma to the buttocks, repeated mechanical stressors (e.g. running) pelvic instability and excessive local pressure (e.g. sitting), especially in thin or cachectic patients. [25 p. 446]

Psoas syndrome presents with low back pain, especially in the lumbar region with radiation down the posterior thigh only to the knee. The Jones tenderpoint associated with this syndrome is about one inch medial to the anterior superior iliac spine. **Answer A**

Posterior facet syndrome presents with low back pain, which radiates to the buttocks and sometimes the calf or ankle. Physical examination generally reveals motion restriction of one or more vertebral segments, limited spinal range of motion, local paravertebral spasm and tenderness. Pain is typically exacerbated with lumbar extension. There would be no characteristic Jones tenderpoint at the piriformis muscle, and no neurologic deficit. [25 p. 446] **Answer B**

Cauda equina syndrome is compression of the nerve roots of the cauda equina. Typical symptoms are saddle anesthesia, decreased deep tendon reflexes, decreased rectal tone, and loss of bowel and bladder control. **Answer C**

Sacroiliac joint syndrome usually presents with pain at the sacroiliac joint area, restricted sacral motion, and associated spasm of one or more of the muscles attaching to the sacrum. Pain is typically at the SI joint itself, not in the middle of the buttock. **Answer E**

65. **Answer D:** Since the patient has piriformis syndrome caused by repeated irritation of the piriformis muscle due to his prolonged sitting. Treatment should be directed at the piriformis muscle for maximum effectiveness. [25 p. 446]

Treatment of the psoas muscle would be indicated for psoas syndrome. **Answer A**

Treatment directed at the posterior facet capsule would be appropriate for posterior facet syndrome. **Answer B** [25 p. 445]

Treatment for sacroiliac joint would be indicated for sacroiliac joint syndrome. **Answer C** [25 p. 445]

Immediate surgical decompression of the lumbar spine is the appropriate management of cauda equina syndrome. **Answer E**

66. **Answer E:** Counterstrain would be the most appropriate and effective treatment for this patient, especially directed at the piriformis muscle. The patient is 42 years old, cachectic, has recently undergone chemotherapy, and is possibly osteopenic. Gentle treatment would therefore be preferred. [25 p. 447]

High velocity low amplitude would be contraindicated in a patient who may be osteopenic (see above). **Answer A**

The purpose of sacral rocking is to relax the muscles of the lumbosacral junction. It typically is indicated in patients with tight lumbar paraspinals. Although sacral rocking would not be entirely inappropriate, it is not the best answer. For a further explanation of sacral rocking and its uses see Appendix A. **Answer B**

Answer C has no known techniques specific for the piriformis that would be as effective, and therefore would not be the most appropriate treatment.

Craniosacral treatment would be a gentle treatment, but it would not be the most appropriate treatment because it would not directly release the key somatic dysfunction of the piriformis muscle spasm. **Answer D**

67. **Answer A:** The patient is cachectic, and doesn't have enough physical padding to prevent the mechanical irritation of the piriformis. He should take more frequent breaks from sitting and add a cushion to his chair to reduce the trauma of sitting and eventually receive nutritional counseling to help him regain his normal weight to prevent this condition.

Losing weight and sitting in a hard chair would make the condition worse, and encourage constant irritation of the piriformis muscle. **Answer B**

Gaining weight takes time and would help, but taking frequent breaks from sitting and moving around offers help immediately. While the cushion on the chair will help sitting for 15 hours a day, not taking sufficient breaks would mostly still aggravate an already irritated piriformis muscle. **Answer C**

If the patient loses weight the condition would still occur and is therefore not the best combination.

Answer D

Gaining weight takes time and a hard chair would aggravate his condition, even with frequent breaks.
Answer E

Case 68-71

68. Answer E: This is a classic presentation of chronic coccygodynia. Coccygodynia is used to describe persistent pain at the coccyx. The etiologies are many, some of which include infection, osteomyelitis, fractures, postnatal injuries, and other types of trauma. [25 p.453] Symptoms include proctalgia fugax (rectal pain from levator ani spasm), pain upon sitting, pain with bowel movements, constipation, and dyspareunia. [25 p.453] Physical exam reveals a characteristic tenderness at the tip of the coccyx and spasm of adjacent muscles.

Postpartum depression is unlikely, since her child was born three years ago. **Answer A**

Although the patient has a piriformis tenderpoint, her main complaint is tenderness at the tip of the coccyx. In addition, piriformis syndrome is often associated with pain that radiates down the thigh. **Answer B**

Cauda equina syndrome is compression of the cauda equina nerve roots. It presents with saddle anesthesia, decreased deep tendon reflexes, decreased rectal tone, and loss of bowel and bladder control. **Answer C**

Sacroiliac joint syndrome usually presents with pain at the sacroiliac joint area, restricted sacral motion, and associated spasm of one or more of the muscles attaching to the sacrum. Answer D

69. Answer E: Since this patient has coccygodynia, treatment of the sacrococcygeal joint with mobilization would be the most appropriate management, since it would address most of her complaints. Other osteopathic techniques used for coccygodynia include a pelvic diaphragm release.

A GI consult would not manage and prevent recurrence of her main problem. **Answer A**

Psychiatric consultation would help this patient's depression, but not remove its organic etiology. **Answer B**

Immediate surgical consultation is the appropriate management of cauda equina syndrome. **Answer C**

Sacroiliac joint injection would be an appropriate management for sacroiliac joint syndrome. **Answer D**

70. Answer E: The Jones tenderpoint for the piriformis is located ½ way between the inferior lateral angle of the sacrum and the greater trochanter within the belly of the piriformis muscle. [26 p.122]

The Jones tenderpoint for the psoas is about one inch medial to the ASIS. **Answer A**

Answers B, C, and D are all located in the upper half of the buttock, distributed from just lateral of the ASIS following around and below the iliac crest. They are not located in the middle of the buttock.

71. Answer B: The typical counterstrain treatment position for the piriformis muscle is with the patient prone, the hip and knee flexed and the thigh abducted and slightly externally rotated.

Case 72-73

72. Answer E: This patient has an acute otitis media, and Galbreath's technique is indicated as appropriate adjunctive therapy. Galbreath's technique is a soft tissue manipulation technique used to increase drainage of middle ear structures via the Eustachian tube.

Answers A, B, C, and D are effective lymphatic techniques, but would not directly affect the ear, and hence would not be the most effective adjunctive therapy.

73. Answer D: The treatment of choice for acute otitis media would be to address the underlying eustachian tube dysfunction. Eustachian tube dysfunction has been associated with cranial somatic dysfunction, especially internal rotation of the temporal bone; therefore, treatment of the temporal bone would be the most effective. [35 p.10]

Although treatment of other cranial bones would help improve all cranial functions, none would be as effective as treating the temporal bone in a case of otitis media. **Answers A, B, C, and E**

Case 74-75

74. Answer E: This patient most likely has a gastric adenocarcinoma with metastatic spread to the periumbilical lymph node (Sister Mary Joseph's nodes). Gastric cancers can cause upper abdominal discomfort varying in intensity from a vague, postprandial fullness to a severe, steady pain. Anorexia, often with slight nausea is common. [43 p.1384]

Peritonitis and pancreatitis usually presents with acute abdominal or pelvic tenderness. It will not typically result in a palpable periumbilical lymph node. **Answers A and B**

Ectopic pregnancy usually presents with abdominal pain, amenorrhea, and vaginal bleeding. It also does not result in a palpable periumbilical lymph node. **Answer C**

Rectosigmoid cancer usually causes GI bleeding, this will result in a positive stool guiac. Classically, colon cancer does not result in a palpable periumbilical lymph node. **Answer D**

75. Answer B: This patient has gastric cancer. This would cause viscerosomatic changes to occur at the T5 - T9 spinal levels.

T4 typically does not receive sympathetic innervation from structures below the diaphragm. **Answer A**

T10, T12 and L2 receive sympathetic innervation from the middle and lower GI tract. **Answers C, D and E**

Case 76-77

76. Answer B: Spondylolisthesis is the anterior displacement of a vertebra in relation to the one below. Spondylolistheses are graded 1 through 4. A grade two is a 25-50% slippage.

Grade 1 spondylolisthesis is a 0-25% slippage. **Answer A**

Grade 3 spondylolisthesis is a 50-75% slippage. **Answer C**

Grade 4 spondylolisthesis is a 75-100% slippage. **Answer D**

Grade 5 spondylolisthesis does not exist. **Answer E**

77. Answer B: Approximately half of patient's with documented spondylolisthesis are asymptomatic. Therefore, the above patient may be experiencing back pain from another source (such as myofascial lumbar strain, facet joint pain, or pain from a herniated disc) and her spondylolisthesis is just an unrelated finding. Usually if the patient is experiencing pain from the spondylolisthesis a bone scan will show increased metabolic activity at the site of the pars interarticularis. This implies that the fracture is new and the likely source of the pain. Over time the fracture will heal (most likely resulting in a non-union) and the bone scan will become negative.

An MRI (magnetic resonance imaging) and CT scan cannot determine the age of a fracture. **Answers A and C**

Lateral lumbar x-rays will determine the grade of spondylolisthesis but not the age of the spondylolisthesis. **Answer D**

Electromyography will only determine if there is nerve root compression, the patient may have nerve root compression from another source. **Answer E**

Matching 78-82

78. Answer E: According to the osteopathic dictionary, direct myofascial release involves engaging the restrictive barrier of the myofascial tissues. The tissue is loaded with a constant force until tissue release occurs. [1 p.1133]

79. Answer A: According to the osteopathic dictionary, counterstrain is an indirect treatment that is based on a series of tenderpoints. It considers the somatic dysfunction to be a continuing, inappropriate strain reflex. It attributes its therapeutic effects by using a specific point of tenderness related to this dysfunction followed by specific directed positioning. [1 p.1133]

80. Answer D: According to the osteopathic dictionary, articulatory treatment is a low velocity/moderate to high amplitude technique where a joint is carried through its full motion with the therapeutic goal of increased freedom range of movement. [1 p.1133]

81. Answer C: According to the osteopathic dictionary, HVLA is a direct technique, which uses high velocity/low amplitude forces. It is also called mobilization with impulse treatment. [1 p.1134]

82. Answer B: According to the osteopathic dictionary, direct muscle energy treatment describes the form of osteopathic manipulative treatment in which the patient attempts to voluntarily move the body against the physician's applied resistance; after the patient relaxes, the physician then takes the body towards the restrictive barrier and repeats until the restriction is resolved. [1 p.1133]

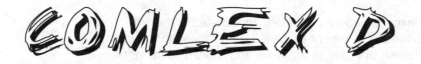

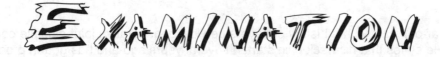

COMLEX D EXAMINATION

1. You are consulted to see a severely debilitated 87-year-old male with complaints of mid thoracic pain. He was in the intensive care unit for 3 weeks and was transferred to a medical/surgical bed yesterday. He has a history of coronary artery disease, congestive heart failure and prostate cancer with vertebral metastasis. His back pain is localized to the mid thoracic region and seems to be musculoskeletal in nature. Which osteopathic manipulative techniques would be best suited to relieve this patient's symptoms?

    A) Muscle energy treatment with the spine extended
    B) Thoraco-abdominal diaphragm release
    C) High velocity low amplitude
    D) Pedal (Dalrymple) pump
    E) Direct myofascial release

2. A patient has a tenderpoint at the right articular process of C5. What is the typical treatment position for the head and neck in order to treat this tenderpoint using counterstrain?

    A) Flexed, sidebent to the left, and rotated to the left.
    B) Extended, sidebent to the left, and rotated to the left.
    C) Flexed, sidebent to the right, and rotated to the right.
    D) Extended, sidebent to the right, and rotated to the right.
    E) Flexed, sidebent to the left, and rotated to the right.

3. An 85-year-old male with a history of severe cervical degenerative joint disease comes to your office. He states that his neck pain started several years ago and has gotten progressively worse. The pain radiates into the upper extremity and fingertips. Pain is worsened with cervical spine extension. What are some of the findings you would expect to see when examining the cervical spine?

    A) Boggy, edematous paraspinal musculature with full range of motion of the cervical spine.
    B) Warm and moist skin texture with some erythema. Sharp, painful paraspinal musculature, and decreased range of motion of the cervical spine.
    C) Hypertonic paraspinals with severe, sharp pain with palpation. And a compensated spinal curve in the thoracic spine.
    D) Dry skin, and a moderate amount of paraspinal tenderness with ropy and fibrotic cervical musculature.
    E) Decreased range of motion of the cervical spine with an uncompensated spinal curve.

4. In a patient with neck and upper thoracic pain, you notice that the fifth cervical vertebrae is extended and rotated right. Ribs 1-5 on the left lag behind with deep inspiration. The thoracic vertebrae, T1 - T5, have a lateral convexity to the right. The transverse processes of these vertebrae are posterior on the right, except for T3, which has a posterior transverse process on the left. Which of the following statements is true regarding diagnosis and treatment?

   A) The above patient has an exhalation dysfunction, and initial treatment should be directed toward rib 1.
   B) T3 is sidebent left, rotated right and the patient would be asked to rotate their torso to the right when correcting this somatic dysfunction using a muscle energy (direct) technique.
   C) The above patient has an inhalation dysfunction and an HVLA thrust can be directed at the rib angle of rib 5 to correct this dysfunction.
   D) C5 will resist translation to the right while the head is in the flexed position. Therefore, the head should be placed in the flexed, sidebent left and rotated left position when positioning for a direct muscle energy technique.
   E) T1 - T5 are neutral, sidebent left rotated right. These vertebrae should be placed in right sidebending and left rotation when employing a direct type of treatment.

5. In a patient with chest wall tenderness, rib 5 has limited inhalation motion around an anterior-posterior axis. The best statement that describes the somatic dysfunction of rib 5 is?

   A) The shaft of rib 5 will approximate the shaft of rib 4 at the mid-clavicular line.
   B) Rib 5 will feel more prominent anteriorly.
   C) The shaft of rib 5 will approximate the shaft of rib 6 in the mid-axillary line
   D) Rib 5 has a pump-handle exhalation dysfunction
   E) The angle of rib 5 will feel more prominent.

6. Which one of the following statements regarding the transverse processes of the cervical spine is true?

   A) They are located posterior to the articular pillars.
   B) They are typically used as palpatory landmarks for osteopathic physicians to induce translation at the cervical spine.
   C) The posterior tubercle of the transverse process serves as the origin of the anterior scalene.
   D) The vertebral artery courses through the transverse processes C1 - C7.
   E) They are located immediately posterior to the zygapophyseal joints.

7. A 74-year-old female is complaining of severe left-sided neck pain. The pain is located at the base of the neck and radiates into her left upper extremity. She demonstrates limited neck range of motion especially with extension. Symptoms and radiation of pain are worsened with passive extension and left sidebending of the neck. Flexion of the neck decreases the pain. Neurological examination is significant for decreased sensation from the lateral elbow to the thumb and left biceps weakness. Reflexes are 1+ in the left biceps; all other reflexes in the upper and lower extremities are normal. Structural examination reveals C4 to be flexed and sidebent left. Given the above information, which of the following is the best statement?

    A) A left posterior-lateral disc herniation at C5 impinging the C5 and C6 nerve roots is the most likely cause of this patient's symptoms.

    B) Degenerative changes and hypertrophy involving the Joints of Luschka and zygapophyseal joints is the most likely cause of this patient's nerve root compression symptoms.

    C) AP x-ray of the cervical spine will most likely show joint space and foraminal narrowing.

    D) The somatic dysfunction at C4 is the most likely cause of this patient's symptoms

    E) Cervical spinal canal stenosis is the most likely cause of this patient's symptoms.

8. While examining a patient, you notice that a child has a somatic dysfunction of rib 5 on the right side. The rib seems to lag with inhalation and move easily into exhalation. Which of the following is the best statement concerning the effected rib?

    A) This patient will have limited cephalad motion of rib 5 at the mid-axillary line

    B) This patient will have a tenderpoint in the pectoralis minor muscle

    C) This patient will display a winging of his scapula

    D) The fourth thoracic vertebrae is non-neutral sidebent right and rotated right

    E) The fourth thoracic vertebrae is non-neutral sidebent left and rotated left

9. Which of the following regarding the thoracic vertebrae is true?

    A) The upper thoracic vertebrae have larger vertebral bodies than the lower thoracic vertebrae.

    B) T4, T5, and T6 have spinous processes that project the most inferiorly so that the spinous process of T5 is level with the transverse process of T6.

    C) T10, T11, and T12 have spinous processes that project horizontally, so that the spinous process of T10 is level with the transverse process of T10.

    D) The accessory vertebral vein courses through the foramen transversarium of the T1 vertebrae.

    E) The inferior demifacet of the vertebral body of T3 articulates with rib 4.

10. A 28-year-old medical student comes to your OMT clinic with complaints of low back and buttock pain. The pain originates from the lumbar spine and radiates into the right groin. Upon inspection the pelvis appears to be shifted to the left. Structural examination reveals L2 and L5 FS_RR_R. Three anterior tenderpoints are noted: one approximately 1 cm lateral to the pubic symphysis on the right superior ramus, one at the right AIIS and the other approximately one inch medial to the ASIS on the right. Range of motion of the hip is normal except for right hip extension and internal rotation, which is decreased. The lumbosacral junction springs freely. She has a positive seated and standing flexion tests on the right. Her left ASIS is more superior when compared to the right. Which of the following statements is true?

A) This patient has a right sacral torsion on a left oblique axis.
B) This patient has a shortened right iliopsoas.
C) The tenderpoint near the pubic symphysis identifies a somatic dysfunction at L2.
D) The left lateral Sim's position is the treatment position to correct the sacral dysfunction.
E) This patient has a posteriorly rotated innominate on the right.

11. In a patient with a posterio-lateral disc herniation at the L3-L4 level, weakness is most likely to be present in which of the following muscles?

A) Extensor hallucis longus
B) Flexor hallucis longus
C) Anterior tibialis
D) Hamstrings
E) Peroneus longus

12. A 30-year-old male runner presents with left-sided low back pain and left hip pain. The pain started yesterday after an 8 mile run. It is sharp but does not radiate into the lower extremities. On examination, you notice tenderness over the left SI joint, a positive seated flexion test on the left, the sacral sulcus on the left is anterior, while the right ILA is posterior and inferior. Based on the information given what is the most likely diagnosis?

A) Left sacral rotation on a left oblique axis (L on L)
B) Left sacral rotation on a right oblique axis (L on R)
C) Right sacral rotation on a left oblique axis (R on L)
D) Right sacral rotation on a right oblique axis (R on R)
E) Unilateral sacral flexion on the right (USFR).

13. A 62-year-old female has neck pain. On examination she has limited rotation of the neck. She is most likely to have a dysfunction at which structure?

A) The sphenoid
B) The occiput
C) The atlas
D) The axis
E) C3

COPYRIGHT 2009

14. Which of the following dysfunctions has been most associated with a vertical downward force on the sacrum at the SI joint.
    A) Innominate anterior
    B) Innominate posterior
    C) Innominate inferior shear
    D) Forward sacral torsion
    E) Unilateral sacral flexion

15. Which one of the following statements is true?

    A) Abduction of the ulna is associated with an increased carrying angle and restricted adduction of the wrist
    B) Cubitus varus is often seen in Turners syndrome.
    C) Falling forward on an outstretched pronated forearm could result in a radial head somatic dysfunction that is associated with restricted forearm supination.
    D) A complication of a scaphoid wrist fracture is avascular necrosis of the distal fragment
    E) Wrist flexion is associated with ventral glide of the carpal bones

16. 65-year-old female presents with intermittent numbness of the first three and ½ digits of her right hand. Symptoms have been present for one year and were not associated with trauma. Symptoms are worsened with driving her car and typing on her computer. On examination, there is decreased sensation over the first three and ½ digits. Tinel's sign is positive at the wrist. There is no weakness or atrophy of the thenar muscles. She has been taking Tylenol with little relief. Her other medications include Nifedipine 10mg QD and Alendronate 70mg once weekly. The most appropriate treatment would include:

    A) Myofascial release to the carpal tunnel followed by HVLA to the cervical spine.
    B) Cervical and thoracic HVLA to alter sympathetic tone in the upper extremity and splinting the wrist during aggravating activities.
    C) Myofascial release to the carpal tunnel, rib raising and wrist splinting
    D) Cervical myofascial release and steroid injection into the carpal tunnel
    E) Rib raising, NSAID's and referral to a hand surgeon

17. A 17-year-old male has a fibular head somatic dysfunction. On examination, the affected ankle tends to plantar-flex and invert more than the unaffected ankle and the proximal fibular head resists anterior glide. What is the biomechanical mechanism that resulted in this type of fibular head somatic dysfunction?

    A) Ankle eversion and external rotation forces the talus to push the lateral malleolus posterior, consequently the proximal fibular head will move anterior due to the natural reciprocal biomechanics of the fibula.
    B) Ankle supination pulls the distal fibular head anterior, consequently the proximal fibular head will move posterior due to the natural reciprocal biomechanics of the fibula.
    C) Ankle eversion and external rotation stretches the gastrocnemius/soleus complex thus pulling the proximal fibular head posterior
    D) Ankle supination stretches the anterior tibialis thus pulling the proximal fibular head anterior.
    E) Ankle plantar-flexion and inversion stretches the peroneus longus tendon thus pulling the proximal fibular head posterior.

18. Dysfunction of which cranial bone is most associated with tinnitus and vertigo?

    A) Temporal
    B) Parietal
    C) Occiput
    D) Ethmoid
    E) Sphenoid

19. Occipital or temporal restriction is least likely to affect which of the following?

    A) Tongue control in the newborn
    B) Peristalsis in the lower 2/3 of the esophagus
    C) Sense of smell
    D) Venous drainage of the cranium
    E) Visual accommodation

20. A patient with an upper respiratory tract infection is having difficulty clearing his secretions. Which of the following treatments would most effectively thin this patient's secretions?

    A) Frontonasal suture spread
    B) Sphenopalatine ganglion intraoral treatment
    C) CV4 decompression
    D) Redoming the diaphragm
    E) Thoracic inlet release

21. Which osteopathic manipulative treatment is the method of choice when attempting to enhance arteriolar lung perfusion and reduce autonomic hyperactivity associated with pneumonia?

A) The occipital decompression
B) Muscle energy C3 -C5
C) The thoraco-abdominal diaphragm release
D) HVLA to T2 - T4
E) Rib Raising

22. A patient with an anterior wall myocardial infarction is likely to have paraspinal musculoskeletal changes at which of the following levels?

   A) C2 and the cranial base on the left
   B) T1-T4 on the left
   C) T5-T7 on the right
   D) T9-T12 on the left
   E) L1-L2 on the right

23. Supraventricular tachyarrhythmias that have been associated with hypersympathetic activity are most likely to arise from:

   A) Right sided sympathetic fibers originating from T1 - T4
   B) Left sided sympathetic fibers originating from T2 - T5
   C) Left vagus nerve
   D) Pre-ganglionic fibers originating from the cervical chain ganglia
   E) Stimulation of the oculocardiac reflex

24. A 66-year-old diabetic male with severe PVD was admitted to the Veterans Administration hospital for an infected foot ulcer. After failed conservative management, the patient had a below the knee amputation. Post-operatively, the patient developed adult respiratory distress syndrome. The patient was hospitalized for several weeks and eventually transferred to a long-term care facility. He has not been able to get out of bed and is starting to complain of back pain. Which one of the following treatment protocols is best suited for this patient's back pain.

   A) Thoracoabdominal diaphragm release to improve lymphatic return followed by muscle energy to the pelvis and lumbar somatic dysfunctions.
   B) Indirect treatments to the lumbar fascia followed by direct gentle low velocity moderate amplitude techniques
   C) Rib raising to improve costal motion followed by gentle high velocity low amplitude treatment.
   D) Myofascial release pelvic diaphragm, followed by isometric exercises to strengthen the lumbar spine
   E) Low velocity moderate amplitude techniques, followed by concentric exercises to strengthen the lumbar spine

25. A 30-year-old male patient complains of sudden attacks of chest pain, perspiration, and palpitations. Vital signs are, HR: 78, BP: 160/110, temperature: 98.8 F, and respirations: 16. Lab results reveal elevated urinary metanephrine. At what spinal level would you expect to find a viscerosomatic reflex?

   A) Occiput
   B) Atlas
   C) T8
   D) T10
   E) L2

26. Which of the following techniques best evaluates posterior motion of the clavicle at the sternum?

    A) Patient prone, index fingers on the anterior aspect of the clavicular head near sternum, patient shrugs shoulders
    B) Patient supine, index fingers on the superior aspect of the clavicular head near sternum, patient depresses the shoulders
    C) Patient supine, index fingers on the superior aspect of the clavicular head near sternum, patient shrugs shoulders
    D) Patient supine, index fingers on the anterior aspect of the clavicular head near sternum, patient protracts the shoulders
    E) Patient supine, index fingers on the anterior aspect of the clavicular head near sternum, patient retracts the shoulders

27. A 54 year old male complains of epigastric abdominal pain that he describes as severe. The pain radiates into the back and gets worse with walking and lying down. The patient reports nausea and vomiting and sweating. The results indicate an elevated serum amylase and lipase. At what spinal levels would there be an acute viscerosomatic reflex?

    A) C3-C5
    B) T1-T4
    C) T5-T9
    D) T10-T11
    E) T12 - L2

28. A 58-year-old female complains of a throbbing headache, blurred vision, and intermittent jaw pain. Physical examination reveals tenderness in the right temporal area of the head. At what spinal levels would you expect to find the tissue texture changes related to a viscerosomatic reflex?

    A) T1-T3
    B) T4-T6
    C) T7-T9
    D) T10-T12
    E) T12-L2

29. A patient complains of mid-thoracic back pain for 3 days. What is the proper position of the patient's spine when starting the evaluation of the thoracic spine?

    A) Flexed
    B) Extended
    C) Sidebent
    D) Neutral
    E) Rotated

30. A 23-year-old female with elevated maternal serum alpha fetal protein underwent a caesarian section. The neonate has a midline skin covered fluid filled sac on his back. On physical examination there is active movement of the upper extremities and hip flexors. On rectal exam, there is a relaxed anal sphincter. What is the most likely diagnosis?

    A) Cavernous hemangioma
    B) Osteosarcoma
    C) Thoraco-lumbar spina bifida meningocoele.
    D) Low lumbar spina bifida meningocoele
    E) Low lumbar spinal bifida meningomyelocoele

31. During palpation of the sacrum you detect cranial sacral motion at the rate of 12 cycles per minute. Around which sacral axis does craniosacral motion occur?

    A) Inferior transverse
    B) Oblique
    C) Middle transverse
    D) Sagittal
    E) Superior transverse

32. A patient presents with symptoms of thoracic outlet syndrome. X-rays of the cervical spine are normal. Which of the following statements is correct regarding testing for this syndrome?

    A) Adson's test is positive when the neurovascular compromise occurs between the first rib and the clavicle.
    B) Wright's test is positive when the neurovascular compromise occurs as it passes under the pectoralis minor muscle at the coracoid process.
    C) Military posture test is positive when the neurovascular compromise occurs with tight or hypertrophied scalene muscles.
    D) The hyperextension test is positive when the neurovascular compromise occurs between the first rib and the clavicle.
    E) Costoclavicular syndrome test is positive when the neurovascular compromise occurs as it passes under the pectoralis minor muscle at the coracoid process.

33. A patient slipped on ice and fell, landing on the left hand. The patient complains of elbow and wrist pain. Physical exam reveals that there are small lacerations on the palmar surface of the right hand from the fall. There is no swelling and just mild generalized tenderness in the right wrist. The forearm prefers pronation and the radial head is restricted in anterior glide. The most likely diagnosis is:

    A) Posterior radial head dysfunction
    B) Anterior radial head dysfunction
    C) Lateral epicondylitis
    D) Medial epicondylitis
    E) Flexion dysfunction of the wrist

34. A patient was climbing up a ladder and slipped down two rungs, landing all his weight on the left forefoot. The patient is complaining of left ankle pain. The left foot is restricted in plantar flexion. Inversion and eversion of forefoot is normal. Based on the above information what is the most likely diagnosis?

   A) Plantar flexion dysfunction of the talus on the left
   B) Somatic dysfunction of the transverse arch of the foot
   C) Posterior talar dysfunction on the left
   D) Anterior fibular head dysfunction on the left
   E) Posterior fibular head dysfunction on the left

35. A patient complains of pain and spasm in his left arm. The patient was doing bicep curls and the gym and pulled his left biceps. Due to the severity of the pain, a reciprocal inhibition technique is chosen for treatment. Which of the following would be an example of this type of technique?

   A. The left elbow is extended to the restrictive barrier and the patient is asked to contract the biceps muscle against resistance.
   B. The left elbow is flexed away from the restrictive barrier and the patient is asked to contract the triceps against resistance.
   C. The right elbow is extended and the patient is asked to contract the right biceps against resistance.
   D. The right elbow is flexed and the patient is asked to contract the right triceps against resistance.
   E. The left elbow is flexed away from the barrier and the patient is asked to contract the biceps against resistance.

36. A patient has chronic left foot pain. The pain is located on the medial aspect of the first metatarsal. Physical exam reveals a lateral deviation of the proximal phalanx of the first toe. The patient denies any trauma to the foot. What is the most likely diagnosis?

   A) Hallux rigidus
   B) March fracture
   C) Morton neuroma
   D) Hallux valgus
   E) Corn

37. The median nerve is formed form which of the following spinal nerve roots?

   A) C5-C6
   B) C5-C7
   C) C5-T1
   D) C7-T1
   E) C2-C5

Case 38-41

A 24-year-old female comes to your office with nausea, vomiting, severe abdominal pain and a low-grade fever. On examination, pain is localized to the right lower quadrant. Rebound tenderness and guarding is present.

38. Local peritoneal irritation from this patient's primary problem is likely to cause somatic dysfunction of which muscle?

   A) Iliopsoas
   B) Iliocostalis
   C) Quadratus lumborum
   D) Rectus abdominus
   E) Piriformis

39. To confirm the above diagnosis using Chapman's reflexes, one would find a small discrete tender nodule at:

   A) The tip of the 12th right rib
   B) In the rectus abdominus halfway between the ASIS and the umbilicus
   C) One cm lateral to the L1 spinous process
   D) The right transverse process of L2
   E) Rib angle of the right 12th rib

40. Abnormal visceral afferent input is likely to result in increased autonomic activity causing somatic dysfunction at which level?

   A) C5
   B) T5
   C) T9
   D) T12
   E) L2

41. Which of the following techniques are useful in reducing abnormal autonomic activity associated with the above diagnosis?

   A) Occipito-atlantal decompression
   B) Manipulation of C3 - C5
   C) Celiac Ganglion Release
   D) Superior Mesenteric Ganglion Release
   E) Sacral inhibition

Case 42-44

An 83-year-old female with severe COPD is having difficulty breathing. You evaluate her costal motion by asking her to take a deep breath while your hands are over her chest wall. You find limited range of motion in ribs 2-6 on the left during expiration. A 5-degree levoscoliosis involving the T2 - T6 vertebral segments is present.

42. This type of palpatory assessment is called:

    A) Inherent respiration motion testing
    B) Gross motion testing
    C) Segmental motion testing
    D) Vertebral motion testing
    E) Passive motion testing

43. The most effective initial treatment that would restore costal motion would be directed at?

    A) Rib 2
    B) Rib 6
    C) Thoracic vertebrae
    D) Thoracic inlet
    E) Anterior scalene

44. Which of the following treatments would be contraindicated in the above patient?

    A) Rib raising
    B) Thoracic pump
    C) Pectoral traction
    D) Craniosacral treatment
    E) Seated facilitated position release

Case 45-49

A 76-year-old male is complaining of right-sided neck pain. The pain radiates from the base of his neck to his right elbow. On examination, he has severely diminished right rotation; all other planes of motion are near normal. There is a tenderpoint located below the clavicle immediately lateral to the manubrium. He has a diminished biceps reflex, and paresthesias over the right thumb without evidence of muscle weakness. Cervical extension and sidebending causes pain to radiate into the right arm.

45. Which cervical structure(s) is (are) most likely to have resulted in this patient's decreased range of motion?

    A) Occiput
    B) Atlas
    C) Third cervical segment
    D) Joints of Luschka in the upper cervical spine
    E) Fifth cervical segment

46. Which of the following is true regarding the biomechanics of the joints of Luschka?

    A) They are located posterior to the intervertebral foramina.
    B) They are superio-lateral projections from the superior articular processes.
    C) They help support cervical discs and protect nerve roots from disc herniation.
    D) They are very susceptible to pannus formation in rheumatoid arthritis.
    E) They limit flexion and extension of the cervical spine.

47. What is the most likely etiology of this patient's referred pain?

    A) Osteoarthritis of the cervical spine resulting in plexopathy.
    B) Hypertrophy of ligamentum flavum causing nerve root compression
    C) Herniated nucleus pulposus causing nerve root compression
    D) Bulging disc resulting in nerve root irritation
    E) Degenerative changes to the joint of Luschka and hypertrophy of the zygapophyseal joint causing nerve root compression

48. Compression of which nerve root or segment of the brachial plexus is most likely resulting in this patient's symptoms?

    A) C4 nerve root
    B) C6 nerve root
    C) C7 nerve root
    D) Superior trunk of brachial plexus
    E) Posterior cord of the brachial plexus

49. The location of the tenderpoint indicates that there may be somatic dysfunction of:

    A) The acromioclavicular joint
    B) The first rib
    C) The second rib
    D) The upper thoracic vertebrae
    E) The sternocleidomastoid

Case 50-52

A 46-year-old male with chronic back pain returns to your office for follow-up. You have been treating him successfully with osteopathic treatment for one month. He states that his back pain is slightly improved since last visit. On examination of the patient today you find the following: L2 FR_LS_L, right innominate anterior, left on left sacral torsion.

50. Which of the following techniques would be the least time consuming for improving the L2 dysfunction?

   A) Myofascial release
   B) Counterstrain
   C) Muscle energy technique
   D) Facilitated positional release
   E) Functional technique

51. What palpatory finding would be expected with the above dysfunctions?

   A) The left sacral sulcus is deep
   B) The backward bending test (sphinx test) is positive
   C) The left ASIS is caudad when compared to the right
   D) Lumbar curve convex to the right
   E) Shorter leg on the right side

52. What is the correct treatment position when treating the sacral dysfunction with a muscle energy technique?

   A) Left lateral Sims position
   B) Right lateral Sims position
   C) Lying on his left side with torso turned to the right
   D) Lying on his right side with torso turned to the left
   E) Prone with left leg off table

Case 53-57

A 25-year-old graduate student comes into your office complaining of severe left-sided neck pain radiating to the shoulder. The pain began a few days after finals' week, during which the patient spent nearly 100 hours working at his desk. Deep tendon reflexes are normal, and Adson's test is negative. During your structural examination, you notice spasm in the posterior scalene muscle. You also note that the occiput and C5 translate equally to the right and left when the head is flexed, however when the head is extended, translation to the right is restricted and translation to the left is normal.

53. Which of the following is the correct diagnosis of the somatic dysfunction at C5?

    A) C5 Flexed, rotated left and sidebent right
    B) C5 Flexed, rotated left and sidebent left
    C) C5 Flexed, rotated right and sidebent right
    D) C5 Extended, rotated right sidebent right
    E) C5 Extended, rotated left and sidebent left

54. The occipital condyles are restricted in:

    A) Extension, right sidebending, and left rotation
    B) Extension, right sidebending, and right rotation
    C) Extension, left sidebending, and right rotation
    D) Flexion, left sidebending, and right rotation
    E) Flexion, right sidebending, and left rotation

55. Spasm in the posterior scalene muscle would be most associated with which rib dysfunction?

    A) 1st Rib inhalation dysfunction
    B) 2nd Rib inhalation dysfunction
    C) 1st Rib exhalation dysfunction
    D) 3rd-5th Ribs inhalation dysfunction
    E) 3rd-5th Ribs exhalation dysfunction

56. In order to properly perform Adson's test, which of the following must occur?

    A) The patient turns their head to the opposite side of the shoulder being tested.
    B) Flexion of the elbow
    C) Palpation of the radial pulse
    D) Internal rotation of the shoulder
    E) The arm must be freely allowed to drop

57. Which of the following organs are most affected by an autonomic imbalance at the upper cervical spine?

    A) Adrenal glands
    B) Ovaries
    C) Kidneys
    D) Uterus
    E) Urinary bladder

Case 58-62

A 53-year-old obese male with a 10-year history of Type II diabetes mellitus presents to your office complaining of low back pain radiating to the right buttocks. The pain started 3 - 4 weeks ago and has gradually increased. The PSIS's are equal and the lumbosacral spring test is positive. The right sulcus is deeper, and the right ILA is deeper. An anterior lumbar tenderpoint is found on the right and L5 is rotated to the right. Patellar and Achilles reflexes are 1+ bilaterally with no gross sensory deficits. Muscle testing is 5/5 throughout. X-rays of the lumbar spine reveal degenerative changes only.

58. Which of the following findings is most likely to be present in this patient?

   A) A short leg on the left
   B) Positive standing flexion test on the right
   C) Lumbar curve convex to the right
   D) Positive seated flexion test on the left
   E) Symmetry restored at the sacral sulci with lumbar extension

59. Which of the following is the correct sacral diagnosis?

   A) Left sacral torsion on right oblique axis
   B) Right sacral torsion on left oblique axis
   C) Left sacral torsion on a left oblique axis
   D) Left unilateral sacral flexion
   E) Right unilateral sacral extension

60. Given the sacral diagnosis and lumbar rotation, what is the somatic dysfunction present at L5?

   A) Neutral, sidebent right, rotated right.
   B) Neutral, sidebent left, rotated right
   C) Flexed rotated right, sidebent right
   D) Flexed rotated right, sidebent left
   E) Extended, rotated right, sidebent left

61. Which of the following findings is most likely to be associated with sacral dysfunctions?

   A) Spasm of the rectus abdominus
   B) Positive Ober's test
   C) Piriformis tenderpoint
   D) Tight hamstrings
   E) Quadratus lumborum tenderpoint

62. Which of the following is true regarding the above patient?

   A) Treatment should be directed at L5 first
   B) The L5 dysfunction can be treated using muscle energy with the patient in the left lateral Sim's position
   C) HVLA is absolutely contraindicated in this patient due to the likelihood of disc herniation
   D) The lumbar tenderpoint is treated with the hips extended
   E) Due to the presence of type II diabetes mellitus and the decreased deep tendon reflexes, muscle energy is absolutely contraindicated

Case 63-66

You are examining a 32-year-old secretary who complains of numbness and tingling in both hands. The symptoms are isolated to the palmar surface of the thumb, index and middle fingers. The symptoms are worse at night. On examination, there is no atrophy or weakness noted at the thenar eminences. There are no radiographic abnormalities and deep tendon reflexes are 2/4 bilaterally.

63. Which of the following diagnostic tests is the most sensitive for carpal tunnel syndrome?

    A) Bone scan
    B) Thermography
    C) Magnetic resonance imaging
    D) Tinel's, Phalen's and Prayer tests
    E) Nerve conduction and electromyographic studies

64. Which of the following structures run though the carpal tunnel?

    A) Palmaris longus tendon
    B) Flexor carpi ulnaris
    C) Radial nerve
    D) Flexor pollicis longus tendon
    E) Adductor pollicis

65. A symptom associated with an increased pressure in the carpal tunnel is:

    A) Weakness in finger abduction and adduction
    B) Loss of sensation of the fifth digit
    C) Weakness in thumb adduction
    D) Weakness in thumb opposition
    E) Loss of sensation on the dorsum of the hand

66. Manipulation of which structure(s) will have the greatest impact on hypersympathetic tone in this patient's upper extremity?

    A) C5-C7
    B) T2-T7
    C) The carpal tunnel
    D) The clavicle
    E) The sacrum

Case 67-70

A 77-year-old female with coronary artery disease is complaining of left sided tinnitus. The noise is described as a low-pitched roaring. Physical examination reveals tympanic membranes intact bilaterally and the temporomandibular joint has no clicks or pops. She has a history of a myocardial infarction one-year ago and takes 325mg of aspirin per day.

67. What is the most likely cause of this patient's tinnitus?

   A) Cerumen impaction
   B) Acute labyrinthitis
   C) Eustachian tube dysfunction
   D) TMJ dysfunction
   E) Salicylate toxicity

68. Tinnitus has been most associated with dysfunction of which cranial bone?

   A) Frontal bone
   B) Parietal bone
   C) Occiput
   D) Temporal bone
   E) Hyoid bone

69. Tinnitus that has been associated with a low-pitched roar is due to:

   A) Imbalance of the supra-hyoid muscle
   B) Temporomandibular disc disruption
   C) External rotation of the temporal bone
   D) Barotraumas of the tympanic membrane
   E) Hypersecretion of cerumen

70. The most appropriate craniosacral technique would be:

   A) Frontal lift
   B) Vault hold
   C) Parietal lift
   D) V-spread
   E) Temporal rocking

Case 71-72

A 12-year-old female runner complains of knee pain when running or going up and down stairs. Physical examination reveals tenderness and mild swelling at the tibial tubercle. X-rays of the knee show soft tissue swelling and a thickening of the ligamentum patellae.

71. The most likely diagnosis is:
    A) Osteochondritis dissecans
    B) Patello-femoral syndrome
    C) Patellar tendonitis
    D) Sever's disease
    E) Osgood-Schlatter disease

72. Osteopathic treatment should be directed at which following?
    A) Iliotibial tract
    B) Adductors
    C) Quadriceps
    D) Semimembranosus tendon
    E) Gastrocnemius

Case 73-75

A patient with singultus for two days presents to your office asking for osteopathic manipulative treatment. The patient had a laproscopic cholecystectomy one week ago. His first singultus attack occurred just after the surgery in the recovery room.

73. The most likely etiology of he singultus is:
    A) Tympanic membrane irritation
    B) Reflux esophagitis
    C) Pneumonia
    D) Diaphragmatic irritation
    E) Pharyngitis

74. The most appropriate treatment for the etiology of the singultus is:
    A) Ear lavage to remove irritation
    B) Proton pump inhibitor
    C) Antibiotics
    D) Appendectomy
    E) Thoraco-abdominal diaphragm treatment

75. The singultus returns several days later. On exam you expect to find tissue texture changes at which spinal level?

    A) C1-C2
    B) C3-C5
    C) T1-T4
    D) T9-T12
    E) L1-L3

Case 76-77

A patient diagnosed with Crohn's disease had a colonoscopy, which found a stricture in the Ileocecal area.

76. At what spinal level would you expect to find palpatory changes related to a viscerosomatic reflex?

  A) C3-C5
  B) T1-T4
  C) T5-T9
  D) T10-T11
  E) L2-L3

77. The above patient would have a Chapman's reflex point in which one of the following locations?

  A) Right proximal area of the iliotibial tract
  B) Right distal area of the iliotibial tract
  C) Left proximal area of the iliotibial tract
  D) Left distal area of the iliotibial tract
  E) Left greater trochanter

Case 78-80

A 72-year-old patient complains of numbness and tingling in his right arm and hand. The patient denies any trauma. X-ray of the cervical spine reveals degenerative changes consistent with arthritis and intervertebral foraminal stenosis.

78. Degenerative changes of which vertebral area is the most likely cause of this patient's nerve root compression symptoms?

    A) Ligamentum flavum
    B) Posterior longitudinal ligament
    C) Annulus fibrosus
    D) Nucleus pulposus
    E) Uncovertebral and zygapophyseal joints

79. Which one of the following tests would clinically confirm this patient's nerve root compression?

    A) Wallenberg's test
    B) Spurling's test
    C) Underberg's test
    D) Adson's test
    E) Yergason's test

80. The patient also has weakness with wrist flexion and forearm pronation. Which nerve is most likely affected?

    A) Axillary
    B) Musculocutaneous
    C) Ulnar
    D) Radial
    E) Median

Case 81-82

A 24-year-old patient complains of low back pain for two days. The patient has never had back pain before and has no numbness, tingling, or radiation of pain from the back. Structural exam reveals L5 FRLSL, the left sacral sulcus is shallow, the left ILA is superior, and the lumbosacral area moves anteriorly upon compression.

81. The most likely diagnosis is:

    A) Right on right sacral torsion
    B) Left on right sacral torsion
    C) Right on left sacral torsion
    D) Left unilateral sacral extension
    E) Right unilateral sacral flexion

82. The patient has the same lumbar and sacral findings. What would the diagnosis be if the lumbosacral area resists compression?

    A) Right on right sacral torsion
    B) Left on right sacral torsion
    C) Right on left sacral torsion
    D) Left unilateral sacral extension
    E) Right unilateral sacral flexion

Directions: For each numbered item (characteristic) select the one lettered heading (treatment type) most closely associated with it. Each lettered heading may be selected once, more than once, or not at all.

A. Direct treatment
B. Indirect treatment
C. Direct and Indirect treatment
D. Soft tissue technique

83. HVLA
84. STILL technique
85. Facilitated positional release
86. Spencer technique
87. Counterstrain
88. Petrissage
89. Indirect muscle energy
90. Positional treatment
91. Post-isometric muscle energy
92. Inhibitory pressure technique

COMLEX D
ANSWERS

COMLEX D Answers

1. Answer E: Hospitalized patients typically respond better with indirect techniques or gentle direct techniques. Often these types of patients cannot withstand aggressive treatment. There are a variety of direct myofascial techniques that a physician can do that will not interfere with his fragile medical status.

Muscle energy (regardless of the position of the spine) is contraindicated in patients with low vitality such as patients in the intensive care unit. **Answer A**

Techniques geared toward improving lymphatic return are relatively contraindicated in patients with advanced stages of cancer. In addition, the thoracoabdominal diaphragm release and pedal pump are less likely to decrease this patient's mid-thoracic pain since it seems to be musculoskeletal in nature and not directly related to lymphatic congestion. **Answers B and D**

High velocity low amplitude is contraindicated in patients with bone metastasis because this may cause a pathologic fracture to the spine. **Answer C**

2. Answer A: Tenderpoints on articular processes are anterior tenderpoints. Tenderpoints on spinous processes (or just lateral to them) are posterior tenderpoints. Anterior tenderpoints are treated in flexion. Treatment position for most cervical tenderpoints (including C5) would be to sidebend and rotate away from the side of the tenderpoint. Thus, putting all the information together, a right anterior cervical tenderpoint should be treated in flexion, sidebending to the left and rotating to the left. **Answers B, C, D, and E**

3. Answer D: The above patient has degenerative joint disease of his cervical spine. The condition has been present for several years and has been getting progressively worse. When you examine this patient you would expect to find chronic changes. There are some key phrases used to describe chronic somatic dysfunctions they are: cool dry skin, absent/decreased edema or erythema, flaccid, ropy and fibrotic tissues, and pain that may be burning, achy or dull in nature.

Boggy and edematous paraspinal musculature is associated with acute somatic dysfunctions. In addition, severe cervical degenerative joint disease is usually associated with a decreased range of motion. **Answer A**

Warm and moist skin texture with some erythema is associated with acute somatic dysfunctions. **Answer B**

Hypertonic paraspinals with severe, sharp pain upon palpation are associated with acute somatic dysfunctions. **Answer C**

An uncompensated spinal curve is associated with acute somatic dysfunctions. Chronic somatic dysfunctions are associated with compensated spinal curves. If a somatic dysfunction produces a spinal curve, over time other areas of the spine will tend to compensate with opposite spinal curves in attempt to straighten the body. **Answer E**

4. Answer D: The patient in the above question has the following dysfunctions 1) an exhalation dysfunction of ribs 1 - 5, 2) T1 - T5 neutral sidebent left and rotated right, except for T3 which is sidebent left, rotated left (sagittal component of T3 is not mentioned), 3) C5 extended rotated right and sidebent right. Translation to the right will induce left sidebending. Since C5 is sidebent right, it will resist left sidebending. When using a direct muscle energy technique, C5 should be positioned against the barrier. C5 then must be flexed rotated left and sidebent left.

Even though the patient has a group exhalation dysfunction, initial treatment should be directed at the thoracic spine. As a general rule, the somatic dysfunction of the thoracic vertebrae is treated before treating rib dysfunctions. **Answer A**

Based on the above findings T3 is sidebent left, rotated left. **Answer B**

The above patient has an exhalation dysfunction of ribs 1-5, because these ribs lag behind with inhalation. **Answer C**

T1, T2, T4 and T5 are sidebent left rotated right (not T3). **Answer E**

5. Answer C: If rib 5 has limited inhalation motion, there is an exhalation dysfunction present. Bucket handle motion occurs around an anterior-posterior axis. Even though rib 5 moves primarily in pump-handle fashion; there is still some bucket-handle motion (for a further explanation of bucket-handle dysfunctions of the upper ribs see Greenman's Principles of Manual Medicine). In a bucket-handle exhalation dysfunction the rib shaft (of rib 5) will approximate the shaft of the rib below (rib 6) in the mid-axillary line.

The shaft of rib 5 will approximate the shaft of rib 4 at the mid-clavicular line in a pump-handle inhalation dysfunction. **Answer A**

Rib 5 will feel more prominent anteriorly in a pump-handle inhalation dysfunction. **Answer B**

Rib 5 has a bucket-handle exhalation dysfunction. Pump-handle movement is around a transverse axis. **Answer D**

The rib angle will not feel more prominent in bucket-handle dysfunctions. Rib angle changes are usually reserved for pump-handle dysfunctions. **Answer E**

6. Answer C: Transverse processes have an anterior and posterior tubercle. The posterior tubercles serve as the origin of the scalenes.

They are located anterior to the articular pillars. **Answer A.**

The articular pillars are typically used as palpatory landmarks for osteopathic physicians to induce translation at the cervical spine. **Answer B**

The vertebral artery courses through the transverse processes C1 - C6. Small accessory vertebral veins go through the foramen transversarium of C7. [3 p.331] **Answer D**

They are located immediately anterior to the zygapophyseal joints. **Answer E**

7. Answer B: The above patient is likely to have cervical stenosis. Cervical stenosis can involve the spinal canal, the intervertebral foramen or both. Since she has decreased sensation at C5 (lateral elbow) and C6 (thumb), weak biceps and decreased biceps reflex, she is most likely to have intervertebral foraminal stenosis and nerve root compression at the C5 and C6 levels. The most common cause of nerve root compression in the neck are degenerative changes involving the joints of Luschka and facet (zygapophyseal) joint hypertrophy.

Since this patient's symptoms decreased with neck flexion she may not have a herniated disc. In addition, a herniated disc involving one level usually affects one nerve root not two. Also, the nucleus pulposus tends to desiccate by the age of 50 and it is therefore, it is less likely to cause of her symptoms. **Answer A**

Even though this patient is likely to have joint space and foraminal narrowing, an AP x-ray does not show the intervertebral foramen. Intervertebral foramen are best seen on oblique views. Answer C

Somatic dysfunction does not usually cause neurologic deficits. **Answer D**

Cervical spinal canal stenosis will result in lower extremity neurological deficits. Usually the patient will be hyper-reflexic in the lower extremities. **Answer E**

8. Answer A: The above patient has an exhalation dysfunction of rib 5 (you name the dysfunction in the direction it wants to go). Although rib 5 primarily moves in a pump-handle fashion, there still is some bucket-handle movement associated with it. Bucket-handle movement is most easily palpated in the mid-axillary line. Therefore, there will be some restriction of cephalad motion of rib 5 in the mid-axillary line.

The pectoralis minor originates at the coracoid process and inserts onto ribs 3 -5. A tenderpoint in this muscle could be due to a somatic dysfunction of ribs 3 - 5, but not always. The tenderpoint that is more specifically related to rib 5 would be either in the mid-axillary line (anterior) or on the rib angle (posterior) **Answer B**

Scapular winging is related to weakness in the serratus anterior and can be due to injury to the long thoracic nerve. It is not necessarily related to a somatic dysfunction of rib 5. **Answer C**

Although a rib dysfunction and thoracic dysfunction can easily be seen together, specific thoracic dysfunctions are not associated with specific rib dysfunction. **Answers D and E**

9. Answer E: Rib 4 will articulate with the transverse process and superior demifacet (on the vertebral body) of T4 and the inferior demifacet of T3.

Vertebral bodies get increasingly larger from the cervical spine to the lumbar spine. **Answer A.**

Based on the "rules of 3's." The first 3 thoracic vertebrae have spinous processes that project horizontally. The following set of 3 (T4, T5, T6), project more inferiorly, and the next set of 3 (T7, T8, and T9), project most inferiorly, and the last set of 3 (T10, T11, T12), project in such a way that T10 follows the rules of T7 - T9, T11 follows the rules of T4 - T6, and T12 follows the rules of T1 - T3. For more details see chapter 3 Thoracic Spine and Ribcage. **Answers B and C**

The vertebral artery courses through the foramen transversarium of C1 - C6. T1 does not have a foramen in its transverse process. **Answer D**

10. Answer B: The iliopsoas is a hip flexor and leg external rotator. Spasm of the iliopsoas will limit hip extension and internal rotation. Additional indicators of a right psoas dysfunction is a pelvis that is shifted to the left, the tenderpoint one inch medial to the right ASIS and a high (L2) lumbar type II somatic dysfunction.

Since the lumbosacral junction springs freely, the patient could not have a backward sacral torsion (right on left or left on right). As a matter of fact, there is not enough information in the question to diagnose a torsion. **Answer A**

The tenderpoint at the AIIS correlates to the L2 somatic dysfunction. **Answer C**

The left lateral Sim's position will correct a sacral torsion. There is not enough information in the above question to diagnose a torsion. **Answer D**

There is not enough information to diagnose an innominate dysfunction. In order to differentiate an innominate rotation vs. an innominate shear in the above question, the location of the PSIS's must be given. **Answer E**

11. Answer C: Anterior tibialis. The above patient has a disc herniation at the L3/L4 level. This will most likely impinge the L4 nerve root. The innervation of the anterior tibialis is from the L4 and L5 nerve roots (deep peroneal nerve).

The innervation of the extensor hallucis longus is from the L5 and S1 nerve roots (deep peroneal nerve). **Answer A**

The innervation of the flexor hallucis longus is from the S2 and S3 nerve roots (tibial nerve). **Answer B**

The innervation of the hamstrings is from the L5 - S2 nerve roots (tibial division of sciatic nerve and peroneal division of the sciatic nerve - short head of biceps). **Answer D**

The innervation of the peroneus longus is from the L5 - S2 nerve roots (superficial peroneal nerve). **Answer E**

12. Answer D: In sacral rotation on an oblique axis the seated flexion test (the test that checks for sacral dysfunction) is positive on the opposite side of the axis. In this case the oblique axis is on the right. A left deep sulcus with a posterior/inferior ILA indicates right rotation. Thus the patient has a right sacral rotation on a right oblique axis.

In left sacral rotation on a left oblique axis, a right sacral rotation on a left oblique axis and a unilateral sacral flexion on the right, the seated flexion test would be positive on the right, therefore it is easy to immediately eliminate those answers. **Answers A, C and E**

Left sacral rotation on a right oblique axis would present with different palpatory findings. The sacral sulcus would be posterior (or shallow) on the left and the right ILA would be anterior/superior. **Answer B**

13. Answer C: As a general rule, when referring to segmental motion (or restriction) it is traditional to refer to motion (or restriction) of the segment above in a functional vertebral unit (two vertebrae). For example, when describing the motion (or restriction) of C1, it is the motion of C1 on top of C2. As the neck rotates, most of the rotation comes from the atlas rotating around the dens of the axis (i.e. the AA joint - C1 on C2). So therefore, restriction with neck rotation will most likely stem from the atlas.

The sphenoid bone is not directly related to rotation restriction of the neck. **Answer A**

Due to the orientation of the occipital condyles on the atlas, this joint (the occipito-atlantal joint) typically prefers flexion and extension. **Answer B**

The axis (C2) and C3 do have a fair amount of rotation, however most of the rotation of the neck comes from the atlas. **Answers D and E**

14. Answer E: A unilateral sacral dysfunction has been associated with trauma at the SI joint. The downward force at the sacrum or an upward force from the leg results in a shearing effect at the SI joint. This force causes the sacrum to be pushed caudad, while the innominate is pushed cephalad. Due to the configuration of the SI joint, the sacral base will move anterior as well as caudad and the ILA will move posterior as well as caudad. [28 p.466]

An innominate anterior is often due to tight quadriceps such as the rectus femoris. **Answer A**

An innominate posterior is often due to tight hamstrings. **Answer B**

An inferior innominate shear has been associated with a vertical downward force on the innominate, not the sacrum. **Answer C**

Forward sacral torsions have not been associated with a specific type of trauma. **Answer D**

15. Answer C: Falling forward on an outstretched pronated forearm is a common cause of a posterior radial head somatic dysfunction. This somatic dysfunction is associated with restricted supination of the forearm.

Abduction of the ulna is associated with an increased carrying angle and restricted abduction of the wrist. **Answer A**

Cubitus valgus is sometimes seen in Turners syndrome. **Answer B**

The vascular arrangement of the scaphoid is that the main vessel enters the distal pole and runs through to the proximal pole. Thus, proximal pole fractures of the scaphoid have a high incidence of avascular necrosis of proximal segment. [52] **Answer D**

Wrist flexion is associated with dorsal glide of the carpal bones. Conversely, wrist extension is associated with ventral glide of the carpal bones. [28 p.624] **Answer E**

16. Answer C: The patient most likely has carpal tunnel syndrome. Conservative measures are most appropriate for initial treatment. These include wrist splints, NSAID's and OMT. OMT should be directed at correcting upper thoracic and rib somatic dysfunction and rib raising to decrease sympathetic tone.

The patient is taking Fosamax (Alendronate) 70mg weekly indicating that the patient has osteoporosis. Therefore, HVLA is contraindicated. **Answers A and B**

Although a steroid injection may be helpful, a more conservative approach such as OMT, splinting and a trial of NSAIDS should be tried first. Since this patient is elderly and diabetic, there is a higher chance of infection with joint injection. **Answer D**

Referral to a hand surgeon is appropriate after conservative treatment has failed. **Answer E**

17. **Answer B:** The above patient has a posterior fibular head somatic dysfunction. This somatic dysfunction is associated with ankle sprains in which the foot is inverted and plantar-flexed and internally rotated. The biomechanical mechanism is: [28 p.686] Ankle supination (inversion + plantar-flexion and internal rotation) tightens the anterior talofibular ligament. This taut ligament pulls on the distal fibular head anterior and the natural occurring reciprocal motion of fibula moves the proximal fibular head posterior.

The proposed mechanism for an anterior fibular head is: Ankle pronation (eversion, dorsiflexion and external rotation) forces the talus and tissues to push directly against the distal fibular head, thus pushing it posterior. Consequently the proximal fibular head will move anterior due to the natural reciprocal biomechanics of the fibula. **Answer A**

Ankle eversion and external rotation (components of pronation) will not cause a posterior fibular head dysfunction. **Answer C**

Ankle supination will not cause an anterior fibular head somatic dysfunction. **Answer D**

Although ankle plantar-flexion and inversion stretches the peroneus longus tendon, it is not the proposed mechanism by which a posterior fibular head occurs. **Answer E**

18. **Answer A:** Vertigo and tinnitus is often associated with cranial nerve VIII dysfunction. Although somatic dysfunction of the sphenoid, occiput and temporal bones can affect cranial nerve VIII, vertigo and tinnitus is most associated with the temporal bone dysfunction.

The parietal bone is not associated with any specific symptom. **Answer B**

The occiput is associated with dysfunctions in cranial nerves VIII - XII. Although dysfunction of cranial nerve VIII can be due to occiput dysfunction, specifically tinnitus and vertigo is attributed to temporal bone dysfunction. **Answer C**

The ethmoid is associated with CN I dysfunction, which will produce an altered sense of smell. **Answer D**

Dysfunction of the sphenoid can cause dysfunction of several cranial nerves (CN I - CN VIII) and result in a variety of symptoms. However, sphenoid dysfunction is not specifically related to tinnitus or vertigo. **Answer E**

19. **Answer C:** Sense of smell is controlled by the olfactory nerve (CN I). An altered sense of smell has been associated with sphenoid, frontal and ethmoid dysfunction.

Occipital or temporal restrictions can alter many physiologic functions. Poor tongue control and poor suckling in the newborn has been attributed to occipital condylar compression. **Answer A**

Occipital or temporal bone dysfunction, especially at the occipito-temporal suture at the jugular foramen, can effect cranial nerves IX, X and XI. The vagus nerve controls peristalsis of the lower 2/3 of the esophagus. **Answer B**

The internal jugular vein drains about 85% of the blood from the cranium. Restriction of the occiput or temporal bones at or near the jugular foramen could affect venous drainage from the cranium. **Answer D**

Temporal bone restriction has been associated with cranial nerve III dysfunction. Preganglionic parasympathetic fibers of cranial nerve III arise from the Edinger-Westphal nucleus (in the midbrain) and project to the ciliary muscle, which will control visual accommodation. **Answer E**

20. **Answer B**: Hypersympathetic activity to the respiratory epithelium increases the number of goblet cells in the respiratory tract. This encourages the production of profuse, thick secretions. Sphenopalatine ganglion treatment stimulates parasympathetic activity and reduces the number of goblet cells and increases the proportion of ciliated columnar cells. [35 p.29] Rib raising to the upper thoracic region will also help normalize sympathetic tone and help reduce the number of goblet cells, thus thinning out secretions. [35 p.26]

Frontonasal suture spread encourages the ethmoid bone to move freely. This encourages natural pumping action through the craniosacral mechanism and improves sinus drainage. [35 p.28] However, it will not change the consistency of the secretions. **Answer A**

CV4 decompression technique primarily enhances the amplitude of the CRI. It will not effectively thin this patient's secretions. **Answer C**

Redoming the diaphragm improves lymphatic drainage, venous return and improves immune function. It certainly has a role in treatment of the upper respiratory tract infection, however it will not change the consistency of the secretions. **Answer D**

Thoracic inlet release will improve lymphatic return from the structures form the head and neck. However, it will not change the consistency of the secretions. **Answer E**

21. **Answer E**: Pneumonia has been associated with hypersympathetic activity. Reducing hypersympathetic activity would also enhance arteriolar perfusion. Rib Raising is the method of choice. It will reduce sympathetic tone, enhance perfusion, decrease epithelial hyperplasia (# of goblet cells), improve lymphatic return and increase costal wall motion.

Occipital decompression will influence parasympathetic activity. Parasympathetic hyperactivity is not associated with pneumonia. **Answer A**

Muscle energy to C3 - C5 is not the method of choice when affecting the sympathetic tone of the lungs. **Answer B**

Although the thoraco-abdominal diaphragm release is an integral part of the OMT protocol for pneumonia, treatment of the diaphragm is not the method of choice when affecting the sympathetic tone of the lungs. **Answer C**

The lungs receive sympathetic innervation from paraspinal sympathetic ganglia at T2 - T7. Although manipulation of these segments may alter sympathetic tone, it is not the treatment of choice. **Answer D**

22. Answer B: A patient with an anterior wall myocardial infarction will have paraspinal musculoskeletal changes at T1 - T4 on the left. [39]

C2 and cranial base dysfunctions have been associated inferior wall MI's. [35 p.60] This is thought to be due to vagal hypertonicity. **Answer A**

Paraspinal musculoskeletal changes from T5 - L2 typically will occur from visceral dysfunction below the diaphragm. **Answers C, D and E**

23. Answer A: Sympathetic innervation of the heart has its origins in the cord segments T1 - T5. Fibers originating on the right innervate the right heart and sinoatrial (SA) node. Hypersympathetic activity predisposes to supraventricular tachyarrhythmias. [35 p.53]

Left sided sympathetic fibers (form T1 - T5) innervate the atrioventricular (AV) node. Hypersympathetic activity predisposes to ectopic foci and V-Tach. [35 p. 54] **Answer B**

The left vagus nerve innervates the AV node and hyperactivity predisposes to AV blocks. [35 p. 55] **Answer C**

Although the heart does receive fibers from the cervical chain ganglia, these fibers are post-ganglionic. [35 p. 54] **Answer D**

The oculocardiac reflex (pressure on the globe of the eye) will reflexively slow the heart by activating vagal efferent fibers. [35 p. 55] **Answer E**

24. Answer B: The elderly patient in the above question is recovering from a debilitating illness. He has peripheral vascular disease and likely has coronary artery disease as well. As noted in the Foundations of Osteopathic Medicine elderly patients and hospitalized patients typically respond better with indirect techniques or gentle direct techniques. An example of gentle direct techniques is articulatory techniques (a.k.a. low velocity, moderate amplitude techniques).

Due to the patient's current condition he would not be able to tolerate HVLA or muscle energy. Although rib raising will increase costal motion and the thoracoabdominal diaphragm release would improve lymphatic return, it would do little for his low back pain. **Answers A and C**

Isometric or concentric exercises may put too much demand on a decompensated heart. **Answers D and E**

25. Answer D: This patient has a pheochromocytoma, which is a catecholamine-producing tumor, of which 90% are found in the adrenal medulla. A viscerosomatic reflex would be found at the T10 spinal level.

The occiput and atlas influence parasympathetic activity in most of the viscera via the vagus nerve, however there are no parasympathetic fibers descending into the adrenal medulla. **Answers A and B**

T8 would receive sympathetic innervation for the upper GI tract. **Answer C**

L2 would receive innervation from the lower GI tract, uterus and cervix, penis, clitoris and legs. **Answer E**

26. Answer D: The clavicle moves in three different directions. First, it moves superior and inferior with shrugging and depressing the shoulder. Second, it moves anterior and posterior with retraction and protraction of the shoulder. Third, it rotates anteriorly and posteriorly with internal and external rotation of the arm when it is abducted at 90°. *28 p.163* Protracting the shoulder will cause the lateral end of the clavicle to move anterior. This will cause the medial end to move posterior.

The clavicle cannot be properly evaluated in the prone position. **Answer A.**

Patient supine, index fingers on the superior aspect of the clavicular head near sternum, patient depresses the shoulders. This will move the clavicle superior at the sternum. **Answer B**

Patient supine, index fingers on the superior aspect of the clavicular head near sternum, patient shrugs the shoulders. This will move the clavicle inferior at the sternum. **Answer C**

Patient supine, index fingers on the anterior aspect of the clavicular head near sternum, patient retracts the shoulders. This will move the clavicle anterior at the sternum. **Answer E**

27. Answer C: This patient has pancreatitis, which is an inflammation of the pancreas. The pancreas would cause a viscerosomatic reflex at T5-T9 spinal levels.

C3 - C5 spinal segments are not involved in a viscero-somatic reflex in pancreatitis. **Answer A**

T1-T4 receives sympathetic innervation from the head and neck. **Answer B**

T10 - T11 receive sympathetic innervation from the middle GI tract. **Answer D**

T12 - L2 receive sympathetic innervation from the lower GI tract. **Answer E**

28. Answer A: This patient most likely has temporal arteritis, which would cause a viscerosomatic reflex change at the T1-T3 spinal levels.

T4-T6 spinal levels are associated with the viscerosomatic reflex from the lungs and esophagus. **Answer B**

T7-T9 spinal levels are associated with the viscerosomatic reflex from the upper GI tract. **Answer C**

T10-T12 spinal levels are associated with the viscerosomatic reflex from the middle GI tract and the gonads. **Answer D**

T12-L2 spinal levels are associated with the viscerosomatic reflex from the lower GI tract. **Answer E**

29. Answer D: The proper way to start the evaluation of the thoracic spine is to perform static palpation in the neutral position. If asymmetry is found, then evaluate the sagittal plane in flexion and extension (Answers A and B). If the asymmetry is not resolved in flexion or extension, then it is a neutral dysfunction.

Answers A, B, D, and E are not usually used when starting an evaluation of the thoracic spine.

30. Answer E: An elevated maternal serum alpha fetal protein is associated with neural tube defects. Neurological deficits are most common in meningomyelocoele. A relaxed anal sphincter indicates injury to the lower spinal cord (around the cauda equina). This lesion may occur anywhere along the neuroaxis, but is most commonly found in the lumbosacral area. Treatment is surgery within several days.

Cavernous hemangiomas are tumors that are cystic, firm, or compressible, and the overlying skin may appear normal in color or have a bluish hue. These lesions are usually found on the face, scalp, back, and anterior chest. They are not associated with neurological deficits. **Answer A**

Osteosarcomas are primary malignant bone tumors that occur during the first 13 years of life. They most commonly occur in the distal femur, proximal humerus, and proximal tibia. **Answer B**

Spinal bifida in the thoraco-lumbar junction may present with upper motor neurological findings such as spasticity, not flaccidity. In addition, the child would not have active hip flexion. **Answer C**

Although it is possible to have a neurological deficit in meningocoele, it is not common. **Answer D**

31. Answer E: Pulmonary respiration and craniosacral motion occur about the superior transverse sacral axis.

The innominates rotate about an inferior transverse sacral axis. **Answer A**

There are two oblique sacral axes that are used in the mechanics of walking or in somatic dysfunctions of the sacrum. **Answer B**

Postural motion occurs about a middle transverse sacral axis. **Answer C**

Sacral margin somatic dysfunctions rotate about a sagittal axis. **Answer D**

32. Answer B: Although some authors do not believe it is possible to locate the area of neurovascular compression with provocative maneuvers (Adson's, Wrights and Military posture test), some osteopathic practitioners [28] believe it is possible. These authors state that Wright's test (also known as hyperextension test) will be positive if the neurovascular compression occurs beneath the pectoralis minor muscle at the coracoid process.

Adson's test is thought to be positive if the neurovascular compression occurs between the anterior and middle scalenes. **Answer A**

Military posture test and costoclavicular syndrome test are two names for the same test and are positive for neurovascular compression between the clavicle and the first rib. **Answers C and E**

The hyperextension test (also known as Wright's test) will be positive if the neurovascular compression occurs between the pectoralis minor muscle at the coracoid process. The hyperextension test is somewhat of a misnomer because the test is performed with the arm in hyperabduction with some extension. **Answer D**

33. Answer A: A posterior radial head dysfunction would cause the forearm to prefer pronation, and the radial head would resist anterior glide. Falling on a pronated forearm causes this dysfunction.

An anterior radial head dysfunction would cause the forearm to prefer supination and the radial head would resist posterior glide. Falling backward on a supinated forearm can cause this dysfunction. **Answer B**

Lateral epicondylitis is a strain of the extensor muscles of the forearm near the lateral epicondyle. It is usually due to overuse of the wrist extensors and not typically associated with trauma. **Answer C**

Medial epicondylitis (also known as golfer's elbow) is a strain of the flexor muscles of the forearm near the medial epicondyle. It is usually due to overuse of the wrist flexors and not typically associated with trauma. **Answer D**

A flexion dysfunction can result from a fall on the back of the hand. The wrist would be restricted in extension. **Answer E**

34. Answer C: The talus normally glides anterior on the tibia with plantar-flexion and glides posterior with dorsiflexion. In a posterior talar dysfunction, the talus glides posteriorly and is restricted in anterior glide. The foot prefers dorsiflexion.

In a plantar flexion dysfunction of the talus, the talus glides anteriorly and is restricted in posterior glide. The foot prefers plantar-flexion. **Answer A**

Somatic dysfunction of the transverse arch typically presents with plantar surface pain and restriction with the navicular, cuboid or cuneiform bones, not tibiotalar restriction. **Answer B**

In a fibular head somatic dysfunction, there will be restriction at the proximal fibular head. There is no mention of such a restriction; therefore these are not the best answers. **Answers D and E**

35. Answer B: This patient has a flexion dysfunction of the left biceps. Reciprocal inhibition can be done using a direct method or an indirect method. [28 p.311, 28 p.680] To correct this dysfunction using an indirect reciprocal inhibition technique, the elbow is flexed away from the restrictive barrier, and the patient is asked to contract the triceps muscle. This causes a relaxation of the biceps muscle via a reciprocal inhibition reflex arc. To correct this dysfunction using a direct reciprocal inhibition technique (which is not one of the choices), the elbow is extended toward the restrictive barrier, and the patient is asked to contract the triceps muscle.

If the left elbow is extended to the restrictive barrier and the patient is asked to contract the biceps muscle against resistance, then this is direct post-isometric relaxation muscle energy. **Answer A**

If the right elbow is extended and the patient is asked to contract the right biceps against resistance, then this is an example of crossed extensor reflex muscle energy. **Answer C**

Answers D, and E are not correctly performed muscle energy treatments for a biceps spasm.

36. Answer D: Hallux valgus (also known as a bunion), is a lateral deviation of the proximal phalanx of the first toe associated with soft tissue changes, pain, swelling, and inflammation at the aspect of the head of the first metatarsal, which is angled medially. [25 p. 336-337]

Hallux rigidus is osteoarthrosis of the first metatarsophalangeal articulation. Joint motion is severely limited, but not typically medially deviated. There is no first toe push off, and localized pain is present at that joint. **Answer A**

March fracture is a stress fracture, usually involving the shaft of the second or third metatarsals. **Answer B** [25 p. 336]

Morton's neuroma is a fibroneuromatous reaction between the heads of the third and fourth metatarsals. [25 p. 336] **Answer C**

Soft corns are hyperkeratotic lesions found between the toes, usually the fourth and fifth toes; they are extremely painful. Hard corns are associated with hammer or claw toes. **Answer E** [25 p. 337]

37. **Answer C**: The median nerve is derived from the spinal nerve roots of C5-T1.

The axillary nerve is derived from nerve roots C5-C6. **Answer A**

The musculocutaneous nerve is derived from nerve roots C5-C7. **Answer B**

The ulnar nerve is derived from nerve roots C7-T1. **Answer C**

C2-C4 are not involved in the brachial plexus. [3 p. 515] **Answer E**

Case 38-41

38. **Answer A:** The above patient has an acute appendicitis. Appendicitis can cause psoas syndrome. [28 p.484] This is probably due to the close proximity of the iliopsoas to the appendix.

The iliocostalis lies posterior to the iliopsoas and quadratus lumborum and therefore is less likely to be irritated in acute appendicitis. **Answer B**

Although the quadratus lumborum is a muscle in the posterior abdominal wall, it is not typically irritated in appendicitis. This is probably because the appendix often lies below the pelvic rim. **Answer C**

The rectus abdominus, although a muscle in the abdomen, due to its position in relation to the appendix it is an unlikely candidate to be irritated in appendicitis. **Answer D**

The piriformis is far enough removed from the peritoneum that local irritation will not directly cause dysfunction. **Answer E**

39. **Answer A:** Small fascial contractions (i.e. Chapman's reflexes) represent viscero-somatic reflexes. The anterior Chapman's point for acute appendicitis is located at the tip of the 12th right rib. This is probably the most tested Chapman's reflex on the COMLEX exams.

Halfway between the ASIS and the umbilicus describes McBurney's point, it is a surgical landmark. It is not associated with Chapman's reflexes in appendicitis. **Answer B**

One cm lateral to the L1 spinous process is the location of the Chapman's point for the kidneys. **Answer C**

The right transverse process of L2 is the location of the Chapman's point for the abdomen and bladder. **Answer D**

The rib angle of the 12th rib is not a location of a Chapman's point. [1 p.939] **Answer E**

40. Answer D: Appendicitis will most likely cause a somatic dysfunction at T12. Although T10 - -T11 receive input from and supplies visceral efferents to the middle GI tract (specifically from the jejunum to the transverse colon), several authors [1, 28] specifically list T12 to be associated with the appendix. Therefore T12 is the best answer.

C5 will not receive abnormal visceral afferent input from appendicitis. **Answer A**

T5 - T9 supplies the upper GI tract (stomach through the duodenum). **Answers B and C**

L2 receives input from the lower GI tract. **Answer E**

41. Answer D: Appendicitis is associated with hypersympathetic activity, specifically at T12. Therefore the most optimal technique will reduce hypersympathetic tone at T12. The purpose of the superior mesenteric ganglion release is to calm sympathetics from segments T9 - T12.

The purposes of the occipito-atlantal decompression, manipulation of C3 - C5, and sacral inhibition is to alter parasympathetic tone. Appendicitis is not associated with hyperparasympathetic activity. **Answers A, B and E**

The purpose of the celiac ganglion release is to calm sympathetics from segments T5 - T9. **Answer C**

Case 42-44

42. Answer B: Gross motion testing is evaluating range of motion over a body region. Since motion is being assessed over the chest wall this is gross motion testing.

Inherent respiratory motion is craniosacral motion. Cranial motion is not being evaluated in this patient. **Answer A**

Segmental motion testing is motion testing at the single vertebral or rib level. **Answer C**

The physician's hands are not in a position to accurately assess vertebral motion or position. **Answer D**

This is an example of active motion testing, not passive motion testing. In active motion testing, the patient induces the motion. In passive motion testing, the physician induces joint motion. **Answer E**

43. Answer C: Usually rib dysfunctions are caused by thoracic dysfunctions; therefore treatment should first be directed at the thoracic spine before treating rib somatic dysfunctions. A 5 degree levoscoliosis of T2 - T6 indicates that these segments are sidebent right indicating possible somatic dysfunction.

One would not treat rib 2 in this case for the above reason. In addition, rib 2 is not the key rib in this inhalation dysfunction. **Answer A**

Rib six would only be treated in this case if the thoracic spine were symmetric. Although a 5-degree scoliosis may be normal, it cannot be assumed. **Answer B**

Although treating the thoracic inlet could be included in the overall treatment in this patient, it would not be the most effective treatment in restoring rib motion. **Answer D**

Since the anterior scalene is attached to rib one only, this should not even be considered. **Answer E**

44. Answer B: This patient likely has osteoporosis; the thoracic pump is contraindicated in patients with osteoporosis.

This patient could tolerate rib raising since it is a gentle articulatory technique. **Answer A**

This patient would also tolerate pectoral traction. It would help relieve any lymphatic congestion, especially in those patients who cannot tolerate the thoracic pump. **Answer C**

This patient would also tolerate craniosacral treatment since it is a gentle technique. **Answer D**

The seated facilitated positional release technique requires passive sidebending and rotation then applying a compressive force. This treatment is gentle and well tolerated in the elderly. **Answer E**

Case 45-49

45. Answer B: Fifty percent of cervical rotation stems from the atlanto-axial joint (the atlas on the axis). If the patient has decreased rotation, this joint would be the most likely affected segment.

The occipito-atlantal joint (the occiput on the atlas) has greatest motion in flexion and extension. **Answer A**

The third and fifth cervical segments have varying proportions of all spinal movements. However, the rotation component is not as much as the atlanto-axial joint. Therefore, a restriction in rotation is less likely to occur at these segments. **Answer C and E**

The joints of Luschka plays role in cervical sidebending, not rotation. **Answer D**

46. Answer C: The joints of Luschka are the articulations of the superior uncinate processes and the superadjacent vertebrae. [29 p.373] These joints have also been called uncovertebral joints. [29 p.5] They help support the lateral side of the cervical discs and protect cervical nerve roots from disc herniation. [28 p. 210, 29 p.79]

They are located immediately anterior to the intervertebral foramina. **Answer A**

The uncinate processes are superior lateral projections originating from the posterior lateral rim of C3 - C7 vertebral bodies, not the superior articular processes. **Answer B**

Pannus formation is inflammatory exudates overlying the lining layer of synovial cells inside a joint. Most authors agree that the joints of Luschka are not true synovial joints therefore it is not susceptible to pannus formation. **Answer D**

The lateral location of the joints of Luschka in the cervical spine would indicate that these joints would not limit flexion and extension, however they play a role in cervical sidebending. **Answer E**

47. Answer E: The most common cause of cervical nerve root pressure is degeneration of the Joints of Luschka plus hypertrophic arthritis of the zygapophyseal (facet) joints. [28 p.214] This typically leads to cervical foraminal stenosis. On physical examination pain is exacerbated with spinal extension.

Osteoarthritis of the cervical spine does not typically result in plexopathy. Plexopathy is another term for neuropathy of a plexus, in this case the brachial plexus. [49] **Answer A**

Hypertrophy of the ligamentum flavum is more likely to cause central canal stenosis rather than foraminal stenosis. **Answer B**

Since this patient is experiencing a reproduction of his radicular pain with cervical extension, a herniated disc causing nerve root compression is less likely. **Answer C**

Although bulging discs are common, often they are asymptomatic. However, if this patient were to have nerve root irritation from a bulging disc, typically the pain would be reproduced with flexion, not extension. **Answer D**

48. Answer B: A diminished biceps reflex would indicate C5 or C6 nerve root pathology. Diminished sensation over the thumb area indicates that this problem is more likely to be the C6 nerve root.

Symptoms are not reproduced with cervical extension in plexopathy. In addition, the patient would have numbness over a greater distribution of the upper extremity. **Answers D and E**

49. Answer B: The anterior rib one tenderpoint is located below the clavicle immediately lateral to the manubrium. Authors have associated this with a depressed first rib. [1 p.815, 25 p.272, 40 p.65]

The AC joint tenderpoint is located slightly medial to the distal end of the clavicle. **Answer A**

The anterior rib 2 tenderpoint is located 6-8cm lateral to the sternum on rib 2. Authors have associated this with a depressed second rib. [1 p.815, 25 p.272, 40 p.65] **Answer C**

Anterior thoracic tenderpoints indicate intervertebral dysfunction. These tenderpoints are located on the sternum or manubrium, not next to it. The anterior first thoracic tenderpoint is located in the midline in the suprasternal notch. The second is midline at the manubrio-sternal joint (angle of Louis). And the third is one-inch below the manubrio-sternal joint. **Answer D**

The anterior seventh cervical tenderpoint is associated with sternocleidomastoid dysfunction, [40] it is located above and behind the clavicle and lateral to the attachment of the SCM. **Answer E**

Case 50-52

50. Answer D: Facilitated positional release is the least time consuming of all the treatments listed. It takes approximately a few seconds to set up the patient correctly and about 3 to 4 seconds to apply the treatment.

It may take several seconds to have a release in muscle tension with myofascial release techniques. **Answer A**

Most counterstrain points are held for approximately 90 seconds (120 seconds for the ribs). **Answer B**

In lumbar muscle energy techniques the patient is placed in a precise position and then asked to actively contract against resistance for 3-5 seconds for 3-5 times. **Answer C**

Functional technique requires the patient to be placed in a position that produces the least amount of palpable tension. The patient is then asked to take a deep breath and hold briefly. This will take longer than facilitated positional release. **Answer E**

51. Answer D: The lumbar curve is convex to the right in a left on left sacral torsion.

The right sacral sulcus is deep in a left on left sacral torsion. **Answer A**

The backward bending test (sphinx test) is negative with forward sacral torsions (left on left and right on right). **Answer B**

The left ASIS would be cephalad compared to the right. **Answer C**

There will be a longer leg on the right side in a right innominate anterior. **Answer E**

52. Answer A: A left on left sacral torsion is treated in the left lateral Sims position. In this position the patient is lying on his left side with his torso turned to the left so he is face down. (See fig 15.7)

A right on right sacral torsion is treated with the patient in the right lateral Sims position. In this position the patient is lying on his right side with his torso turned to the right so he is face down. **Answer B**

A right on left sacral torsion is treated with the patient lying on his left side with torso turned to the right. (See fig 15.8) **Answer C**

A left on right sacral torsion is treated with the patient lying on his right side with torso turned to the left. **Answer D**

This is not a treatment position for sacral torsions. **Answer E**

Case 53-58

53. Answer C: Translation to the right induces left sidebending and translation to the left induces right sidebending. Since C5 translation to the right is restricted when the head is extended, this segment is restricted in left sidebending when the head is extended. Therefore, C5 is sidebent right. Since C5 follows type II mechanics (sidebending and rotation to same side), it will be rotated to the right.

54. Answer C: Translation to the right induces left sidebending and translation to the left induces right sidebending. The OA joint is the movement of the occipital condyles (or the occiput) on the atlas. Occipital translation to the right (left sidebending) is restricted when the head is in extension. Since the OA joint follows type I mechanics, (sidebending and rotation to opposite sides), it will be restricted in right rotation. Therefore, the OA is restricted in left sidebending and right rotation.

55. Answer B: The posterior scalene originates from the transverse process of C4 - C6 and inserts onto the second rib. Tenderness of this muscle would be most associated with a rib 2 dysfunction.

Tenderness in the anterior scalene may be associated with a rib 1 dysfunction. **Answers A and C**

Tenderness in the pectoralis minor may be associated with dysfunctions of ribs 3-5. **Answers D and E**

56. Answer C: Adson's test detects thoracic outlet syndrome. Thoracic outlet syndrome is a compression of the neurovascular bundle at the thoracic outlet. The shoulder being tested is extended, slightly abducted and the arm is externally rotated while the physician palpates the radial pulse. The patient takes a deep breath and turns his head toward the side being tested. Please see Chapter 18 special tests for a full description on how to perform the test.

See above. **Answer A**

The elbow is extended with Adson's test. **Answer B**

See above. **Answer D**

The arm is freely allowed to drop in the drop arm test. **Answer E**

57. Answer B: Out of the choices listed the ovaries would be most affected from an autonomic imbalance of the upper cervical spine. Function of the vagus nerve may be influenced by somatic dysfunction of The OA, AA and C2 joints. The vagus nerve innervates the ovaries and testicles. For a full description of the vagal nerve innervation, see chapter 10 Facilitation.

The adrenal glands are innervated solely by the sympathetic nervous system. **Answer A**

Although the kidneys do receive innervation from the parasympathetic system, it has little effect. [35 p.126] **Answer C**

All pelvic organs except the ovaries and testes receive parasympathetic innervation from the pelvic splanchnic nerve. **Answer D**

The pelvic splanchnic nerve controls the parasympathetic functions of the urinary bladder. **Answer E**

Case 58-62

58. Answer D: The patient in the above case has a sacral somatic dysfunction. The sacrum has rotated left on a right oblique axis. This will result in a positive seated flexion test on the left (seated flexion test positive on the opposite side of the axis).

A short leg on the left is more likely to occur with innominate dysfunction. Since the PSIS's are equal, there is no innominate dysfunction. **Answer A**

A positive standing flexion test is more likely to occur with innominate dysfunction, this patient does not have an innominate dysfunction. **Answer B**

A left on right sacral torsion will result in a lumbar curve that is convex to the left. **Answer C**

Answer E is describing a negative backward bending test; in a left sacral rotation on a right oblique axis, the backward bending would be positive. **Answer E**

59. Answer A: Since the lumbosacral spring test is positive, part or the entire sacral base has moved posterior. The sacral sulcus on the right is deeper; therefore the left is more shallow and must have moved posterior. Out of the choices given, the only diagnosis that fits the above findings is a left sacral torsion on a right oblique axis.

In a right torsion on a left oblique axis the right sulcus would be shallow and the left would be deep. **Answer B**

In a left sacral torsion on a left oblique axis, the lumbosacral spring test is negative. **Answer C**

In a left unilateral sacral flexion, the left sacral sulcus would be deeper and the lumbosacral spring test is negative. **Answer D**

In a right unilateral sacral extension, the right sulcus would be shallow. **Answer E**

60. Answer C: Since L5 rotated to the right and the sacrum has rotated to the left, there is a sacral torsion present. In sacral torsions, specific L5 findings will be present. Following the rules of L5 on the sacrum: The sacrum is rotated left therefore L5 is rotated right (given in the question). The sacrum has a right oblique axis, therefore L5 is sidebent right. Following Fryette's law II, if L5 is sidebent and rotated to the right it must be non-neutral (flexed or extended).

Theoretically L5 cannot be neutral, sidebent right, rotated right due to Fryette's laws. **Answer A**

If L5 were neutral, sidebent left, rotated right, a left on left sacral torsion would be present. **Answer B**

Theoretically L5 cannot be flexed, rotated right, sidebent left due to Fryette's laws. **Answer D**

Theoretically L5 cannot be extended, rotated right, and sidebent left due to Fryette's laws. **Answer E**

61. Answer C: Piriformis tenderpoints are often associated with sacral dysfunctions. [25 p.235] They are also associated with sciatic irritation due to the close proximity to the sciatic nerve.

Spasm of the rectus abdominus is associated with superior pubic shear. **Answer A**

A positive Ober's test is associated with a tight iliotibial band. **Answer B**

Tight hamstrings are more likely to produce an innominate dysfunction, specifically a posterior rotated innominate. **Answer D**

A quadratus lumborum tenderpoint is more likely to produce lumbar sidebending dysfunction and/or rib 12 dysfunction. **Answer E**

62. Answer A: Treatment should be directed toward L5 first. Sacral dysfunctions will often spontaneously resolve with treatment of L5.

A left on left sacral torsion (not L5) can be treated using muscle energy with the patient in the left lateral Sim's position. **Answer B**

The above patient is unlikely to have a disc herniation because the onset of pain is gradual and the decreased reflexes are most likely due to diabetic neuropathy. Therefore, HVLA would not be contraindicated. **Answer C**

Anterior lumbar tenderpoints are typically treated with the hips flexed. **Answer D**

Muscle energy is only contraindicated in patients with low vitality, such as ICU patients and post-surgical patients. **Answer E**

Case 63-66

63. **Answer E:** The sensitivity of nerve conduction and electromyographic studies is reported to be 87% - 98%. Nerve conduction studies will identify if any conduction block has resulted from damage to the myelin or axon of the median nerve. Needle electromyography will identify if this damage is severe enough to have caused denervation.

Carpal tunnel syndrome is a neuropathic problem and will not show up on a bone scan or thermography. **Answers A and B**

Tinel's, Phalen's and Prayer tests are all used to aid in the diagnosis of carpal tunnel syndrome. However, the sensitivity and specificity for these tests vary from as low as 10% in some studies to as high as 80% in other studies. **Answer C**

Although MRI is able to show soft tissue structures, it is not adequate for identifying nerve compression at the carpal tunnel. **Answer D**

64. **Answer D:** There is one nerve and 9 tendons that run though the carpal tunnel. They are: Median nerve, 4 tendons of the flexor digitorum superficialis, 4 tendons of the flexor digitorum profundus and the flexor pollicis longus tendon

The flexor carpi ulnaris inserts onto the pisiform bone and does not enter the carpal tunnel. **Answer B**

65. **Answer D:** Carpal tunnel syndrome could result in muscle weakness in all muscles innervated by the median nerve in the hand. These are: abductor pollicis brevis, opponens pollicis, and part of the flexor pollicis brevis.

Sensation to the fifth digit, finger abduction and adduction (interossi) and thumb adduction (adductor pollicis) are supplied by the ulnar nerve. **Answers A, B and C**

The radial and ulnar nerves supply sensation to the dorsum of the hand. **Answer E**

66. **Answer B:** Sympathetic control of the upper extremity is supplied by T2-T8 spinal segments. Therefore, manipulation to T2 - T7 would have the greatest impact on hypersympathetic tone.

Although the upper extremity receives innervation from cervical spine, the sympathetic vasomotor fibers originate in the upper thoracic spine. **Answer A**

Manipulation directed at the carpal tunnel, the clavicle or sacrum would not directly impact the sympathetic tone in the upper extremity. **Answers C, D and E**

Case 67-70

67. Answer C: Patients with structural adhesions affecting the Eustachian tube may complain of hearing loss, recurrent otitis media, vertigo and/or tinnitus. [35 p.15]

On physical examination, the tympanic membranes are visualized; therefore cerumen impaction is not likely. **Answer A**

Acute labyrinthitis will result in severe vertigo. It is less likely to cause tinnitus. [35 p.11] **Answer B**

Temporomandibular joint dysfunction is less likely because there were no clicks or pops of the jaw. **Answer D**

Salicylate toxicity will result in bilateral, not unilateral tinnitus. [35 p.11] **Answer E**

68. Answer D: It is well established that cranial dysfunction is associated with tinnitus, [56 p.389-90] however the temporal bone has been most associated with tinnitus. [35 p.11] It is also associated with hearing loss and vertigo. [35 p. 9]

69. Answer C: External rotation of the temporal bone is associated with low-pitched roaring tinnitus. Fixed internal rotation has been associated with a high-pitched tinnitus. [35 p.9]

Imbalance of the supra-hyoid muscle is associated with hyoid bone dysfunction. **Answer A**

Temporomandibular disc disruption would cause a temporomandibular joint dysfunction. **Answer B**

Barotrauma to the tympanic membrane could cause a tympanic membrane perforation. **Answer D**

Hypersecretion of cerumen could theoretically cause cerumen impaction. **Answer E**

70. Answer E: In patients with cranial somatic dysfunction who also are experiencing vertigo tinnitus the goals of OMT include achieving a balance between the temporal bones, normalizing the C.R.I. and removing areas of dural strains. [35 p.14] In the above patient this would be best achieved by temporal rocking.

The frontal and parietal lifts are not the most appropriate technique for treating tinnitus. **Answers A and C**

The vault hold is most commonly used as a hold for assessment of cranial rhythm dysfunctions. **Answer B**

The V spread is used to remove restriction of sutures. **Answer D**

Case 71-72

71. Answer E: This is a classic presentation of Osgood-Schlatter's disease. This traction apophysitis of the tibial tubercle results from microtrauma. It occurs around puberty and is caused by overuse. Athletic activity combined with a recent growth spurt results in a detachment of cartilage fragments from the tibial tuberosity. [32 p.624-6]

Osteochondritis dissecans is a common condition characterized by subchondral bone necrosis and sometimes by complete or partial separation of articular fragments. The most common site is the lateral aspect of the medial femoral condyle. Pain is not usually present at the tibial tubercle. **Answer A**

Patello-femoral syndrome is an overuse syndrome. It is the most common patello-femoral disorder. The principal symptoms are anterior knee pain and a grating sensation aggravated by activities involving knee flexion (e.g. climbing stairs, running). Pain is typically present on the posterior surface of the patella, not at the tibial tubercle [32 p.361] **Answer B.**

Patellar tendonitis is an inflammation of the patellar tendon usually caused by overuse. It results in pain at the insertion of the quadriceps tendon or at the patellar tendon at the insertion into the patella, rather than at its more inferior insertion on the tibial tubercle. [32 p.356] **Answer C**

Sever's disease is a traction apophysitis of the calcaneus resulting from microtrauma. At the site where the Achilles tendon joins the calcaneus, there can be avulsion and inflammation due to overuse. [32 p.562-3] **Answer D**

72. Answer C: The quadriceps are involved in knee extension, an overuse of which is the source of the pain. Treatment of these muscles would directly affect the patellar tendon, causing a reduction of the traction of tension on the tibial tuberosity.

Treatment of the iliotibial tract is indicated in hip and lateral knee pain that may result in iliotibial tendonitis. **Answer A**

Treating the adductors would be indicated in an adductor strain; it would not be indicated for Osgood-Schlatters disease. **Answer B**

Treatment of the semimembranosus tendon would be appropriate after treatment of the quadriceps. The quadriceps would have a more direct effect on the patellar tendon and tibial tuberosity. **Answer D**

Treatment of the gastrocnemius would be indicated for Sever's disease. **Answer E**

Case 73-75

73. Answer D: Diaphragmatic irritation is a common reaction to a laproscopic cholecystectomy and is a known etiology of singultus. Singultus is another term for hiccups. [12 p. 488-489]

Answers A, B, C, and E are all possible etiologies of singultus, but are not part of the case history, and therefore are less likely causes. [12 p.488-489]

74. Answer E: The cause of this patient's singultus is diaphragmatic irritation as a result of his laproscopic cholecystectomy. This is the only choice that addresses the diaphragm.

Ear lavage could be used to treat tympanic membrane irritation. **Answer A**

Proton pump inhibitor would be indicated for reflux esophagitis. **Answer B**

Antibiotics are indicated for bacterial pneumonia. **Answer C**

Appendicitis is a cause of singultus; an appendectomy is the indicated treatment. **Answer D**

75. Answer B: Irritation of the hemidiaphragm or Glisson's capsule of the liver causes phrenic pain that is referred to C3-C5. [35 p.81]

C1-C2 has parasympathetic influences via the vagus nerve. Singultus is more likely to effect the phrenic nerve. **Answer A**

T1-T4 receives sympathetic stimulation from the head and neck. **Answer C**

T9-T12 receives sympathetic innervation from the middle GI tract. **Answer D**

L1-L2 receives sympathetic innervation from the lower genitourinary tract. L3 does not usually have sympathetic innervation, since the spinal cord only extends to L2. **Answer E**

Case 76-77

76. Answer D: The middle GI tract receives sympathetic innervation from T10 - T11. The middle GI tract begins at the jejunum and terminates at the end of the transverse colon.

C3 - C5 spinal segments are not involved in a viscero-somatic reflex in Crohn's disease. **Answer A**

T1-T4 receives sympathetic innervation from the head and neck. **Answer B**

T5-T9 receives sympathetic innervation from the upper GI tract. **Answer C**

The spinal cord stops at L2; there is no sympathetic innervation originating below this level. **Answer E**

77. Answer A: The Chapman's point for the iliocecal area is located on the right proximal femur at the greater trochanter within the iliotibial tract.

The Chapman's point for the right half of the transverse colon is located on the right distal femur in the iliotibial tract. **Answer B**

The Chapman's point for the sigmoid colon is located on the left proximal femur at the greater trochanter in the iliotibial tract. **Answers C and E**

The Chapman's point for the left half of the transverse colon is located on the left distal femur in the iliotibial tract. **Answer D**

Case 78-80

78. Answer E: Degenerative changes within the uncovertebral joints (a.k.a. joints of Luschka) plus hypertrophic arthritis of the intervertebral synovial joints (a.k.a. facet or zygapophyseal joints) are the most common cause of cervical nerve root compression. [28 p.214]

Degenerative changes within the ligamentum flavum, posterior longitudinal ligament, annulus fibrosus, and nucleus pulposus all are contributing factors for nerve root compression, however it is less likely. **Answers A, B, C, and D**

79. Answer B: Spurling's test aims to close down cervical intervertebral foramina. If there is any intervertebral foraminal stenosis, nerve compression would occur and pain would radiate down the arm.

Wallenberg's test and Underberg's test are used to test for vertebral artery insufficiency. **Answers A and C**

Adson's test is used to test for thoracic outlet syndrome. **Answer D**

Yergason's test is used to determine the stability of the biceps tendon in the bicipital groove. **Answer E**

80. Answer E: The median nerve and ulnar nerve innervates the wrist flexors, however only the median nerve innervates the pronator teres and pronator quadratus.

The axillary nerve innervates the deltoid and teres minor muscles. **Answer A**

The musculocutaneous nerve innervates the biceps, brachialis and coracobrachialis muscles. **Answer B**

The ulnar nerve does innervate some wrist flexors however it does not innervate wrist pronators. **Answer C**

The radial nerve innervates muscles around the elbow, and the wrist and finger extensors. **Answer E**

Case 81-82

81. Answer E: The patient has a right unilateral sacral flexion. The static findings are a deep right sulcus (meaning a left shallow sulcus) and an inferior and slightly posterior right ILA (meaning a superior and slightly anterior left ILA) with a negative lumbosacral spring test.

A right on right torsion has a deep left sulcus and a posterior, slightly inferior ILA on the right, and a negative lumbosacral spring test (the lumbosacral area moves anteriorly on compression). **Answer A**

Left on right sacral torsion, a right on left sacral torsion and a left unilateral sacral extension would have a positive lumbosacral spring test with different static findings. **Answers B, C, and D**

82. Answer D: If the lumbosacral area resists springing (a positive lumbosacral spring test), then this indicates that the sacral base has moved posterior. In a left unilateral sacral extension, the left sulcus would be shallow and the left ILA would be superior.

A right on right torsion has a deep left sulcus and a posterior, slightly inferior ILA on the right, and a negative lumbosacral spring test (the lumbosacral area moves anteriorly on compression). **Answer A**

A left on right sacral torsion would have a positive lumbosacral spring test with a deep right sulcus and a posterior and slightly inferior ILA on the left. **Answer B**

A right on left sacral torsion would have a positive lumbosacral spring test with a deep left sulcus and a posterior and slightly inferior ILA on the right. **Answer C**

A right unilateral sacral flexion would have a negative lumbosacral spring test. **Answer E**

Matching

83. **Answer A:** HVLA is a direct treatment, which uses high velocity/low amplitude forces. It is also called mobilization with impulse treatment or thrust technique. [1 p. 1134]

84. **Answer C:** Still technique is characterized as a specific non-repetitive articulatory technique that is indirect then direct. [56 p.1242]

85. **Answer B:** Facilitated positional release is an indirect treatment that describes a system of indirect myofascial release treatments developed by Stanley Schiowitz, D.O. The area being treated is placed into a neutral position, decreasing tissue and joint tension in all planes. Then an activating force (compression or torsion) is added. [1 p. 1133]

86. **Answer A:** The Spencer technique is a series of direct manipulative procedures. It was designed to prevent or decrease soft tissue restrictions about the shoulder. [1 p. 1133]

87. **Answer B:** Counterstrain is an indirect treatment that is based on a series of tenderpoints. It considers the somatic dysfunction to be a continuing, inappropriate strain reflex. It attributes its therapeutic effects by using a specific point of tenderness related to this dysfunction followed by specific directed positioning. [1 p. 1133]

88. **Answer D:** Petrissage is a soft tissue treatment technique that utilized deep kneading or squeezing action to express swelling. Although it can also be considered a direct technique, more importantly it addresses the soft tissues. [1 p. 1134]

89. **Answer B:** Indirect muscle energy is an indirect treatment. The physician imitates the dysfunction, by positioning away from the restrictive barrier, and then instructs the patient to contract equally against the offered counterforce. This process is repeated until the restrictive barrier is resolved.

90. **Answer A:** Positional treatment is a direct segmental technique in which a combination of leverage, patient ventilatory movements, and a fulcrum are used to achieve mobilization of the dysfunctional segment. It may be combined with springing or thrust technique. [1 p. 1133]

91. **Answer A:** Post-isometric relaxation muscle energy technique is a direct form of muscle energy in which the area being treated is moved toward the restrictive barrier.

92. **Answer D:** Inhibitory pressure technique is the application of pressure to soft tissues to produce relaxation by reducing reflex activity.

REFERENCES

1. American Osteopathic Association: <u>Foundations for Osteopathic Medicine.</u> Baltimore, Williams and Wilkins, 1997.

2. DiGiovanna, E., Schiowitz, S.: <u>An Osteopathic Approach to Diagnosis and Treatment.</u> Philadelphia, J.B. Lippencott Co., 1991.

3. Moore, K.L.: <u>Clinically Oriented Anatomy</u>. Third Edition. Baltimore, Williams and Wilkins, 1992.

4. Brashear, Jr, H.R., Raney, Sr, R.B.: <u>Handbook of Orthopaedic Surgery.</u> Tenth Edition. St. Louis, C.V. Mosby Co., 1986.

5. Magee, D.J.: <u>Orthopedic Physical Assessment</u>. Second Edition. Philadelphia, W.B. Saunders Co., 1992.

6. Hoppenfeld, S.: <u>Physical Examination of the Spine and Extremities</u>. Norwalk, Appleton-Century-Crofts, 1976

7. Borenstein, D.G., Wiesel, S.W., Boden, S.D.: <u>Low Back Pain</u>. Second Edition. Philadelphia, W.B. Saunders Co., 1995

8. Berkow, R.: <u>Merck Manual</u>. Sixteenth Edition. Rahway, Merck Research Laboratories, 1992

9. Buckwalter, J.A., Weinstein, S.L.: <u>Turek's Orthopaedics: Principles and their Applications</u>. Fifth Edition. Philadelphia, J.B. Lippincott Co.

10. Rubin, A., Stallis, R.: Evaluation and Diagnosis of Ankle Injuries. *American Family Physician.* 1996;54(5):1609-1618

11. Magoun, H.I.: <u>Osteopathy in the Cranial Field.</u> Kirksville, The Journal Printing Co., 1976

12. Dambro, M.R.: <u>Griffith's Five-Minute Clinical Consult 2000</u>. Eighth edition. Lippincott, Williams and Wilkins 2000

13. Fix, J.D.: <u>Neuroanatomy</u>. Second Edition. Baltimore, Williams and Wilkins, 1995

14. Greenman, P.E.: <u>Principles of Manual Medicine.</u> Second Edition. Baltimore, Williams and Wilkins, 1996

15. Patterson, M.M.: A model mechanism for spinal segmental facilitation. *JAOA.* 1976;76:62/121-72/131.

16. Berne, R., Levy, M: <u>Physiology</u>. Third edition. St. Louis, Mosby, 1993.

17. Guyton, A.: <u>Textbook of Medical Physiology</u>. Eighth Edition. Philadelphia, W.B. Saunders 1991.

REFERENCES

18. Adams, R., Victor, M.: <u>Principles of Neurology</u>. Fifth Edition. New York, McGraw Hill, 1993.

19. Owens, C.: <u>An Endocrine Interpretation of Chapman's Reflexes</u>, 1937. Reprinted by the Academy of Applied Osteopathy, May 1963.

20. Travell, J.G., Simons, D.G.: <u>Myofascial Pain and Dysfunction</u>. Vol I. Baltimore, Williams and Wilkins, 1983.

21. Travell, J.G., Simons, D.G.: <u>Myofascial Pain and Dysfunction</u>. Vol II. Baltimore, Williams and Wilkins, 1983.

22. Simons, D.G.: <u>Muscle Pain Syndromes</u>. Journal of Manual Medicine. 1991:6:3-23

23. Chaitow, L.: <u>Soft Tissue Manipulation</u>. Ellington, Great Britian, Thorston Publishing, 1987.

24. Olsom, W.H., et al.: <u>Handbook of Symptom-Oriented Neurology</u>. Second edition. St. Louis, Mosby-Year Book Inc., 1994.

25. DiGiovanna, E., Schiowitz, S.: <u>An Osteopathic Approach to Diagnosis and Treatment</u>. Second Edition. Philadelphia, J.B. Lippencott Co., 1997.

26. Yates, H.A., Glover, J: <u>Counterstrain: A Handbook of Osteopathic Technique.</u> Tulsa, Y-Knot Publishers, 1995.

27. Chung, K.W.: <u>Gross Anatomy</u>. Third Edition. Baltimore, Williams and Wilkins, 1995.

28. Kuchera, W.A., Kuchera, M.L.: <u>Osteopathic Principles in Practice. Second Edition (revised),</u> second printing, Columbus, Greyden Press, 1993.

29. Bland, J.H.: <u>Disorders of the Cervical Spine: Diagnosis and Medical Management</u>. Second Edition. Philadelphia, W.B. Saunders, 1994

30. Boden, SD et.al.: Orientation of lumbar facet joints: Association with Degenerative Disc Disease. *Journal of Bone and Joint Surgery*. March 1996: 78-A(3) p.403 - 411.

31 Deyo, R.A., Diehl, A.K., Rosenthal M.: How many days of bed rest for acute low back pain? A randomized clinical trial. <u>New England Journal of Medicine</u>. Oct 1986: 23;315(17):1064-70

32. Snider, R.K.: <u>The Essentials of Musculoskeletal Care</u>. American Academy of Orthopedic Surgeons, 1997

33. Kimberly, P.E., Funk, S.L.: <u>Outline of Osteopathic Manipulative Procedures: The Kimberly Manual.</u> Millennium Edition. Walsworth Publishing Co, 2000

34 Carey, C.F., Hans, H.L., Woeltje, K.F.: <u>The Washington Manual of Medical Therapeutics</u>. 29th edition. Lippencott-Raven, 1998

35. Kuchera, W.A., Kuchera, M.L.: <u>Osteopathic Considerations in Systemic Dysfunction.</u> Second Edition (revised). Columbus, Greyden Press, 1994

36. Frymann, V.M.: <u>The Collected Papers of Voila M. Frymann, DO: Legacy of Osteopathy to Children.</u> Indianapolis, American Academy of Osteopathy, 1998

37. Blood, S.D. Treatment of the sprained ankle. *JAOA.* July 1980; 79:680-692

38. Teirney, L.M.: Current 2001 Medical Diagnosis and Treatment. 40th edition. McGraw-Hill, 2001

39. Rosero, H., et. al: Correlation of palpatory observations with anatomic locus of acute myocardial infarction. *JAOA.* Feb 1987: 87:119

40. Jones, L.H.: Jones Strain-Counterstrain. Jones Strain-Counterstrain inc., Boise, 1995

41. Hoffman, J.R., et. al.: Validity of a set of clinical criteria to rule out injury to the cervical spine in patients with blunt trauma. N*ew England Journal of Medicine.* July 2000:343(2).

42. Klippel, J.H.: Primer on Rheumatic diseases. 11th edition. Atlanta, Arthritis Foundation, 1997.

43. Isoolbaohor, K.J., et. al.: Harrison's Principles of Internal Medicine. 13th edition. New York. McGraw-Hill Inc. 1994

44. Mitchell, F.L., Moran P.S., Pruzzo N.A..: An Evaluation and Treatment Manual of Osteopathic Muscle Energy Procedures. First Edition. Mitchell, Moran & Pruzzo Associates, 1979

45. Still, A.T.: The Philosophy and Mechanical Principles of Osteopathy, 1892, Kirksville, Osteopathic Enterprises, 1986.

46. Webster, G.V." Sage Sayings of A.T. Still. Indianapolis, American Academy of Osteopathy, Reprinted 1991

47. Gray's Anatomy. 38th Edition. New York Edinburgh London Tokyo Madrid and Melbourne, Churchill Livingston, 1995.

48. Rivera-Martinez, S, Capobianco, J.D.: Osteopathic treatment of nephrotic syndrome, *American Academy of Osteopathy* Journal, Fall 2001:11(3)

49. Anderson, D.M.: Dorland's Illustrated Medical Dictionary. 28th Edition. Philadelphia, WB Saunders, 1994

50. Marino, R.J.: International Standards for Neurological Classification of Spinal Cord Injury. 6th edition. American Spinal Injury Association, 2002

51. Silverstein F.E., et. al.: Misoprostol reduces serious gastrointestinal complications in patients with rheumatoid arthritis receiving non-steroidal anti-inflammatory drugs. *Annals of Internal Medicine* 1995:123:241-249

52. Reid, D.C.: Sports Injury: Assessment and Rehabilitation. New York, Churchill-Livingstone, 1992

53. Magee, D.J.: Orthopedic Physical Assessment. Third Edition. Philadelphia, W.B. Saunders Co., 1997.

54. Malanga, GA., Savarese, RG., "Rehabilitation of Upper Extremity Nerve Injuries": Peripheral Nerve Injuries in the Athlete. Champaign, Human Kinetics. 2002

55. Capobianco, J.D., Protopapas, M.G., Rivera-Martinez, S: Understanding the combined motion of the C3/C4 vertebral unit: A further look at Fryette's model of cervical biomechanics. *American Academy of Osteopathy Journal.* Fall 2002:12(3) p. 15-29

56. American Osteopathic Association: <u>Foundations for Osteopathic Medicine</u>. 2nd Edition. Baltimore, Lippencott, Williams and Wilkins, 2002

57. Eiff, MP: <u>Fracture Management for Primary Care</u>. Philadelphia, W.B. Saunders, 1998

58. Thorpe, RG: Manipulative procedures in Lumbosacral Problems, *Osteopathic Annals*, August 1974

59. Goldberg, S: <u>Clinical Anatomy Made Ridiculously Simple</u>. MedMastor. Inc., 1984

60. Teirney, L.M.: <u>Current Medical Diagnosis and Treatment 2002</u>. 41st Edition. McGraw-Hill Publishing, 2002

Calcaneus 78, 80
Calculus, ureteral 30
Caliper motion (see Ribs, *motion of*)
Canal
    Hypoglossal 92
    Optic 91
Cancer 9, 29, 126, 174,175, 176
    In acquired scoliosis 38
    Metastasis 146
    Prostate 30
Capate bone 64
Capobianco D.O., John 15, 121
Cardiac (see Heart)
Cardiovascular function in scoliosis 38, 39
Carpal bones 64
Carpal tunnel syndrome 66-67, 161-162
Carpometacarpal joints 64
Carrying angle 65
Cauda equina syndrome 29, 33, 146
Cecum (see Colon, *cecum*)
Central nervous system 85, 86, 99, 145
Cephalgia 92 (see also Headache)
Cerebral palsy
    In neuromuscular scoliosis 38
Cerebrospinal fluid 85, 122, 124
Cervical nerve root compression (see Nerve
    root, *cervical* and Radiculopathy)
Cervical rib 62
Cervical spine
    Anatomy 13
    Articular pillars 13, 130
    C2 connections to vagus 107
    Counterstrain techniques 130
    Dural attachments 86
    Examination 159
    Facilitated positional release 133
    Foramen 13
    Stenosis 14, 15
    HVLA of 147-148
    Joints
    Facet 7, 14, 16
    Hypertrophy 14, 16
    Luschka 14, 16
    Ligaments 14
    Manipulation 9 (see also specific treatment types)
    Motion of 15
    Motion testing 15
    Muscle energy of 137
    Muscles of 13
    Nerve root compression 14, 16
    Nerves 14
    Pain (see Pain, cervical)
    Stenosis 16
    Translation testing 15
    Transverse processes 13
Cervico-thoracic diaphragm 118
Cervico-thoracic junction 119
Cervix (dilation) 108
Chapman D.O., Frank 113
Chapman's reflexes (points) 113

Lymphatic effects 124, 173
Treatment 9, 107, 173
Chest cage (see Ribcage)
Childbirth 89, 93, 108
Cholecystitis 101
Chondromalacia patellae 168
Chronic
    Pain (see Pain, *chronic*)
    Somatic dysfunction 9
    (see also Tissue, *chronic*)
Chronic obstructive pulmonary disease 126,
    175
Cirrhosis 124, 126
    Lymphatic effects 123
Clavicle 13, 59, 62, 130, 131, 174
    Motion of 61
Claw hand 68
Clonus 177
Cobb angle 38
Coccygeus muscle 44
Coccyx 43
Colitis 126
Colon
    Ascending 103-105
    Cecum 103-105
    Chapman's points 113-114
    Descending 108
    Parasympathetic innervation 103, 108
    Sigmoid 30, 103-105, 108
    Splenic flexure 105
    Sympathetic innervation 104, 107
    Transverse 103-105
    (see also Gastrointestinal)
Common compensatory pattern 119
Common peroneal nerve 76
Compartment syndrome 77
Compensation
    Spinal
        In scoliosis 39
        In somatic dysfunction 3
Compression
    Nerve root (see Nerve root and
        Radiculopathy)
    Strain (see craniosacral)
Condylar compression 92, 107
Condylar decompression 107
Condyles, occipital 15
Congenital
    Scoliosis 38
    Spinal malformation 28
Congestive heart failure 126, 175, 176
Constipation
    Osteopathic treatment 108
Contraction, muscle
    Concentric 7
    Eccentric 7
    Isometric 7, 135
    Isotonic 7

K

Kidney
> *Autonomic effects on 102*
> *Chapman's point 113*
> *Parasympathetic innervation 103*
> *Sympathetic innervation 104*
> *(See also Genitourinary)*

Kirksville Krunch
> *Thoracic spine 149-150*
> *Rib 151*

Klumpke's palsy 63

Knee
> *Anatomy 73*
> *Deformity 76*
> *Examination 166-168*
> *Joints of 74*
> *Ligaments 74, 166*
> *Menisci 74, 166, 167*
> *Motion of*
> *Muscles 73*

Knocked-Kneed 76

Konstancin exercises 39

Korr PhD., Irvin 106

Kupffer cells 125

Labor pain
> *Osteopathic treatment 108*

Lachman's test 167

Lacrimal glands 103

Lamina (see specific spine area)

Laminectomy 31

Landmarks
> *Anatomic 19, 28*

Lasegue's test 162

Lateral epicondylitis 67

Lateral femoral patella tracking syndrome
  (see Patello-femoral syndrome)

Lateral longitudinal arch 78

Lateral masses (see Cervical spine, *articular* *pillars*)

Lateral strain (see Craniosacral)

Latissimus dorsi muscle 20, 59, 140, 179

Leg length
> *Apparent (functional) 38, 39*
> *Discrepancy, causes of 39*
> *In innominate dysfunction 45-46*
> *True (anatomic) 39*
> *(see also Short leg syndrome)*

Lens (eye) 102

Levator ani muscle 44

Levoscoliosis 37

Lift technique (craniosacral) 93

Lift therapy (see short leg syndrome)

Ligaments
> *Acromioclavicular 61*
> *Alar 13*
> *Ankle 78-80*
> *Anterior cruciate 74, 77, 166,167*
> *Anterior talofibular 79, 124, 168*
> *Calcanofibular 79*
> *Calcaneonavicular 80*
> *Capitus femoris 73*
> *Cervical 14*
> *Coracoacromial 61*
> *Coracoclavicular 61*
> *Deltoid 80*
> *Fibular collateral (lateral collateral) 74, 168*
> *Iliofemoral 73*
> *Iliolumbar 44*
>> *Stress and 39, 44*
> *Injury 77*
> *Ischialfemoral 73*
> *Lateral collateral (knee) 74, 168*
> *Ligamentum flavum 31*
> *Medial collateral (knee) 74, 77, 168*
> *Of Treitz 105*
> *Pelvic*
>> *Accessory 44*
>> *True 43*
> *Plantar 80*
> *Posterior cruciate 74, 166*
> *Posterior longitudinal 27, 30, 31*
> *Posterior talofibular 79*
> *Pubofemoral 73*
> *Sacroiliac 39, 43*
> *Sacrospinous 44*
> *Sacrotuberous 44*
>> *Tension of in dysfunction 44*
> *Sprain*
>> *Degrees of 77*
> *Spring (see Calcaneonavicular)*
> *Talofibular*
>> *Anterior 79*
>> *Posterior 79*
> *Tibial collateral (medial collateral) 74, 77, 168*
> *Transverse 13, 146*

Liver
> *Autonomic effects on 102*
> *Lymphatic drainage 122*
> *Parasympathetic innervation 103*
> */spleen pump 125, 176*
> *Sympathetic innervation 104*

Localization, in muscle energy 136

Long thoracic nerve 60, 63

Lordosis, lumbar 31, 166

Loss of motion
> *In somatic dysfunction 2*

Louis, angle of 19

Low velocity, moderate amplitude
  techniques (see Articulatory techniques)

Lower extremity
> *Anatomy 73, 78*
> *Joints 73, 78*

M

N

Spleen/liver pump 125
Spondylolisthesis 31-32
Definition 31
Diagnosis 31
Etiology 31
Grading31, 32
Radiographic diagnosis 32
Signs 31
Treatment 31
Spondylolysis
Definition 32
Etiology 32
Pars Interarticularis 32
Radiographic diagnosis 32
Spondylosis 32
Spontaneous release by positioning (see Counterstrain)
Sprain
Ankle 79
Degrees of 77
Spray and stretch technique 115
Spring test (a.k.a. Lumbosacral spring test) (see Lumbosacral spring test)
Springing technique (see Articulatory technique)
Spurling's test 16, 159
Standing
*Flexion test (see **Flexion test**)*
*Postural x-rays (see **X-rays**)*
Stenosis (see specific spine areas)
Step-off sign 31
Sternoclavicular joint
Dysfunction of 61
Motion of 61
Sternocleidomastoid muscle 13, 92, 114, 130
Sternum 13, 19, 21, 131
Stomach
Parasympathetic innervation 103
Sympathetic innervation 104
Strachan 48
Straight leg raise test 30, 162
Strains/sprains
Neck 9, 16, 146
Lumbar 30
Craniosacral 89-91
Stretching 30
Still point 93
Stroke (see Cerebrovascular accident)
Structural spinal curve 37
Subclavian
Artery 60, 62
Vein 60, 62, 122
Subluxation
Innominate (see Innominate, *somatic dysfunction*)
Sub-occipital muscle spasms 16
Subscapular nerve
Upper 179
Lower 179

Subscapularis muscle 59, 179
Subtalar joint 78
Suckling in the newborn 92, 107
Superior gluteal nerve 184
Superior orbital fissure (see Fissure)
Superior transverse axis 86, 87
Supination
Of foot 74, 79
Of forearm 64, 66, 143, 161
Supinator muscle 64, 181
Supraclavicular fossa 178
Suprascapular nerve 179
Supraspinatus muscle 59, 179
Tears of 63
Supraspinatus tendonitis 62
Supraventricular tachyarrhythmias 101, 114
Surgery
In cauda equina syndrome 33
In compartment syndrome 77
In herniated discs 30
In scoliosis 39
Laminectomy 31
Sutherland, William 85, 86
Swan-neck deformity 67
Sweat glands 102
Sympathetic nervous system
Of the lymphatic system 123
Key concepts 105
Treatments 106-107, 155, 173-174
Visceral innervation 104
Vs. parasympathetic 102
Synchondrosis
*Cranial (see **Sphenobasilar**)*
Syncope
Systemic dysfunction
Synovial joints

T

Talocalcaneal joint (see Subtalar joint)
Talocrural joint 78
Talofibular joint 75 (see also Fibular head, motion)
Talus bone
Motion of 76, 78
Technique (see specific techniques)
Temporal bone 91, 92, 93, 124
Temporomandibular joint
Dysfunction 93
Tenderpoints, counterstrain 129-133
Characteristics 129
In relation to viscero-somatic reflexes 130
Maverick point 130
Vs trigger point 115

V